Michael W. Zellmann-Rohrer and Edward O. D. Love
Traditions in Transmission

Archiv für Papyrusforschung
und verwandte Gebiete

Begründet von
Ulrich Wilcken

Beiheft 47

De Gruyter

Traditions in Transmission

The Medical and Magical Texts of a Fourth-Century Greek and Coptic Codex (Michigan Ms. 136) in Context

by
Michael W. Zellmann-Rohrer
and Edward O. D. Love

De Gruyter

ISBN 978-3-11-077875-5
e-ISBN (PDF) 978-3-11-077891-5
ISSN 1868-9337

Library of Congress Control Number: 2022931135

Bibliographic information published by the Deutsche Nationalbibliothek
The Deutsche Nationalbibliothek lists this publication in the Deutsche Nationalbibliografie; detailed bibliographic data are available on the Internet at http://dnb.dnb.de.

Printing and binding: CPI books GmbH, Leck

www.degruyter.com

Contents

Acknowledgements

In the course of a collaboration that began over lunch in Oxford in 2016, on a book that was substantially completed in 2020, the authors have accumulated not a few debts of gratitude to other colleagues and friends. Zellmann-Rohrer thanks in particular Pablo Alvarez and his colleagues at the University of Michigan Library for assistance in consulting the codex that is our principal, and Julia Hamilton, Barbara Richter, and Andreas Winkler for advice on Egyptian language matters. Love is grateful to Cat Warsi, Elizabeth Fleming, and Franciso Bosche-Puche for their assistance in consulting Crum's papers in the archive of the Griffith Institute, Dagmar Budde for her references on the Edfu Mammisi texts, Victoria Altmann-Wendling for her help with certain Graeco-Roman hieroglyphic texts, Joachim Friedrich Quack for sharing his working editions of the unpublished magical texts in Demotic, Korshi Dosoo for numerous productive discussions on §§9–10, and ultimately to Mark Smith for first reading §§9–10 with him during his MSt Coptic classes. Bärbel Kramer is also thanked for her care in typesetting the results.

Berlin & Würzburg, October 2021

MZR: *Dedicated to the memory of William Hoyt Worrell*

…

EODL: *Dedicated to Gesa*

Because I wouldn't be anywhere without Coptic

Preface

In the course of the last generation, there has been a significant increase in the study of the category of text conventionally and conveniently characterized as "magic" for its own sake, from collected text editions of the primary sources[1] and collected studies of "Ancient Magic",[2] to specific studies of the magical traditions preserved in sources in the Egyptian,[3] Greek,[4] and Aramaic and Hebrew languages.[5] It is in this context that this monograph appears, planned as both a text edition and study of those texts in their wider context of medical and magical practices from late Roman and Byzantine Egypt and the broader Mediterranean area. The product of a collaborative application of Egyptian-Coptic and Greek philology, this book is also contemporary with two ongoing projects that have sought to re-establish the text editions of the entire corpus of Greek and Coptic magical texts from Egypt, in which both authors have participated and whose methodology has set an example for the present work. The first is the project *The Transmission of Magical Knowledge in Antiquity*, funded by the Neubauer Collegium for Culture and Society of the University of Chicago, which is (re)publishing all of the Greek-language "formularies", that is, "master copy" handbooks on papyrus, from Egypt[6] alongside a selection of those in Demotic and Old Coptic[7] in a series titled *The Greek and Egyptian Magical Formularies*. The second is the project *The Coptic Magical Papyri*, funded by the *Excellent Ideas* program of the Julius-Maximilians-Universität Würzburg, which is (re)publishing all magical texts in Coptic in both an online and freely

[1] From those of the so-called Greek and Demotic Magical Papyri (*PDM* and *PDM*) in Betz 1986, to the corpus of Coptic magical texts in Meyer and Smith 1994.

[2] See Faraone and Obbink 1991; Schäfer and Kippenberg 1997; Jordan, Montgomery, and Thomassen 1999; Meyer and Mirecki 1995; 2002; Shaked 2005; Bohak, Harari, and Shaked 2011; Edmonds 2019; Frankfurter (ed.) 2019.

[3] See Ritner 1993; Dieleman 2005; Love 2016.

[4] For the Classical and Late Ancient periods, Faraone 1999 and Johnston 2008; for the Byzantine and later phases, Zellmann-Rohrer 2018 and 2019a.

[5] See Bohak 2008; Harari 2017; Zellmann-Rohrer 2021.

[6] The Egyptian focus is broadened by the inclusion, for comparative perspectives, of one copper lamella from Sicily and one agate gemstone from the Black Sea region.

[7] The former, those conventionally termed the *Demotic Magical Papyri* (*PDM*) and the latter P.Brit.Mus. EA 10808 (bibliography below). It has not been possible to include in the scope of this project the dozens of contemporary manuscripts inscribed with magical texts in hieratic and Demotic that have come to light since the publication of the *PGM* by Preisendanz et al. nearly a century ago. These will instead appear in four volumes, edited by Joachim Friedrich Quack.

available database and in print form. These projects, as this monograph, are a testament to the need to bring together colleagues of not only different philological proficiencies, but also from different scholarly traditions, e.g. Coptology and Egyptology, Classics and Greek Papyrology, as well as Anthropology and History of Religion, in order to study the vast body of textual sources, which, while coming from an Egyptian context, evidence a diversity of cultural and religious backgrounds. We therefore hope that this monograph is of interest to colleagues in all of these disciplines, which are increasingly being brought together in the study of magical traditions from the ancient world.

Introduction

In the Fayum region of Egypt, perhaps its capital city Arsinoe-Crocodilopolis (Coptic ⲡⲉⲓⲟⲙ, the modern Medinet el-Fayyum), sometime in the fourth century of the common era, a copyist undertook a small project: the slender, roughly palm-sized codex that resulted (Plates 1–8), whether for his own use or produced on commission, may not have occupied him long, but the copying, and its expansion by others, has left a substantial and long-lasting witness to an interesting moment in the history of religion and bilingualism in Egypt. On fine parchment in an elegant handwriting that would not have been out of place in the more luxurious literary tomes of the day, this writer set about copying a small collection of technical literature with a focus on healing. The properly bilingual contents present 31 recipes, four entirely in Greek, 24 in Coptic, and two in a mixture of the two. These recipes comprise magical rituals for healing and broader personal advancement, pharmacological and related medical recipes, as well as advice for the management of a household. The finished product shows firm roots in both traditional Egyptian religion and ritual as well as medical practices of Hellenic culture more recently introduced to Egypt. Faithful and comprehending copying of archaic, even poetic Coptic invocations featuring the Egyptian gods Amun and Thoth share pages with an incantation constructed from the verses of one of Greece's foremost poets, Homer, invocations of Judaeo-Christian angels and the supreme deity, alongside more prosaic medical recommendations.

While precision on how the copy came about, and who the commissioner and user were, are lacking in the absence of direct indications, the codex has light to shed here too. The manuscript is a counterpoint, in terms of its preference for shorter and less elaborate rituals and concern with practical healing and medical treatment as opposed to mystical revelation or aggressive magic, to the better-known bilingual "Theban magical library".[8] The conjunction of pharmacology, ritual healing and ritual recipes of broader scope suggests the practice of a professional, whether an all-around ritual practitioner or a physician providing further services as a sideline. In addition to the care shown in its production, the manuscript continued to be valued and used. Over time, two later hands seem to have filled out originally blank pages in the pre-made codex.

---

[8] For this dossier, see Dosoo 2016a; for a broad statistical perspective on the magical papyri of Graeco-Roman Egypt, showing that healing procedures were in fact the best represented category, see id. 2016b.

Despite its promise, the codex has yet to figure prominently in the burgeoning discipline of the study of ancient magic.[9] The impetus for the new edition offered here is the hope of bringing it to wider knowledge. The re-publication was planned in the first instance as a collaborative effort in Egyptian and Greek philology, to do justice to the textual complexity of both the Coptic and Greek portions. A more extensive commentary than previously offered also seeks to situate the codex in the increasingly developed discipline of ritual and magic in Late Antiquity, as well as Graeco-Roman and Coptic medicine.

The edition is introduced by discussion of previous scholarship on the codex, its provenance, palaeographic, codicological, and linguistic data. Two more substantive essays follow on the bilingual aspect of the codex in the context of pre-Coptic Egyptian exemplars, and its healing prescriptions in the context of medicine in Late Antiquity. Finally, the principles of the new edition are explained, and the contents of the codex and their phases of copying are presented in outline. The edition itself is followed by a translation, line-commentary on philological points, and excurses on larger interpretive questions for select sections.

Previous Studies

The first edition was furnished by the Michigan Coptologist William H. Worrell in 1935, with translation and brief notes, incorporating advice received from the Coptologist Walter E. Crum.[10] The manuscript had previously figured briefly in a long correspondence between Worrell and Crum, stretching back at least to 1907, and touching at several points on Crum's work on his *Coptic Dictionary*.[11] Worrell had asked for advice in his edition of other magical texts, those that he would publish as the so-called "Coptic wizard's horde".[12] Already in November of 1931, Worrell sent Crum "a photostat of my unrevised pen copy of our No.

[9] For references see the Preface; the present edition compensates for the absence of this codex from the plan of the *Greek and Egyptian Magical Formularies* series, following on its omission from the revised corpus of Preisendanz and Henrichs (*PGM*) and Daniel and Maltomini (*Suppl.Mag.*) for Greek-language texts.

[10] Worrell 1935, 17–37. For further bibliography (summarized below) see also TM 92874.

[11] The correspondence received by Crum is now in the British Library, Add. Ms. 45960, ff. 132–224 and Oxford, Griffith Institute Archive, Crum MSS 8, Crum Notebook 87. For the contents of the former in general, see Bonner 1964; for a specific aspect concerning an exchange among Crum, Worrell, and Harold Idris Bell on the position of Coptic in relation to papyrology, Choat 2013.

[12] P.Mich. inv. 593 in a letter of 12 February 1927 (British Library, Add. Ms. 45960, f. 159); P.Mich. inv. 594, 596, 599, and 603 in others of 11 and 25 November 1927 (ibid. ff. 162, 163); in a third, on 2 June 1928 (ibid. f. 168), references are requested on the biblical Seth (son of Adam) mentioned in this archive.

136 to be used like the other photographic material which you have from us", apparently as material for the *Dictionary*, but with the further request, "If you find errors, or if you decide upon other readings, I should like to have them, together with such notes and comments as you feel like making".[13] Crum was offered credit in the coming publication, which would, Worrell judged, optimistically as it turned out, "not be long in coming". Crum's replies, in the form of "notes" and an annotated hand copy of Worrell's photostat, were acknowledged in December and in January of the following year, as was the reason for delay in publication in November. The manuscript had been in the hands of an anonymous colleague of Worrell's—perhaps the Michigan Classicist and keen student of magical texts, Campbell Bonner, whose opinions are cited in places in notes to Worrell's edition, along with those of the latter's student Elizabeth Stefanski—for the past two years.[14] In August of the next year, Worrell wrote to announce that his edition had been "put into shape", but, mentioning a suggestion of Crum about the meaning of what proves to be a traditional Egyptian divine epithet (ⲛⲟⲣϯⲟⲩ, p. 5/10), admitted that the portion to which it belonged, which he termed a "hymn", had been translated so far only "with great difficulty, and without understanding much", and that he would welcome further "light on the subject".[15]

Since then, the manuscript has attracted the notice of several scholars. The first sustained attention was not in the context of magic, but rather Coptic medicine. Medical excerpts from the codex were translated by Walter C. Till in the course of his study on Coptic medicine, in particular the range of medicinal substances used and pathologies addressed.[16] This survey has now been updated, with mention of the Michigan codex once again, by Tonio Sebastian Richter.[17] Paul E. Kahle adduced the text in his overview of Coptic phonetic and dialectal developments in the publication of texts from Balaʾiza, adding an important

---

[13] 11 Nov. 1931 (British Library, Add. Ms. 45960, f. 186).

[14] 4 Dec. 1931 (Oxford, Griffith Institute Archive, Crum MSS 8, Crum Notebook 87, f. 74), with "[t]hanks for the notes to 136," some clarifications about page-numbering, and answers to queries apparently made by Crum about readings on pp. 12–14 of the codex ("I have written just what I see, without regard to sense"); 8 Jan. 1932 (British Library, Add. Ms. 45960, f. 187), and 21 Nov. 1932 (ibid. f. 191).

[15] 14 Aug. 1933 (British Library, Add. Ms. 45960, f. 197).

[16] §4 = Till 1951a, 132 no. 1; §5 = ibid. 133 no. 2; §7 = ibid. 133 no. 3; §8 = ibid. 133 no. 4; §14 = ibid. 133 no. 5; §§16–17 = ibid. 133 no. 6; §19 = ibid. 133 no. 7; §20 = ibid. 133 no. 8; §21 = ibid. 133 no. 9; §22 = ibid. 133 no. 10; §23 = ibid. 133 no. 11; §24 = ibid. 133 no. 12; §25 = ibid. 133 no. 13; §26 = ibid. 133 no. 14; §27 = ibid. 133 no. 15; §28 = ibid. 133 no. 16; §29 = ibid. 133 no. 17; §30 = ibid. 133–134 no. 18; §31 = ibid. 134 no. 19.

[17] Richter 2014, 189–191 no. 24; 2017, 155.

assessment of its palaeography by the Classicist and pioneer in the study of the codicology of Greek papyri, Colin H. Roberts.[18]

For the study of Coptic magic, the manuscript was made accessible in English translation by Marvin Meyer and in Italian by Sergio Pernigotti.[19] It has also been briefly mentioned in various surveys of Coptic magic, most recently by Roxanne Bélanger Sarrazin,[20] but beyond occasional attention to points of detail—above all from Jacques van der Vliet—,[21] close study in this context was set off by the work of David Frankfurter, who took an interest in the traditional Egyptian content of the incantations numbered §§9–10 in the new edition and their relation to Isiac mythology, an avenue taken up more recently by van der Vliet.[22] Most recently, Korshi Dosoo has considered the traditional Egyptian content of §§3 and 9 within what he identified as the "Christian" context of 4th century CE Egypt, while nevertheless placing them among the latest witnesses of the Graeco-Egyptian magical tradition preserved in Greek or Coptic.[23] While the manuscript is cited by Theodore De Bruyn as "an example of the continuing salience of Graeco-Egyptian incantations and remedies in a bilingual Greek and Coptic milieu",[24] the manuscript has yet to contribute to scholarship on Greek-language magical texts specifically, a situation probably not helped by the decision of the first editor to set the entirety of the text in Coptic characters. A fitting complement to academic studies on the document's medical aspects was its recent inclusion in the exhibition "The Art and Science of Healing, from Antiquity to the Renaissance", put on jointly by the University of Michigan Library and Kelsey Museum of Archaeology.[25]

Provenance

The codex was purchased by the American missionary and doctor David L. Askren, who was active in the Fayum from 1904–1939, in Medinet el-Fayyum on behalf of the University of Michigan.[26] The precise date of the purchase is

---

[18] *P.Bal.* I p. 254.

[19] Meyer and Smith 1994, 83–90 no. 43; Pernigotti 1995, 3715–3718 no. 21.

[20] Bélanger Sarrazin 2017a, 395 no. 164.

[21] Van der Vliet 1991, 228–231.

[22] Frankfurter 2009; id. 2018, 206–208; van der Vliet 2018, 153–160.

[23] Dosoo 2021.

[24] De Bruyn 2017, 80–81.

[25] 10 February–30 April 2017 <http://exhibitions.kelsey.lsa.umich.edu/art-science-healing/coptic2.php> [last accessed 25 October 2021].

[26] Worrell 1935, 17. On Askren's role in the purchasing of papyri and related antiquities on behalf of the University of Michigan see Boak 1959–60; Pedley 2012, 235–236, 271; Nongbri

unknown, but delivery was taken in May of 1924 by Francis W. Kelsey, professor of Classics at Michigan and architect of the University's papyrus collection.[27] For similarly unrecorded reasons, perhaps simply due to its disposition as a mostly intact parchment codex, it was deposited by Kelsey later that year not among the papyri but rather with the Library's medieval manuscripts, where it has remained ever since.[28] Given that a manuscript's provenance is not necessarily one and the same as its context of production and use, as discussed in the section on **Linguistic and Orthographic Features**, below, it is notable that the dialectal features of the Coptic texts are consistent with a Lower Egyptian origin.

Physical Description

This relatively small-format codex was originally formed of four bifolia of light-colored parchment of a good quality. The page dimensions, 12.4 cm in height by 10.5 cm in width,[29] fall into group XI in the typology of Turner, nearly "square" in the sense developed by Schubart, with a width-to-height ratio of 7:8.[30] The text is in a single column, with an outer margin of c. 1.0 cm and inner, top, and bottom margins of c. 0.5 cm. The single quire of the original four bifolia was tacketed with thread still in place in the center of the quire, visible in the inner margin of pp. 7–8. The first folio is now lost and its mate detached. Its outside will have been left blank as the front cover, just as the outside of the last has been left as the back cover. Page numbers were added in the outer margins beginning at p. 1 (ⲁ, lost) and running only to p. 8 (ⲏ). The orientation of sides with respect to flesh and hair follows the expected rule (flesh faces flesh, and hair, hair), the hair being rather closely shaven: pp. 1–2 grain, 3–4 flesh, 5–6 grain, 7–8 flesh, 9–10 grain, 11–12 flesh, 13–14 grain (both the blank outside covers being flesh). The collation may be given as follows:

2014, esp. bibliography at 95 n. 7; Hickey, Maravela, and Zellmann-Rohrer 2015, 158–164 and 174 n. 12; Nongbri 2018, 87–91, 116–122.

[27] Information: accession register, Special Collections.

[28] A letter of Kelsey, dated 4 December 1924, describes this and the rest of a small lot of manuscripts, including an Ethiopic amuletic roll (Ms. 135).

[29] P. 2/3 is slightly shorter, c. 11.8 cm. The height of the first 10 lines of a page, as measured on p. 3, is 5.0 cm.

[30] Turner 1977, 29: attested as early as the third century.

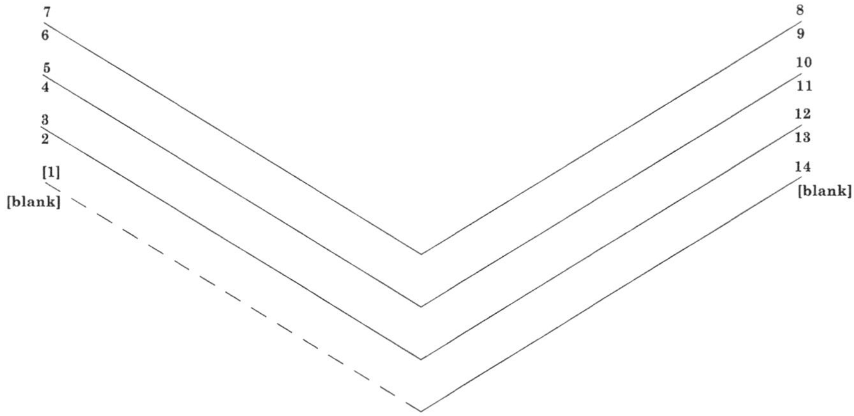

A repair to a hole in the parchment with fish-skin or similar, between manufacture of the substrate and writing, can be seen on the folio with pp. 4/5 (circa l. 17 on the former and 16–17 on the latter). A secondary folding along both the horizontal and vertical may date to a medieval or modern phase of storage.

Palaeography and Dating

The main script is a sloping majuscule bookhand that may be assigned with confidence to the fourth century CE.[31] Letters are formed with no discernible shading. The following forms may be noted: half-uncial ⲁ; ⲃ occasionally with extended baseline;[32] ⲉ with extended crossbar; small ⲟ; ⲥ with extended rightward stroke at top terminus;[33] ⲩ with long vertical and short, high branches; ϥ with long vertical and narrow, angular bow. Certain forms, such as the small ⲟ,

[31] Useful comparanda are: *P.Herm.* 4 (Cavallo-Maehler, *GB* 2a) and 5 (Turner, *GMAW* 70), ca. 320–325 CE; *P.Oxy.* XI 1358 (Cavallo-Maehler, *GB* 1b), early fourth century CE; *P.Oxy.* XI 1352 (Cavallo-Maehler, *GB* 12a), early fourth century CE; *PSI* VIII 958 (Roberts, *GLH* 24a), second half of the fourth century CE (after 381); *T.Kellis Copt.* 2, fourth century CE.

[32] E.g. p. 5.17; cf. *T.Kell.Copt.* 2. This feature also characterizes the earliest-attested Old Coptic hand from the Fayum (specifically, Dime-Soknopaiou Nesos), P.Mich. inv. 6124r–v+6131v (second century CE), ed. Worrell 1941 with Quack 2019b, 62–63.

[33] Cf. *P.Dura* 10 (Roberts, *GLH* 21b), first half of the third century CE.

narrow ⲣ, and tall ⲩ with narrow and uneven branches, point even earlier.[34] There are no signs of the standard features of the later bimodular Coptic uncial (Alexandrian majuscule), particularly the contrast between the oval letters ⲉ ⲑ ⲟ ⲥ, written with narrow forms, and the rest, written broadly.[35]

In his study of the history of the Coptic dialects, Kahle classed the Michigan codex among "a number of texts which are still Egyptian in religion and thought, and which, presumably, were either copied from Demotic direct or were based on copies of such texts" as indeed "[b]y far the most important of these" (with special reference to the sections numbered §§9–10 in the new edition).[36] Kahle judged the text to have been written "at a time when the [Coptic] language was not yet standardized", dating the codex to the mid-fourth century on the advice of Roberts. Out of caution, and in the continued absence of a definitive study of Coptic palaeography, we prefer a broader dating to the fourth century. A sixth century date was offered by the first editor, who noted "the small ⲟ, the flat ⲱ and the broad letters" as evidence for an earlier date, but hesitated over the difficulty of "how an early and practiced scribe could copy a text in his native language with so little comprehension and fidelity". If as it seems this claim refers to the same lengthy Coptic invocations, §§9 and 10 in the present edition, the difficulty may lie more in modern understanding of the text than the infelicity of the scribe.[37] An additional point alleged in favor of a later date, a supposed Bohairicism, was based on a misreading.[38]

Punctuation by middle and low punctus, and by colon, is in use, with only occasional apostrophe; superlineation is used both for phonetic marking and to accompany some divine names and similar in invocations. Section divisions are indicated by ornamental head- and tail-pieces and paragraphoi; that the former are at least in part a secondary addition is indicated by p. 7.16 (§12), where a section-divider has been drawn over a section title. Page numbers are added likely by the main hand, with a single overline.[39]

The codex appears to be the work of three hands, which filled out the premade unit over time (see also the following section **Outline of Content and Phases**). The first phase consists of the first eight pages, in which the hand (1) is consistent, as are features of punctuation-marks and the addition of page

---

[34] Cf. *P.Oxy.* XVII 2098 (*P.L.Bat.* IV 19; Roberts, *GLH* 19b), first half of the third century CE; *P.Oxy.* VII 1015 (Turner, *GMAW* 50).

[35] On this script see Cavallo 1975; Cavallo-Maehler, *GB* p. 23; and Orsini 2008.

[36] *P.Bal.* I p. 254.

[37] An incomplete understanding of Vorlagen transliterated from Demotic by subsequent scribes is also a possibility, and will be considered below.

[38] The abbreviation ⲫ̅ⲧ̅ for ⲡⲛⲟⲩⲧⲉ at p. 3.10 of the present edition; the text here is in fact Greek, and abbreviates the word φύσις: see further the line-commentary.

[39] A similar style of page numeration can be found in the early fourth-century *P.Lond.Lit.* 127 (Cavallo-Maehler, *GB* 3b).

numbers. The continuation through p. 9 and onto p. 10 is probably the work of the same hand (1), which gives the same general impression: although the initial lines of pp. 9–10 are in a comparatively more spacious layout, the final lines of p. 9 resemble the hand of pp. 2–8 closely, while none of the letters show diagnostic differences; on the contrary, the distinctive ⲉ with extended crossbar, ⲥ with extended rightward stroke at top terminus, and tall ⲩ are maintained. The disappearance of the page numbers, however, suggests that this portion is a later addition, as does the situation of §§14 and 15. The latter now intrudes on the former, with which it has no obvious connection. It seems probable that the same writer (hand 1) at first skipped over p. 9, adding §15 instead in an originally blank section of p. 10, but then later decided to add the lengthy §14 beginning directly at the start of the first unwritten page, p. 9, which consequently needed to be fitted around §15 overleaf. Conscious of the discontinuity, this writer (hand 1) provided an aid to readers in the form of the reference sign ~ at the foot of p. 9 and the resumption of §14 on p. 10. That the same scribe was at work in Phases 1–3 is also supported by the consistency of the orthographic and linguistic features within those phases, in comparison to the differences exhibited in Phases 4 (Hand 2) and 5 (Hand 2), discussed in **Linguistic and Orthographic Features**, below.

After this, a new hand (2), roughly contemporary, takes over and continues to fill out the blank space at p. 10/12 with §16 and following, with yet another hand (3) then taking over at p. 13/10 for the final two sections (§§30–31), no more than a century later. These additions by the second and third hands, as also the additions of the first hand on pp. 9–10, are accompanied by a shift in content, with a preponderance of pharmacological as opposed to ritual material, excepting §18 (p. 11), as well as a linguistic shift, the Greek language being restricted to the first phase.[40] Further activity of later hands is represented by the addition of paragraph divisions, at least in the case of §12 (p. 7), where the horizontal dividing line overwrites the original title.

Outline of Contents and Phases

As detailed above in the discussion of palaeographic features, the pre-made codex was filled out by three distinct hands in five phases. Identification of the composition of the pages by three separate hands over time, in combination with analysis of the contents presented here in schematic form, suggests that a core, properly bilingual unit, comparable to the multi-lingual Roman-period ritual handbooks but more medicinal in scope, was progressively supplemented with

[40] The linguistic situation is directly comparable to the bilingual history of composition in the *PGM* III archive discussed in **Transmitting Textual Traditions**, see Love 2017.

Coptic recipes. Both factors speak eloquently against a single (slipshod and unfinished) translation, as was assumed by ed.pr. and subsequent commentators.[41]

A concordance of the page and line numbers of the codex with the sequential line numbers given in Worrell's edition is given in the appendix.

Phase 1 (Hand 1):

§1. p. 2/1–9 (beginning lost). Coptic: spell said over oil; text and signs written on a metal sheet, for healing (against gout?)

§2. p. 2/10–17. Greek: amuletic text written on a silver sheet, against gout

§3. p. 2/17–p. 3/15 (beginning lost). Greek and Coptic: invocation of Isis, against uterine disorder

§4. p. 3/15–19. Greek and Coptic: medical recipe, against splenitis

§5. p. 3/19–21. Coptic: medical recipe, against excessive eyelash growth

§6. p. 4/1–12. Greek: Homeric incantation and prayer to the angel Gabriel, against fever

§7. p. 4/13–15. Coptic: medical recipe, against teething pain

§8. p. 4/16–19. Coptic: medical recipe, against swellings

§9. p. 5/1–p. 6/5. Coptic (no heading): invocation, for fertility, birth, and milk production

§10. p. 6/6–p. 7/11. Coptic (no heading): invocation, alternate version of §9 (?)

§11. p. 7/11–15. Greek (no heading): invocation, against bleeding

§12. p. 7/16–p. 8/4. Coptic: invocation, for favor

§13. p. 8/5–13. Greek: textual amulet, against stomach- and headache

Phase 2 (Hand 1?):

§15. p. 10/1–6. Coptic (no heading): invocation, for general assistance

Phase 3 (Hand 1?):

§14. p. 9/1–17 + p. 10/7–11. Coptic: medical recipe with healing ritual, against dysuria

Phase 4 (Hand 2):

§16. p. 10/12–16. Coptic: medical recipe, against uterine disorder

§17. p. 10/16–19. Coptic: medical recipe, against chronic uterine disorder

---

[41] Worrell remarked, "The original was, in part at least, Greek; and some of the text has been taken over, untranslated" (1935, 17), which was adopted by Meyer in the preface to his translation, "At least a portion of the document has been translated from Greek, and some of the present text ... has been left, untranslated, in Greek" (*ACM* p. 83).

§18. p. 11/1–8. Coptic: healing ritual including textual amulet, against mental illness (demonic possession)
§19. p. 11/9–15. Coptic: household recipe, against pests
§20. p. 12/1–4. Coptic: medical recipe, against skin-sores and mange
§21. p. 12/4–11. Coptic: medical recipe, against skin-sores on the face
§22. p. 12/12. Coptic: medical recipe, against disorder of the testicles (?)
§23. p. 12/13–16. Coptic: medical recipe, against rheum in the eyes
§24. p. 12/16–18. Coptic: medical recipe, against sores on the posterior
§25. p. 12/18–20. Coptic: medical recipe, against toothache
§26. p. 13/1–3. Coptic: medical recipe, against earache
§27. p. 13/3–5. Coptic: medical recipe, against constipation
§28. p. 13/5–8. Coptic: medical recipe, against (general pain causing) crying in children
§29. p. 13/8–10. Coptic: household recipe, against pests

Phase 5 (Hand 3):
§30. p. 13/10–18. Coptic: medical recipe, preparation of a poultice (for wounds?)
§31. p. 14/1–20. Coptic: medical recipe with ritual strictures, against sciatica

Linguistic and Orthographic Features

As the codex is the work of three hands and was compiled in at least five phases (see the preceding sections) from various source texts, themselves the result of previous compilations, the linguistic and orthographic features exhibited in the texts must be treated by hand, phase, and cluster of texts. The following analysis draws upon the conventional terminology, location, and understanding of Coptic dialects[42] in addition to established terminology from linguistics.[43] Throughout, Egyptological conventions are used in referring to the form or stage of the Egyptian language as "Demotic", but the script as "demotic" (as "hieratic" and "hieroglyphs").

[42] An informative summary of both Coptic dialects and their history of research, with references, remains Funk 1988—see esp. the map at p. 182 fig. 6—, in addition to the individual entries in the *Claremont Coptic Encyclopedia* and the continually valid study by Kahle in *P.Bal.* I pp. 193–242.

[43] Esp. "idiolect", referring to the speech, dialect, and by extension written idiom of a single individual, where "idiom" refers to an individual form of expression, from that of a person to that of a dialect or language community, and "idiolectal variation" denotes the ubiquitous variation within a language that exists between each and every speaker. A convenient reference for such terminology is Matthews 2007.

Hand 1 copied p. 2/1 to p. 8/13 (Phase 1) before apparently returning to copy p. 10/1–6 (Phase 2) and p. 9/1–17+10/7–11 (Phase 3). This bilingual copyist copied eight pages of Coptic- and Greek-language text before returning to inscribe two further recipes in Coptic on page 10, and then pages 9 and 10. While there is relatively little diagnostic variation in the Greek against the background of phonetic spellings in contemporary documentary papyri, or in the Coptic against what would later be recognized as standard Sahidic, certain notable features can be highlighted regarding the Coptic.

In §§1–8 and §§11–13 a small number of features are noteworthy: the thorough treatment of /e/ with supralinear strokes to mark syllabic consonants[44] that, in most cases, cover both the preceding and following consonant[45], with one exception of writing with ⲉ and one where the supralinear stroke is unexpectedly omitted[46]; certain orthographies that could suggest southern phonetic features in §§7–8[47]; one instance of an unparalleled reduction of diphthong ⲉⲓ̈ to simple ⲓ in ⲛⲟⲓ̈ⲧ for S ⲛⲟⲉⲓ̈ⲧ (p. 3/17), yet an alternation of these in ⲉⲓⲱⲧ (p. 3/17–18) and ⲓⲱⲧ (p. 6/12), suggesting the orthographies are instead derived from the source texts, rather than the idiolect of Hand 1. For variation within the same section (§1), consider the combination of dittography, haplography, and Egyptianized orthography in (ⲡ)ⲡⲉⲧⲁⲗⲟⲛ (p. 2/3) compared with ⲡⲡⲉⲇⲁⲗⲗⲟⲛ (p. 2/7).

Linguistic features of the Greek portions of this phase may be categorized as phonetic spellings related to vowels and consonants. Vocalic features include occasional conflation of vowel quality, /a/ for /e/ and /e/ for /a/,[48] and a more common conflation of vowel quantity: /ē/ for /i/, /ei/ for /i/, /i/ for /ē/, /ō/ for /o/ and twice /o/ for /ō/.[49] There are also two cases of aphaeresis of an initial vowel, /a/ and /o/.[50] Consonantal features include conflation of /g/ for /k/[51] and possibly

---

[44] Before §§9–§10: ⲧⲁϩⲥ̄⸗ (p. 2/1) compare ⲧⲁϩⲥ̄⸗ of Hand 3 (p. 14/14); ⲉϫ̄ⲛ̄- (p. 2/1) and ⲉϫ̄ⲙ̄- (p. 2/2); ⲙ̄ⲛ̄- (p. 2/3; 2/8); ϩ̄ⲙ̄ϫ (p. 3/18); ϭⲱϫ̄ϥ̄ (p. 3/21); ⲱϣ̄ⲙ̄ (p. 4/17); ⲛ̄ϩⲏⲧ⸗ (p. 4/17); ⲧ̄ⲛ̄ⲛⲟ⸗ (p. 4/18). After §§9–10: ⲛ̄ⲙ̄ⲙⲁ⸗ (p. 7/17) and ⲉϫ̄ⲛ̄- (p. 9/14; 10/3–4 and ⲉϫⲛ̄- (p. 9/15; 10/14). Compare also the reduction of ⲉ/ⲁ to a supralinear stroke in ⲛ̄ϩ̄ⲣ̄ⲛ- (p. 8/2) but not in ⲛⲁϩⲣⲛ- (p. 8/3).

[45] Compare Hand 1 ⲙ̄ⲛ̄- (p. 2/3; 2/8; 9/7; 9/8; 9/10) with Hand 2 ⲙⲛ̄- (p. 10/13; 12/3; 12/10); Hand 1 ϩ̄ⲙ̄ϫ (p. 3/18) with Hand 2 ϩⲙ̄ϫ̄ (p. 12/9; 12/14) and Hand 3 ϩⲙ̄ϫ̄ (13/13; 14/3).

[46] The indefinite article ϩⲉⲛ- (p. 3/19) and ⲛⲡⲉ⸗ (p. 4/14), respectively; note in the latter also a rare instance of absence of assimilation.

[47] ⲛⲁϫⲉ "tooth", "teeth" (p. 4/13–14) compared with Hand 2 ⲛⲁⲁϫⲉ (12/18) and ⲧ̄ⲛ̄ⲛⲟ⸗ (p. 4/18) compared with Hand 2 ⲧⲛⲟ⸗ (p. 12/3; 12/14; 12/17), see *P.Bal.* I pp. 61–62 §13 and 111–112 §80l, respectively.

[48] καφαλλαλγίαν for κεφαλαλγίαν (p. 8/6); ἔτεκαν for ἔτεκεν (p. 3/9).

[49] ἐρίδη for ἐρίδι(ν) (p. 3/13); λείαν for λίαν (p. 2/15); τίν for τήν (p. 3/9); ἀκίνδυν{ω}ων for ἀκίνδυνον (with dittography over a line-break) (p. 3/11–12); ὅ(ρας) for ὥρας (p. 3/17) and ὁς for ὡς (p. 4/1).

[50] ʼβασανίστως for ἀβασανίστως (p. 3/12); τί for ὅτι (p. 7/14).

[51] δόγιμον for δόκιμον (p. 2/10).

/g/ for /t/, if not a graphic confusion of Γ and T,[52] and of /s/ for /d/,[53] doubling of /l/,[54] and weakness of final /n/ before a following consonant[55] and of final /s/ in general,[56] to which a rare, apparent instance of conflation of cases may relate in which the genitive of a feminine noun terminating in /-ēs/ is substituted for the dative in /-ē/,[57] if a general uncertainty about the placement of final /s/ is assumed.

None of these features are diagnostic of a particular region, and the sample size is restricted. More significantly, the phonetic spellings in sum suggest that Greek was *legible* to a writer for whom Coptic was the native and primary language. The variance will have arisen in an internal dictation and does not descend to purely graphic copying of a totally unfamiliar language. The anomalous τρίτε for τρίτον "thrice" (4/4) may be further evidence for the influence of interaction with Greek as a living language, as perhaps related to the process by which Greek personal names in -ος result in -ⲉ terminations in Coptic (see further the commentary).

The Coptic §§9–10 also require independent treatment due to their distinct content to the texts that precede and follow in the codex, exhibiting many notable linguistic and orthographic features in their own right, as well as in comparison to those of the other sections of the texts of this codex.

§9 exhibits a more varied treatment of ⲛ- than elsewhere in the codex, strongly suggestive of orthographies, miscopyings or misunderstandings carried over from its source text: from potential instances of the haplography of ⲛ,[58] to the omission of ⲛ,[59] and its rendering with ⲉ,[60] as well as the absence of assimilation.[61] Likewise, the treatment of ⲉ- is varied, from haplography of ⲉ-,[62] exclusive to §§9–10, to its outright omission.[63] As with §§1–8 and §§11–13, and §10, the thorough treatment of /e/ with supralinear strokes to mark syllabic con-

[52] μήγραν for μήτραν (p. 3/9).

[53] ἰσών for ἰδών (p. 4/2).

[54] καφαλλαλγίαν for κεφαλαλγίαν (p. 8/6).

[55] ἀνατολή for ἀνατολήν (p. 3/9); τό for τόν (p. 4/5).

[56] εἰ for εἰς (p. 2/12) (before vowel); σελήνη (p. 2/12) (before consonant).

[57] θαλάσσης for θαλάσσῃ (p. 3/13).

[58] ⲛ̄ⲧⲏϭⲙⲉ for S ⲙ̄ⲛⲧⲏϭⲙⲉ or even ⲛ̄ⲛⲧⲏϭ ⲙ̄ⲙⲉ (p. 6/13), although neither is technically necessary, and potentially also ⲕⲉⲗⲉⲗⲉ ⲛ̄(ⲛ)ϣⲱⲥ (p. 6/13–14); ϣⲃⲱⲧ ⲛ̄(ⲛ)ⲉⲗⲟⲓ̈ϩ (p. 6/14); ϫⲟⲟⲕⲉϥ ⲛ̄(ⲛ)ⲉⲙⲉ (p. 6/15).

[59] (ⲙ̄)ⲡⲟⲟⲩ (p. 5/16), although not unusual, and ⲣ̄ ⲡⲣⲏⲥ (ⲛ̄)ⲧⲓⲛ (p. 7/6); for the latter omission of the dative, see *P.Bal.* I p. 109 §80f.

[60] ⲉⲛⲧⲱⲃⲉ ⲉⲙⲓⲥⲉ for ⲛⲧⲱⲃⲉ ⲙ̄ⲙⲓⲥⲉ (p. 5/17–18), suggestive of A, see *P.Bal.* I p. 113 §82e.

[61] ⲡⲃⲛ̄ⲧ ⲛ̄ⲡϣⲱ̣ⲡⲉ (p. 6/11–12) and ⲃⲱⲕ ⲛ̄ⲙ̄ⲙⲉⲩⲉ (p. 7/9).

[62] ⲧⲓⲛⲁ (ⲉ)ⲉⲃⲱⲧ (p. 5/6); ⲛ̄ⲛⲉⲧϣⲓⲧ(ⲉ): ⲉⲓ̈ⲧⲣⲉ- (p. 5/11–12); ⲉⲥϯ ⲛⲁⲁⲕⲉ· (ⲉ)ϥⲧⲟⲟⲩ ⲛ̄ⲥⲟⲩ (p. 5/16).

[63] Compare ⲕⲁⲙ (p. 5/5; 5/8) with ⲕⲁⲙⲉ (p. 6/2–3), as well as with §10 ⲕⲁⲙ (p. 7/2) and F ⲕⲉⲙ (p. 6/18).

sonants that, in most cases, cover both the preceding and following consonant is found,[64] with one exception that differs to Hand 1 elsewhere.[65] Variations between orthographies in §9 and §10,[66] as well as in other sections of Phase 1,[67] are also found, strongly suggesting that these orthographies were carried over from their source texts and were not features of the copyist's idiolect. The omission of the attributive marker in the construction of compounds is also found in cases where it would be expected in standardized dialects of Coptic through the use of the construct form of a noun,[68] but also in numerous instances where it would not, due to the absence of a standardized construct form of that noun.[69] The interference of the copyist of Hand 1's idiolect with the source text may be exhibited by the variations between different orthographies of the same word,[70] and may suggest the subsequent adjustment of a source text in a southern dialect (L or A) to S.[71] Numerous misspellings of, miscopyings from, or copyings that lacked understanding of, the source text are also exhibited.[72] The copyist of Hand 1's idiolect, or at least his idiosyncratic orthographic conventions, is exhibited by (ⲟ)ⲟⲩ,[73] ⲱ for ⲟⲟ,[74] ⲱ for ⲱⲱ,[75] ⲟ for ⲱ,[76] and ⲟ for ⲟⲟ,[77] which seem suggestive of a reduced ⲱ and ⲟⲟ diagnostic of Mesokemic. Other lexemes or orthographies appear suggestive of other northern[78] and southern[79] dialects. The

---

[64] ⲙ̅ⲛ̅- (p. 5/1; 5/2); ϣⲙ̅ⲛ̅ⲧ̅- (p. 5/2); ⲥ̅ⲛ̅ⲧⲉ (p. 5/6); ⲛ̅ⲧⲟⲧ⸗ (p. 5/9); ϩ̅ⲛ̅- (p. 5/10; 6/5); ⲱⲧ̅ⲡ̅ (p. 5/11); ⲣ̅-ϣⲁⲩ (p. 5/12); ϣⲁⲧ̅ⲛ̅- (p. 5/12–13); ⲟⲩⲱⲧ̅⸗ (p. 5/13); ϣⲟⲙ̅ⲛ̅ⲧ̅ (p. 5/15); ⲡⲟⲗϭ- (p. 5/17); ϭⲛ̅ⲧ̅⸗ (p. 5/18); ϩ̅ⲙ̅- (p. 5/20); ⲙ̅ⲙⲁⲩ (p. 6/2); ⲥ̅ⲙ̅ⲛ̅- (p. 6/3); ⲥⲙ̅ⲛ̅ⲧ̅⸗ (p. 6/3); ϣⲙ̅ϣⲉ (p. 6/3); ⲣ̅-ⲉⲣⲱⲧⲉ (p. 6/4).

[65] Compare ⲙⲉⲛ (p. 5/17) with Hand 1 elsewhere as ⲙ̅ⲛ̅- (p. 2/3; 2/8; 9/7; 9/8; 9/10).

[66] Compare ⲡⲉϊ- (p. 5/3; 5/4) and ⲡⲁϊ- (p. 5/6) with ⲡⲓ- (p. 6/10) and ⲡⲁϊ- (p. 7/7) in §10.

[67] Compare ⲙ̅ⲡⲉ⸗ (p. 5/18 [twice]; 5/19) with ⲛⲡⲉ⸗ (p. 4/14) in §7.

[68] E.g. ⲧⲟⲩⲣⲏⲥ not ⲧⲏⲟⲩ ⲛ̅ⲣⲏⲥ (p. 5/4).

[69] ϩⲧⲟϩⲁⲧ not ϩⲧⲟ ⲛ̅ϩⲁⲧ (p. 5/8) and ϩⲧⲟⲕⲁⲙ not ϩⲧⲟ ⲛ̅ⲕⲁⲙ (p. 5/8), directly comparable to Demotic *ḥtr-ḥḏ* and *ḥtr-km* (*P.London-Leiden* verso 33/1), neither belonging to the "genderless suffixes" noted by Layton (2000, 89–90 §112, cf. §96 and §114).

[70] Firstly ⲉⲙⲉ "herdsman" (p. 6/15), then ⲁⲙⲉ (p. 6/16) and ⲁⲙ̅ⲉ (p. 6/19–20) as well as ⲉⲃⲱⲧ "Abydos" (p. 5/6) and ⲁⲃⲱⲧ (p. 7/6) in §10.

[71] For the interchangeable and diagnostic nature of ⲉ for ⲁ, see *P.Bal.* I p. 58–59 §7.

[72] ⲣⲏⲣⲉ (p. 5/4) for ⲣⲏⲧⲉ "manner/fashion"; (ⲟⲩ)ⲏⲣ (p. 5/16–17) and ⲟⲩ' (p. 5/17); and the text missing between the end of p. 5/20 and the beginning of p. 6/1.

[73] Compare ϩⲣⲟⲩ (p. 5/1), ϩⲣⲟⲟⲩ (p. 5/1) and ϩⲣⲟⲟⲩ (p. 5/2): in the latter case ⲟ has been added before ⲟⲩ as an emendation, seemingly an adaptation to the most common S orthographic convention from a source text or idiolect that favors reduced ⲟⲩ.

[74] ⲟⲩⲱⲧ̅⸗ (p. 5/13) for S ⲟⲩⲟ(ⲟ)ⲧ⸗, see *P.Bal.* I p. 87 §56B.

[75] ⲧⲱⲃⲉ "brick" (p. 5/17).

[76] Compare ⲧⲟⲛⲟⲩ (p. 3/19) rather than ⲧⲱⲛⲟⲩ.

[77] Compare ⲛ̅ⲧⲟⲧ⸗ (p. 5/9) rather than ⲛ̅ⲧⲟⲟⲧ⸗.

[78] ϣⲓⲧ(ⲉ) for B ϣⲓϯ (p. 5/12) and ⲗⲉⲃⲉⲛ for B/S ⲗⲉⲃⲁⲛ (p. 6/1). Note that Demotic *is* the Lower Egyptian language variety that comprises the dialectal predecessor of Bohairic. Yet compare ⲥⲓⲃⲓⲧ for S ⲥⲓⲃⲧ (p. 5/7), apparently not attested in B but common in Demotic.

grapheme ϯ, not used in Old Coptic yet established in the Fayum already by the end of the 3rd century CE,[80] is found in the divine epithet ⲡⲟⲣϯⲟⲩ (p. 5/10) and ϯⲛⲁⲗⲕⲉ (p. 5/16). In one instance a traditional Egyptian divine name (theonym), ⲏⲥⲉ̄ "Isis" (p. 5/15), is written with a supralinear stroke in the same style as Graeco-Egyptian *voces magicae*.[81]

§10, as §9, exhibits a mixed treatment of /e/, with a secure instance of haplography[82] and—albeit not unexpected—omission,[83] alongside supralinear strokes marking syllabic consonants that, in most cases, cover both the preceding and following consonant,[84] with few exceptions.[85] As in §9, several variant orthographies suggest that they are derived from the source text of §10, rather than the copyist of Hand 1's idiolect.[86] Similarly, the omission of the attributive marker in the construction of compounds is also found in cases where it would not be expected, due to the absence of a construct form of that noun in standardized dialects of Coptic.[87] Numerous misspellings of, miscopyings from, or copyings that lacked understanding of, the source text are also exhibited.[88] The idiolect behind Hand 1, or at least the idiosyncratic orthographic conventions, are perhaps exhibited in F ⲕⲉⲙ (p. 6/18) in contrast to S ⲕⲁⲙ (p. 7/2) in §10 and ⲕⲁⲙ (p. 5/5; 5/8) and ⲕⲁⲙⲉ (p. 6/2–3) in §9; the F penchant for ⲃ over ϥ,[89] given ⲃ instead of ϥ in ⲃⲛⲧ (p. 6/11) which suggests ϥ is added to ⲃ in ϣⲁϥⲃⲉ (p. 4/16), rather than vice versa; ⲡⲏⲧ for the absolute and qualitative form (p. 7/8 [twice]) and (p. 6/19; 7/7) respectively; and free variation between ϭ and ⲕ[90] in ⲧⲏϭ+ (p. 6/18) and ⲧⲏⲕ+ (p. 7/1).

---

[79] ϩⲟⲓ̈ⲙⲉ "wave", "flood" (p. 5/1; 5/2) is closest to L/A ϩⲁ(ⲉ)ⲓⲙⲉ and ⲧⲙⲁⲥⲓ̈ⲟ (p. 5/10–11) appears closer to A ⲧⲙⲁⲥⲉⲓⲟ than S ⲧⲙⲉⲥⲓⲟ.

[80] See *P.Bal.* I pp. 148–149 §127E.

[81] Compare ⲓ̄ⲁ̄ⲱ̄ (p. 8/1), also Hand 1.

[82] ⲁⲩϩⲱⲛ ⲉⲧⲟⲟⲧⲉ (ⲉ)ϩⲧⲣⲟⲩ for ⲉϩⲧⲟⲟⲩⲉ (p. 6/7).

[83] Compare ⲕⲁⲙ (p. 7/2) and F ⲕⲉⲙ (p. 6/18) with ⲕⲁⲙ (p. 5/5; 5/8) and ⲕⲁⲙⲉ (p. 6/2–3) in §9.

[84] ⲧ̄ⲃ̄ⲛⲛⲟⲟⲩⲉ (p. 6/7); ⲡⲱⲣ̄ϣ̄ (p. 6/12); ⲣ̄-ⲥⲏⲃⲉ "to sprout" (p. 6/13); ⲧ̄ⲃ̄ⲛⲏ (p. 7/4; 7/10); ϭ̄ⲛ̄- (p. 7/7).

[85] Compare ⲣ- (p. 6/13; 6/14; 6/15) with ⲣ̄- (p. 7/5; 7/6).

[86] Compare ⲓⲱⲧ (p. 6/12) with ⲉⲓⲱⲧ (p. 3/17–18) in §4; ⲙⲉ⸗ (p. 6/13; 6/14) with A ⲙⲁ⸗ (p. 6/15); ⲡⲓ- (p. 6/10) and ⲡⲁⲓ̈- (p. 7/7) with ⲡⲉⲓ̈- (p. 5/3; 5/4) and ⲡⲁⲓ̈- (p. 5/6) in §9.

[87] ⲉⲥⲟⲩϩⲏⲣ for ⲉⲥⲟⲟⲩ ⲛ̄ϩⲏⲣ (p. 7/2) and ⲉⲥⲟⲩⲕⲁⲙⲉ for ⲉⲥⲟⲟⲩ ⲛ̄ⲕⲁⲙⲉ (p. 7/2–3). These are presumably otherwise unattested construct forms of S ⲉⲥⲟⲟⲩ, or evidence the writing (ⲟ)ⲟⲩ discussed for Hand 1 in §9 above coupled with the omission of the attributive marker. The former explanation is supported by ϩⲉⲱ for S ⲉϩⲉ-ⲱ (p. 7/3). An indication that these orthographies are more likely to derive from their source text is the spelling ⲟⲩⲥⲟⲟⲩ ⲛ̄ⲕⲁⲙⲉ (p. 12/6–7) for ⲟⲩ-ⲉⲥⲟⲟⲩ ⲛ̄ⲕⲁⲙⲉ by Hand 2.

[88] (ⲉ)ϩⲧⲣⲟⲩ (p. 6/7) for ⲉϩⲧⲟⲟⲩⲉ "at dawn" and ϭⲁϩⲏⲧ (p. 7/8) for ⲥⲁϩⲏⲧ "north(ern side)".

[89] See *P.Bal.* I pp. 136–137 §121.

[90] For this comparably southern feature, see *P.Bal.* I p. 147 §126.

In Phase 2, the use of ⲛⲓⲙ ⲡϣⲉ ⲛⲓⲙ (p. 10/5–6) in §15 compared to ⲇ̣ⲇ̣ (p. 8/3) in §12 suggests that the orthographies of the source texts were carried over. In Phase 3, one potential instance of haplography is exhibited, where (ⲙ̅)ⲙ̅ⲏⲛⲉ (p. 9/12) and ⲙ̅ⲙⲏⲛⲉ (p. 10/11) both appear in the same section (§14). The treatment of /e/ with supralinear strokes marking syllabic consonants that, in most cases, cover both the preceding and following consonant, is also common to Phase 3.[91] Either the copyist's idiolect, his idiosyncratic orthographic conventions, or the carrying over of the orthographic conventions of the source texts can be seen in: the omission of ⲟⲩ in ⲟⲩⲟⲩ or reduction of ⲟⲩⲟⲩ to ⲟⲩ,[92] comparable to that in §9, found in (ⲟⲩ)ⲟⲩⲱⲛ (p. 9/11); S/A ϭⲱⲛ (p. 9/9); ⲉⲣⲏⲩ (p. 9/7) alongside ⲉⲣⲏⲟⲩ (p. 9/10); omission of ⲃ in ⲕⲟⲗⲟⲙⲏⲑⲣⲁ from κολυμβήθρα (p. 10/8); and apparent free variation between ⲅ and ⲕ[93] in ⲁⲙⲟⲅ (p. 9/13; 10/9; 10/10) and ⲁⲙⲟⲕ "mouthful (?)" (p. 10/7).

Hand 2 copied p. 10/12 to p. 13/10 (Phase 4). This monolingual phase exhibits the following points of interest and contrast with Phases 1–3 of Hand 1 and Phase 5 of Hand 3. In the treatment of ⲛ-: a difference is exhibited in the writing of the attributive marker between Hands 1, 2, and 3;[94] dittography of ⲛ-, exclusive to Hand 2;[95] omission of ⲛ in the Future II.[96] Comparable to Hand 1, the thorough treatment of /e/ with supralinear strokes to mark syllabic consonants that, in most cases, cover both the preceding and following consonant is found,[97] but, unlike Hand 1, never in ⲙⲛ̅-,[98] while in ϩⲙⲙⲉ (p. 11/13) Hand 3 omits while

[91] ϣⲟⲙ̅ⲛ̅ⲧ̅ (p. 9/2; 9/3; 9/4; 9/11); ⲙ̅ⲛ̅- (p. 9/7; 9/8; 9/10); ϩ̅ⲛ̅ⲕⲉ (p. 9/8); ⲏⲣ̅ⲡ̅ (p. 9/9) compare Hand 2 ⲏⲣⲡ̅ (p. 10/18); ⲙ̅ⲏⲛⲉ (p. 9/12); ⲛ̅ⲙ̅ⲙⲁ⸗ (p. 9/12; 9/16); ϣⲟⲙ̅ⲛ̅ⲧ̅ (p. 9/12); ⲥⲁϣ̅ϥ̅ (p. 9/13); ⲡⲁϩ̅ⲧ̅⸗ (p. 9/14); ϭ̅ⲡ̅- (p. 9/14); ⲣⲁⲧ̅ϥ̅ (p. 9/15–16); ⲕⲟⲧ̅ⲥ̅ (p. 9/16); ⲙ̅ⲛ̅ⲛ̅ⲥⲱⲥ (p. 9/17); ϩ̅ⲙ̅ⲙⲉ (p. 9/17; 10/8); ⲥⲁϣ̅ϥ̅ (p. 10/7; 10/8–9; 10/9–10); ϣⲟⲙ̅ⲛ̅ⲧ̅ (p. 10/10); ϩⲙ̅ⲟⲟⲥ (p. 10/15); ⲱⲥ̅ⲕ̅ (p. 10/17).

[92] For omission, see *P.Bal.* I p. 85 §53; for reduction, see *P.Bal.* I pp. 87–88 §58.

[93] Rare in Coptic words: see *P.Bal.* I pp. 95–96 §71.

[94] Compare ⲛⲉϩ (ⲙ̅)ⲙⲉ (p. 13/12), where the attributive is not essential, by Hand 2, with ⲉⲃⲓⲱ ⲙ̅ⲙⲉ (p. 12/17–18) by Hand 3 and Hand 1 in Phase 3 (ⲙ̅)ⲙ̅ⲏⲛⲉ (p. 9/12) as well as ⲙ̅ⲙⲏⲛⲉ (p. 10/11). Consider also the only instance in the entire manuscript where the attributive is not written with a supralinear stroke, but simply as ⲛ- (p. 12/8).

[95] Albeit across a line break in ϩⲛ̅ϫ̅ⲃ̅ⲥ | ⲛ̅ⲛ̅ϣⲉ ⲛ̅ⲛⲟⲩϩⲉ (p. 10/14–15). Compare also the dittography of ⲧ, not across a line break, in ⲟⲩⲉⲧⲧⲟⲩⲱⲧ+ (p. 12/14) for ⲟⲩⲉⲧⲟⲩⲱⲧ+.

[96] ⲉⲓⲁ- for ⲉⲓⲛⲁ- (p. 12/17); for this characteristic L feature, see *P.Bal.* I p. 105 §129 and pp. 151–158 §§128–129.

[97] ϩ̅ⲙ̅- (p. 10/13; 11/10; 11/14; 12/5); ϫ̅ⲃ̅ⲥ (p. 10/14; 11/12); ϩⲛ̅- (p. 10/14; 12/15; 12/17; 12/18; 13/1); ϩⲓϫⲛ̅- (p. 10/15); ⲏⲣⲡ̅ (p. 10/18); ϩⲟⲗ̅ϭ̅+ (p. 10/18); ⲥⲁϩ̅⸗ (p. 11/8), compare Hand 1 ⲥⲁϩ̅⸗ (p. 2/6); ⲉϫⲛ̅- (p. 11/12); ⲛⲟⲩϫ̅ⲧ̅ (p. 11/15); ϩⲟⲥ̅ⲙ̅ (p. 12/2); ⲥⲁϣϥ̅ (p. 12/6); ⲣⲟϫ̅ϩ̅+ (p. 12/7); ⲥ̅ⲕ̅- for ⲥⲉⲕ (p. 12/8); ⲛⲟϫ̅ⲧ̅ϥ̅ for ⲛⲟⲩϫⲕϥ̅ (p. 12/9); ⲃ̅ⲣ̅ⲣⲉ (p. 12/9); ϩⲙ̅ϫ̅ (p. 12/9; 12/14); ⲣⲟϫ̅ϩ̅⸗ (p. 12/14); ⲕⲛ̅ⲛⲉ (p. 12/16); ⲣⲟϫ̅ϩ̅+ (p. 12/7); ⲁⲛⲧⲏⲗ̅ⲙ̅ (p. 13/4–5).

[98] Compare Hand 2 ⲙⲛ̅- (p. 10/13; 12/3; 12/10) with Hand 1 ⲙ̅ⲛ̅- (p. 2/3; 2/8; 9/7; 9/8; 9/10).

Hand 1 has ϩⲙ̄ⲙⲉ (pp. 9/17; 10/8); ⲉ is written out in one case[99] and omitted in another two.[100] The influence of northern dialects is exhibited,[101] specifically B in §16,[102] §22,[103] and §28[104] and F in §20.[105] Either the copyist's idiolect, his idiosyncratic orthographic conventions, or the carrying over of the orthographic conventions of the source texts can be seen in: expansion to a diphthong ⲉⲓ for ⲓ in ⲡⲁⲉⲓϣⲉ[106] (p. 12/1) for S ⲡⲁ(ⲓ)ϣⲉ and for ⲉ in ϩⲁⲃ[ⲗ]ⲉⲉⲗⲉ̣ⲓ for S ϩⲁⲃⲗⲉⲉⲗⲉ (p. 12/13); ⲉ where S has ⲏ in ⲥⲡⲗⲉⲗⲓⲛ (p. 13/11) for ⲥⲡⲗⲏⲗⲓⲛ; doubling of ⲁ where Hand 1 has ⲁ in ⲛⲁⲁϫⲉ (p. 12/18); raising of /o/ to /e/ in ⲧⲟⲩϫⲉ (p. 11/7) for absolute ⲧⲟⲩϫⲟ;[107] reduction of the consonant cluster ⲗⲗ to ⲉⲗ in ϩⲉⲗⲱ[108] (p. 10/14); ⲃ for ϥ in ⲃⲱ (p. 10/14) and ϫⲁⲧⲃⲉ[109] (p. 11/9); in Greek loanwords, Egyptian /t/ from Greek /d/ is consistently rendered ⲇ, unlike Hand 1 and 3,[110] although Egyptianized vocalizations of Greek loanwords are found,[111] unlike Hand 1. Compare also ψιμύθιον "white lead" spelled ⲥⲓⲙⲓⲑⲓⲟⲛ (p. 13/8–9) by Hand 2, but ⲡⲥⲓⲙⲓⲑⲓⲟⲩ (p. 13/15) by Hand 3. Orthographies that more likely evidence the carrying over of orthographic conventions from source texts comprise: free variation between ϯ- and ⲧⲓ- in ϯ-ⲧⲕⲁⲥ (p. 10/17) and ⲧⲓⲧⲕⲁⲥ (pp. 12/18; 13/1). Consistent and inconsistent orthographies that more likely evidence an idiolect behind Hand 2 comprise: ⲧ for ⲕ after ϫ in ⲛⲟϫⲕ⸗, ⲛⲟⲩϫ̄ⲧ̄⸗ (p. 11/15) and ⲛⲟϫⲧ̄⸗ (p. 13/9) consistently in §19 and §29; ⲧϫ for ⲧϣ in ⲡⲉⲧϫⲱⲛⲉ (p. 11/6), compare ϣⲱⲛⲉ (p. 11/1).

Hand 3 copied p. 13/10 to p. 14/20 (Phase 5), filling the remainder of the premade codex. This monolingual phase exhibits the following points of interest and contrast with Phases 1–3 of Hand 1 and Phase 4 of Hand 2. Comparable to Hands 1 and 2, the thorough treatment of /e/ with supralinear strokes to mark syllabic consonants that, in most cases, cover both the preceding and following

---

[99] Compare ⲉⲣ- (p. 13/4) with Hand 1 ⲣ̄- (p. 7/5; 7/6) and Hand 3 ⲣ̄- (p. 14/15).

[100] Compare (ⲉ)ⲥⲟⲟⲩ (p. 12/6; 12/7) with Hand 1 ⲉⲥⲟⲩ- (p. 7/2 [twice]).

[101] Compare ⲧⲛⲟ⸗ (p. 12/3; 12/14; 12/17) to Hand 1 ⲧ̄ⲛ̄ⲛⲟ⸗ (4/18), the latter being more characteristic of the Theban area: see *P.Bal.* I pp. 111–112.

[102] B ϭⲓⲱⲟⲩ (p. 10/13).

[103] B ⲗⲁⲗⲉ- (p. 12/12).

[104] B ⲁⲧⲕⲁⲥ (p. 13/7).

[105] F ⲁⲛⲏϣ (p. 12/2).

[106] Perhaps under Lycopolitan influence: see *P.Bal.* I p. 78; but the pronunciation of this diphthong is already levelled with /i/ in contemporary Greek.

[107] I.e. the writing of the construct or prenominal form where the absolute would be expected.

[108] Spellings with ⲉ for ⲗ are discussed in *P.Bal.* I p. 97 §74B.

[109] Perhaps under Fayumic influence: see *P.Bal.* I pp. 136–137 §121.

[110] Compare ⲇⲁⲓⲙⲟⲛⲓⲟⲛ (p. 11/2) with Hand 3 ⲧⲟⲕⲓⲙⲟⲛ (p. 14/1).

[111] Compare ⲁⲛⲅⲕⲉⲫⲁⲗⲟⲥ from ἐγκέφαλος (p. 12/7–8) with Hand 3 ⲟⲛⲅⲓⲁ from οὐγκία (p. 14/2; 14/3) and Hand 1 ⲟⲝⲩⲅⲅⲓⲛ from ὀξύγγιον (p. 3/18).

consonant is found,[112] with omissions rare[113] and renderings with ⲉ exclusive to the indefinite article.[114] The idiolect behind Hand 3 may be suggested in: lowering of /i/ to /e/ in ⲥⲉⲟⲟⲩⲛ (p. 14/20) for ⲥⲓⲟⲟⲩⲛ; (ⲟⲩ)ⲟⲩ in (ⲟⲩ)ⲟⲧ̅ϩ̅ (p. 14/4), also exhibited by Hand 1 (if not dittography); ⲱ for ⲱⲱ in ⲧⲱⲃⲉ (p. 14/20), also exhibited by Hand 1; ⲙⲡ⸗ (p. 14/7; 14/17), ⲙ̅ⲡ⸗ (p. 14/8; 14/17), and ⲙⲡ̅⸗ (p. 14/15) with ⲙ̅ⲡⲉ⸗ (p. 5/18 [twice]; 5/19) and ⲛⲡⲉ⸗ (p. 4/14) by Hand 1; reduction of the initial consonant cluster in ⲛ̅ⲥⲁϩⲧⲉ (p. 13/16–17), i.e. ⲛ̅ⲅ̅ⲥⲁϩⲧⲉ, and ⲛⲧⲁⲗⲁ̣ϥ̣ (p. 14/11), i.e. ⲛ̅ⲅ̅ⲧⲁⲗⲁϥ; inconsistent reduction of the final consonant cluster in ϣⲁⲧ̅⸗ (p. 13/17), compare ϣⲁⲛⲧ̅⸗[115] (p. 14/12); and the Fayumic orthographies ⲡⲉⲛⲓⲡⲉ (p. 14/7–8) and ⲧⲁⲗⲁ⸗ (14/11)—compare S ⲧⲁⲗⲟ⸗ (p. 11/12) by Hand 2—; as well as perhaps more northern than not ⲓ[116] (p. 14/17) and ⲡⲓⲣⲟⲩⲧ (p. 14/18). Haplography is attested once,[117] as is dittography.[118] As in Hand 1 and 2, Egyptianized orthographies of Greek loanwords are found,[119] including the doubling of consonant clusters in ⲁⲗⲗⲱⲏ from ἀλόη (p. 14/6) but their reduction in ⲅⲣⲁⲙⲁ from γράμμα (p. 14/5). It is unclear whether these reflect the idiolect of the copyist of Hand 3, his idiosyncratic orthographic conventions, or the source texts. In the case of the orthography ⲡⲥⲓⲙⲓⲑⲓⲟⲩ from ψιμύθιον (p. 13/15), to be compared with ⲥⲓⲙⲓⲑⲓⲟⲛ (p. 13/8–9) by Hand 2, the treatment of the consonant-cluster /ps/ may be explained by the above factors, but the termination in -ⲟⲩ is surely the result of direct transliteration from a Greek genitive form: see the section **Context in the Practice of Medicine and Healing** below and the corresponding place in the line-commentary.

Beyond the archaic features of the two incantations in §§9–10, which have been discussed in detail, the rest of the codex demonstrates a relatively early phase of Coptic in which Greek loanwords are plentiful and the old personal

---

112 ϩ̅ⲙ̅- (pp. 13/10; 14/12); ϩⲙ̅ϫ̅ (pp. 13/13; 14/3); ⲁⲛⲧⲏⲗ̅ⲙ̅ (p. 13/17); ⲟⲩⲟⲧ̅ϩ̅ (p. 14/4); ϩ̅ⲛ̅- (p. 14/6); ⲃ̅ⲛ̅ⲛⲉ (p. 14/7); ⲛ̅ϩⲏⲧ⸗ (p. 14/9); ⲉⲧ̅ⲙ̅ⲙⲁⲩ (p. 14/14); ⲧⲁϩ̅ⲥ̅⸗ (p. 14/14) compare Hand 1 ⲧⲁϩ̅ⲥ̅⸗ (p. 2/1); (ⲟⲩ)ⲟⲧ̅ϩ̅ (p. 14/4); ⲙⲡ̅ⲕ (p. 14/15); ⲣ̅ (p. 14/15); ϣⲟⲙⲛ̅ⲧ̅|ⲧⲉ (dittography) (p. 14/15–16); ⲙⲡ̅ⲅ̅ (p. 14/17); ⲛ̅ⲕⲟⲧ̅ⲕ̅ (p. 14/19); ⲥⲟⲩⲧⲱⲛ̅⸗ (p. 14/19).

113 ⲙⲡⲕⲓ (p. 14/17). Note also that the supralinear stroke is omitted in ⲙⲡ⸗ (p. 14/7) because the circumstantial precedes it, but is written in the next line ⲙ̣̅ⲡ⸗ (p. 14/8) where the circumstantial does not.

114 Compare ϩⲉⲛ- (pp. 13/18; 14/10) with ϩⲛ- (p. 14/10).

115 Compare also ϣⲁⲛⲧ̅⸗ (p. 4/18–19) and ϣⲁⲛⲧⲉ⸗ (p. 7/6–7) by Hand 1 and ϣⲁⲛⲧ⸗ (p. 11/14) by Hand 2.

116 Where Hand 1 and 2 has ⲉⲓ (pp. 5/14; 6/8; 6/15; 10/9; 11/9; 13/17).

117 ⲉϣⲁⲥⲧⲁϩ̅ⲥ̅(ⲥ) (p. 14/4), at the end of a line.

118 Once in the attributive marker at p. 14/16.

119 Compare ⲧⲟⲕⲓⲙⲟⲛ from δόκιμον (p. 14/1) with Hand 2 ⲇⲁⲓⲙⲟⲛⲓⲟⲛ from δαιμόνιον (p. 11/2) (Hand 2) or ⲟⲛⲅⲓⲁ from οὐγκία (pp. 14/2; 14/3) with Hand 2 ⲁⲛⲅⲕⲉⲫⲁⲗⲟⲥ from ἐγκέφαλος (p. 12/7–8) and Hand 1 ⲟⲝⲩⲅⲅⲓⲛ from ὀξύγγιον (p. 3/18).

suffix on nouns is preserved (ⲉⲓⲁ ⲣⲱⲕ, p. 12/19, in place of the younger construction with ⲧⲁⲡⲣⲟ; note also ϩⲏⲧⲕ̅, p. 9/14). In addition to the novel orthographies discussed above, some rare and in part still obscure words offer lexicographical interest, discussed more fully in the line-commentary: ⲁⲙⲟⲅ (pp. 9/13; 10/9; 10/10) and ⲁⲙⲟⲕ "mouthful (?)" (p. 10/7); ⲁⲛⲏϣ ⲙ̅ⲡⲣⲏ of a medicinal plant (p. 12/2); ⲉⲃⲣⲓ-, an otherwise apparently unattested construct form of ⲉⲃⲣⲁ "seed" (p. 9/3; 9/4; 9/5); ⲕⲉⲓ of an obscure household pest (?) (p. 13/8); ⲗⲟⲟⲕⲉ apparently from ⲗⲟⲕ "cup" (pp. 12/9; 13/16); ⲙⲟⲕⲉ+ from ⲙⲓⲕⲉ "to rest" (p. 14/4–5); ⲡⲟⲗϭ-, a construct form of ⲡⲱⲗϫ "to release" (p. 5/17); ⲡⲓⲣⲟⲩⲧ "to come forth" (p. 14/18); ⲡⲁϩ⸗, a prepronominal form of ⲡⲱϩ "to stretch" (p. 9/15); ⲣⲁⲧ̅ϥ̅, a nominalized form of ⲣⲱⲧⲃ "to recline" (p. 9/15–16); ϩⲉⲗⲕⲓⲉⲙⲁ of a medical ingredient (p. 13/14); and a variant of ⲛⲟⲩϫⲕ with /t/ in place of /k/ or /č/: ⲛ̅ⲕⲛⲟⲩϫ̅ⲧ̅ (p. 11/15) and ⲛⲟϫⲧ̅ϥ̅ (p. 13/9). The loanword ⲡⲉⲣⲓⲭⲣⲓⲁ (p. 12/3; 12/10) attests a Greek περιχριάω (-ᾶν) otherwise not found until the late Byzantine period.

Selected Studies

Transmitting Textual Traditions in the Roman Period (1st–4th Centuries CE) (EL)

This study concerns the *language contact situation* that resulted in a bilingualism of spoken and written Egyptian-Coptic and Greek during the late Roman Period (3rd and 4th centuries CE)—the context of the production and first use of the Michigan codex[120]—and how this had changed dramatically from the situation of the early Roman Period (2nd and 3rd centuries CE).[121] Within this process, the trends of *language* and *script shift*, and thereby *intra-* and *interlingual translation*, or even *intra- and interscript transliteration* and *transcription*,[122] that brought about the transmission of a variety of textual traditions across the boundaries of script, language, culture, and place can be understood. As the Michigan codex is a bilingual compilation of recipes in Coptic and Greek, this analytical basis will in turn illuminate aspects of its composition. As discussed in the line-commentary and excurses, some of these recipes betray the hallmarks of translations from Greek (§§5, 21, 24, 28, 29, 30), others contain features strongly suggestive of translations from Greek (§§17, 19, 20, 28), and some perhaps evidence a history of textual transmission that could go back to Old Coptic and ultimately Demotic source texts[123] (§§9 and 10). This variety attests the contemporary situation of bilingualism and biliteracy that was able to bring together wider traditions from the Eastern Mediterranean and reflexes of trad-

---

[120] As noted in **The Compilation of Michigan Ms. 136**, based on the palaeography of the hands, the later additions may have been in the 5th century CE, while there is no reason to exclude that unmarked use may have carried on even later.

[121] The frameworks of approach and the findings presented here are those utilized in and resulting from my doctoral research, now published as Love 2021a and partly summarized in Love 2021b.

[122] In Egyptology, *transcribe* is often distinguished from *transliterate*: to transcribe is to set the sign(s) of one logographic script into those of another logographic script, e.g. a transcription of hieratic in demotic; to transliterate is to set the sign(s) of a logographic script into those of an alphabetic script, e.g. a transcription of hieratic in Old Coptic.

[123] As noted above in **Previous Studies**, Kahle (*P.Bal.* I p. 254) was the first to make this judgement, classifying the Michigan codex among "a number of texts which are still Egyptian in religion and thought, and which, presumably, were either copied from Demotic direct or were based on copies of such texts", noting §§9 and 10 as "[b]y far the most important of these" otherwise principally Old Coptic sources.

itional Egyptian religion. The Michigan codex more particularly straddles the divide between the corpus of magical texts known as the Graeco-Egyptian magical papyri (GEMP) and the corpus of Coptic magical papyri (CMP) proper, evidencing both traditionalist and innovative trends in contemporary scribal and magical traditions. By contextualizing the codex as an outcome of this history of language contact and textual transmission through transliteration and translation, this section aims to understand not only the texts of the Michigan codex in its contemporary milieu of production and use during the 4th century CE, but also the aspects of the history of textual transmission responsible for their extant form. After all, such a codex is a formalized—written up—compilation—"archive"—of texts in its own right, which must have been brought together from different source manuscripts over the course of time.[124]

This study is sub-divided into six sections. (I) comprises an introduction to the frameworks of analysis applied in studying (II) and (III), the evidence for, and scribal traditions of, textual transmission during the early (1st and 2nd century CE) and late (3rd and 4th century CE) Roman Period, respectively. The implications of these analyses of textual transmission for understanding the composers, redactors, and compilers as well as past, prior, and contemporary practitioners of the recipes in the Michigan codex will then be treated in (IV). (V) examines the scholarly consensus on the textual vs. oral transmission of magical texts, particularly those containing divine dramas—often termed "*historiolae*" or "charms"—, and proposes a counterpoint to the predominant thesis of oral transmission based on the evidence of sections (II), (III), and (IV). Consequently, (VI) assesses the scholarly assumptions about the context of the production of the Michigan codex, and the practice of its recipes, by providing a counterpoint to the scholarly consensus of the supposed inexorable Christianization of cultural repertoires during the 4th century CE in the form of a thesis on "Syncretism in the Other Direction". Underpinning the theses and analyses in these sections, the hypothetical source texts of §§9 and 10 that ground their textual transmission among the plurality of cultural repertoires exhibited in the GEMP are interwoven with the excurses to §§9 and 10.

I. Language and Script Communities, Domains, and Variety in the Roman Period

At the outset, a brief note on terminology is necessary. *Mono-/bi-/triliteracy* is termed by analogy to *bilingualism*, in which two distinct languages are utilized

[124] Discussed in **The Compilation of Michigan Ms. 136**.

in different contexts by the same individual/community. Thus, the phenomenon of *bilingualism* exists within, and is maintained by, bilingual *speech communities*—themselves comprised of two *speech communities* of the respective languages. *Mono-/di-/trigraphia* is termed by analogy to *diglossia*, in which two distinct forms of the same language are utilized in different contexts by the same individual/community.[125] Thus, the phenomenon of *diglossia* exists within, and is maintained by, monolingual *speech communities*. By extension, *biliterate script communities* comprise individuals who are *producers* (writers) and *responders* (readers) of two distinct writing systems, e.g. Coptic and Greek, while digraphic *script communities* comprise individuals who are *producers* (writers) and *responders* (readers) of two scripts of the same writing system, e.g. hieratic and demotic.[126]

Drawing from sociolinguistics and linguistic anthropology, the study of spoken, and thus by extension written, languages need not be undertaken in the abstract, but can be studied in a contextualized way as existing within *communities* that are *producers* (speakers/writers) or *responders* (listeners/ readers) of a language.[127] While *speech communities* are constituted and reified by their shared language(s)[128] as well as by responding to (listening) and producing (speaking) aural/oral culture, *script communities* are constituted and reified by their shared literacy/literacies as well as by responding to (reading) and producing (writing) textual culture.[129] Furthermore, the dynamics of speech and writing change according to the *domains* in which they are utilized, and the conventions (e.g. register and formality) which govern those domains. The domain of writing that concerns this section, then, is one which produced ritual

[125] This relates particularly to languages which have a *high* and *low* form: a modern example is *Hochdeutsch* compared to a dialect of German; a Roman Period example is Classical Egyptian written in hieratic or hieroglyphs compared to Demotic written in demotic.

[126] Throughout, Egyptological conventions are used in referring to the form/stage of the Egyptian language as "Demotic", but the script as "demotic" (as "hieratic" and "hieroglyphs").

[127] For an introduction to the domains of speech and their communities, see, for example, Grinevald and Bert 2011; Mullany 2006; Patrick 2002. These frameworks are applied to discuss the phenomenon of (principally but not exclusively written) language contact, shift, tip, and death in the early Roman Period in Love 2021a, summarized in Love 2021b.

[128] A superordinate level of *language community* can also be determined, which would incorporate all speakers of Egyptian and Greek in a linguistically- rather than sociolinguistically-defined community. In a contemporary context, a *language community* can be conventionally understood at the national or supranational level, e.g. all readers of this study are members of a global English language and script community.

[129] Apparently first used by Houston (2008, 231–232), for whom the script community "exists in relation to a writing system; it survives (i.e. as a distinct community) because the system is used and transmitted across generations (i.e. within that milieu)". This concept is developed in Love 2021a, and summarized in Love 2021b.

texts, more specifically, ritual texts for personal benefit—conventionally and conveniently termed "magical". But this domain is not isolated from the others: the processes of language and script *contact* and *shift* that occurred in other domains impacted and defined the written languages and scripts utilized in that *domain* of writing.

Language contact situations, first in terms of spoken, and often subsequently in terms of written, language result almost exclusively in a *superordinate language contact situation* developing between two or more languages.[130] This situation means that one language becomes the *dominant* and the other becomes the *minority* language in any number of its domains.[131] Extended *language contact situations* result not only in code-switching, code-mixing, and the borrowing of loanwords—as from *dominant* Greek to *minority* Coptic—, but also *language shift*, whereby a speech community *shifts* from the *minority* language in one or more domains to the *dominant* language. The consequence of *language shift* is, almost exclusively, *language tip*, whereby productive bilingualism is replaced by reductive monolingualism and ultimately language moribundity and death. Although the processes of intergenerational transmission (learning) are different between spoken and written languages, and therefore within speech and script communities, spoken and written languages are analogous. *Written language shift* does not only occur between different languages, and the writing systems of those languages: it can also be characterized as an *interlingual shift*, i.e. from one language to another. Yet *intralingual shift* can occur within a diglossic language as well, i.e. from one form of a language to another, as can *interscript shift* between two distinct writing systems or within a digraphic writing system, i.e. from one script of a writing system to another.

During the 1st and 2nd centuries CE, before the broad obsolescence of Egyptian writing during the 3rd century CE,[132] language and script use in Egyptian scribal production was the most complex of any period in Egyptian history. A triglossia of Egyptians existed: (i) Spoken Egyptian; (ii) Egyptian written in the administrative, literary, and technical domains (principally Demotic in demotic); and (iii) Egyptian written in the monumental and ritual domains (principally

---

[130] Stable bilingualism is not the same as a language equilibrium resulting from a *co-ordinate language contact situation*. After all, even if language (ii) is not under threat from language (i), if language (i) is spoken and written at University but language (ii) is exclusively spoken at home, language (ii) has already *obsolesced* in the academic domain due to a *superordinate language contact situation* with language (i), i.e. (ii) is the *minority* language, whereas (i) is the *dominant* language.

[131] For a particularly informative study of language death, its stages and its modelling, as utilized in Love 2021a, §3.1, see Batibo 2005.

[132] This brief statement refers to the conclusion reached in Love 2016, §7.5.4, developed and evidenced with new, including unpublished, sources in Love 2021a, summarized in Love 2021b.

Middle/Classical Egyptian in hieroglyphs in the former, and hieratic in the latter domain). Written Egyptian in all of its forms/stages and rendered in all of its scripts was the preserve of priestly *communities of practice*,[133] supplanted in all domains of writing outside of them by Greek, and therefore utilized almost exclusively in the production of textual culture of relevance for the maintenance of such communities. Greek had come to dominate in all domains of writing concerning the administration of Egypt, as well as in the production of textual culture in the ritual, literary, and technical domains that were not embedded within priesthoods. However, while written Egyptian and thereby Egyptian textual culture was primarily associated with those temple and priestly communities, those same communities were also responders and producers of ritual,[134] literary,[135] and technical[136] texts in Greek.

Nevertheless, with few notable exceptions, by the middle of the 3rd century CE this complex situation of biliteracy and multigraphia had given way to an almost all-encompassing monoliteracy and monographia of Greek, dominating all domains of writing.[137] This had no impact on the contemporary situation of bilingualism that existed in Egypt, however, where the vast majority of the population had always been and remained first-language Egyptophones—with a proportion learning Greek for reasons of expedience.[138] Indeed, this stable bilingualism of Egyptian among first-language Egyptophones and Greek among first-language Grecophones, as well as among a proportion of first-language Egyptophones, had already existed for centuries. Nevertheless, the spoken form of Egyptian had the status of *minority* language in several *domains of speech*, just as written forms of Egyptian were the *minority* language in several *domains of writing* during the late Ptolemaic and early part of the Roman Period.[139] The

133 That is, to avoid the non-definition of "priesthoods" by referring to them simply as "priesthoods", they are defined as communities who undertook the maintenance of (a) particular cult(s), and which were constituted through mutual engagement in the undertaking of that joint enterprise which was in turn reified through their shared repertoire of cultural experience. For the *community of practice*, see the introduction by Meyerhoff 2002.

134 Consider the discussion of the translation of Egyptian ritual texts into Greek at Oxyrhynchus, discussed below, which—by extension—is strongly suggestive of the circulation of Greek-language ritual texts in priestly milieux. For this, see in particular Dieleman 2005.

135 Consider, for example, the circulation of Homer in a priestly milieu at Tebtunis, discussed in the excursus to §6. For summaries of the use of Greek in the literary domain at Oxyrhynchus, Tebtunis, and Soknopaiou Nesos, see Love 2021a, §§5.1, 6.1, and 7.1.

136 See the summary of the use of Greek in the technical domain at Oxyrhynchus, Tebtunis, Soknopaiou Nesos, and Narmouthis in Love 2021a, §§5.1, 6.1, 7.1, and 8.1.

137 For the multilingual experience in Egypt from the Ptolemaic to Islamic Period, see the contributions in Papaconstantinou 2009 as well as Fewster 2002; Fournet 2009; Thompson 2009.

138 Bilingualism among the civic elite, clergy, and in the world of commerce has been discussed briefly in Bagnall 2017.

139 This summary is a paraphrase of the study Love 2021a, summarized in Love 2021b.

emergence of Coptic as a written idiom, then, resulted ultimately in a rebalancing of this situation of *agraphia*, in which spoken Egyptian had not been written in any form outside of priestly milieux.[140] With the dating of early non-documentary Coptic manuscripts in the 3rd century CE still contentious, the rate of uptake is hard to judge.[141] Nevertheless, by the 4th century CE, and especially the second half of that century, there are significant collections of manuscripts that evidence the translation of the canonical and apocryphal gospels into Coptic, not to mention broader textual culture ascribed to Christian, Gnostic, and Manichaean milieux. Thus, emerging from the situation of bilingualism in Egypt, the written language of Egyptian-Coptic made contact with written Greek in several, and eventually all, domains of writing, existing first in a *co-ordinate language contact situation*, before supplanting written Greek almost entirely in a *superordinate language contact situation*.[142]

In the domain of magical texts,[143] the shift from Greek as the predominant language of magic during the 3rd and 4th centuries CE to Coptic occurred during the 5th century CE. Notably earlier than in other domains of writing,[144] in the domain of magical texts the *language shift* that began with the advent of Coptic as a written language—with numerous regional varieties—in its own right became a *language tip* at some point in the 4th century, leading to Coptic becoming the *dominant* language in that domain. It is, then, in this context that the production and use of the Michigan codex must be placed—the texts of which themselves exhibit this same language shift, from the Coptic-Greek bilingual phase 1 written by a bilingual copyist to the Coptic monolingual phases 4 and 5 written by two later copyists (see **The Compilation of Michigan Ms. 136** and **Outline of Content and Phases**).

In a recent article on bilingualism and mono-/digraphia at the nexus of magical traditions, the diachronic shift in the languages utilized in the domain of magical texts extant from Egypt, from Egyptian-Greek in the Roman and Byzantine Period through Greek-Coptic in the Byzantine and Islamic Period to

[140] This relates to the well-known statement by Bagnall that "no form of written Egyptian was in everyday use in the second century" (1993, 235)—"an Egyptian wanting to write a letter to a fellow Egyptian had to do so in Greek" (1993, 201). It is mistaken, however, to conclude that "the emergence of Coptic, as it seems, was not preceded by recorded historical development" or that while "a substantial percentage of the inhabitants of Egyptian in the third-fourth centuries [CE] must have spoken a form of Egyptian", "there is no evidence of what this spoken Egyptian might have been like" (Zakrzewska 2015, 186). Consider, for example, the Bigraphic Coptic of Narmouthis treated in Love 2021a, §8.

[141] See now the formative study in Fournet 2020.

[142] For this process in particular, see Richter 2009.

[143] Based on the characteristics noted above.

[144] See in particular Richter 2009.

Coptic-Arabic, was studied.[145] That treatment highlighted the broad typological similarities between the factors relating to language and script shift which influenced bilingual and mono-/digraphic redactions of magical texts in Egypt from the 2nd to 10th/11th century CE, and how this informs the socio-linguistic and also cultural identifies of both practitioners and their clients. Furthermore, beyond surveying the distribution of language and script use in those magical texts, that study investigated principally how bilingualism and monographia facilitated the practicing of those magical texts in monolingual or bilingual *speech communities* and in monoliterate or biliterate *script communities*. Here, then, the corpora of bilingual and monographic texts attested need not be revisited. Instead, selected case studies will be presented as indices of wider phenomena of language and script shift.

This is especially relevant for contextualizing the Michigan codex, which—as noted above—was produced in one or more generations that were experiencing a slight to significant shift from Greek to Coptic in different domains of writing and therefore textual culture production.[146] Nevertheless, although copying (responding) does not require spoken fluency and the recipes themselves are principally monolingual Coptic or Greek, the three copyists who worked on the Michigan codex could well have belong to such *bilingual speech* and *biliterate script* Coptic-Greek communities—however large or small. Considering next the transliteration and translation of textual traditions in the domain of magical texts will inform an understanding of how these textual traditions could have been transmitted across the boundaries of script, writing system, and written language over time. Consequently, this will allow insights into how certain recipes ended up in the Michigan codex, despite coming from diverse and distinct source texts whose histories of textual transmission perhaps spanned generations, languages, and scripts—bridging the GEMP and CMP.

II. Transliterating and Translating Textual Traditions in the Early Roman Period (1st–2nd centuries CE)

The texts of the Michigan codex that have attracted the most attention since its initial publication by Worrell are those containing reflexes of traditionally Egyptian content (§§9 and 10). As discussed below (V), these have been interpreted principally as having been transmitted through oral tradition. And yet such conclusions are premature precisely because the viability of textual transmission has not yet been adequately interrogated since Kahle judged that §§9

145 Love fc. c.

146 Not to mention produced in a century that began minority and may have ended majority Christian.

and 10 were perhaps derived from Demotic source texts.[147] A counterpoint is the diversity of scribal production and redaction during the early Roman Period, which informs the viability of textual transmission from pre-Coptic Egyptian source texts into Coptic magical texts. What needs to be tested, then, is whether there are attested routes of transmission from the textual culture that was the preserve of priestly *communities of practice* and their *script communities* during the early Roman Period to magical texts produced by, and used within, entirely different milieux during the late Roman Period. Specifically, whether it is feasible to consider transmission from the broad obsolescence of Egyptian textual culture production at the beginning of the 3th century CE to the end of that same century, a temporal frame in which it seems likely that the majority of the source texts of the Michigan codex were in circulation, which was itself only compiled in the 4th century CE. After all, no substantial manuscripts dated later than the so-called Demotic magical papyri[148] preserve pre-Coptic Egyptian textual culture.[149] Therefore, although this suggests that the (re)production of Egyptian textual culture broadly ceased, that does not mean that the textual content of those extant manuscripts was not still in circulation for some time after their compilation.[150] Consequently, and as is evidenced in the Old Coptic sections of the bilingual magical texts of the *PGM* III archive[151] and the codex *PGM* IV, it was possible for reflexes of traditionally Egyptian textual content to be transmitted later than the latest textual culture production in hieroglyphs, hieratic, or demotic—that is, across both the boundaries of script (transliteration/ transcription) and language (translation).

As introduced in the preceding section, the triglossia of Egyptians that existed during the 1st and 2nd centuries CE placed particular demands on textual culture production within Egyptian script communities. In order to continue to transmit a plurality of texts of distinct genres which were themselves written in particular forms/stages of the Egyptian language—Middle/Classical Egyptian in hieroglyphs and hieratic and Demotic in demotic—, *interscript shift*—the shift from one script to another, e.g. hieratic to demotic, and—in some, yet rarer cases,

[147] *P.Bal.* I p. 254.

[148] For recent bibliographies of the corpus of the *PDM*, its composition and dating, see Love 2016, 7 n. 21–22; 9 n. 33; 10 n. 39; to which add Dosoo 2016a and Dieleman 2019.

[149] Love 2016, §7.5.4, supplemented in Love 2021a, §§2.2.1.3; 3.2.2.3; 4.1, summarized in Love 2021b, §2.

[150] See the discussion in Love 2016, §§7.3; 7.5.4; 7.6.

[151] For the discovery that the manuscript conventionally termed *PGM* III is in fact two separate papyrus bookrolls which formed a bilingual archive compiled by two different copyists, see Love 2017 and the discussion below (III).

demotic to Old Coptic—became increasingly common.[152] That is to say, centuries and indeed millennia of *language* and *script conventions*, which governed the forms/stages of the Egyptian language and scripts of the Egyptian writing system that could be utilized in particular domains of writing for particular products of textual culture, began to shift. Indeed, *intralingual translation*, often accompanied by *interscript transcription*, e.g. Middle/Classical Egyptian texts in hieratic translated and transcribed into Demotic texts in demotic, were a feature of Egyptian scribal tradition from the Late Period—when such triglossia began to become increasingly pronounced.[153] By the late Ptolemaic Period, every form/stage of the Egyptian language is found written in every script. That is to say, Demotic texts are found transcribed into hieroglyphs[154] and hieratic,[155] while Old,[156] Middle[157]/Classical[158] Egyptian texts are found—as expected—in hieratic, and also transcribed into demotic, or even a hierato-demotic hybrid.[159] Transliterations of Classical Egyptian and Demotic texts into Old Coptic are also attested,[160] but these are much rarer than transcriptions into demotic.

The most crucial consideration in the light of these interscript transcriptions into demotic and intralingual translations into Demotic is that they concern principally the ritual domain of textual culture production. The examples cited are ritual texts practiced in the cult of various deities and their festivals. From the Ptolemaic, and especially during the Roman Period, the rationale behind transcribing language forms/stages of Egyptian which are older than Demotic into demotic was that demotic was the first script learned. Old, Middle, and Classical Egyptian texts transcribed into demotic were therefore readable by a larger proportion of literates than if they had they been transmitted in hieratic or

152 This phenomenon, and its implications, are the focus of Love 2021a, §4, summarized in Love 2021b, §3.

153 This itself succeeded a scribal tradition of intralingual translation from Middle into Late Egyptian, attested from the New Kingdom, see the discussion in Love 2021a, §4.2.

154 E.g. the "Instructions for the Production of the Khoiak Figures of Osiris at Dendera", the first five books of which are written in late Middle Egyptian, the sixth in Late Egyptian, and the seventh in Demotic (Quack 2010, 327–329).

155 E.g. the "Great Decree to the Silent Land" of P.MMA acc. 35.9.21 (c. 332–151 BCE) contains sections that are linguistically Demotic, see Quack 2010, 316.

156 See Smith 2014.

157 E.g. the Ptolemaic stela S.Brit.Mus. EA 711, see Vleeming 1990; 2004; Smith 2009, 665–668 no. 60.

158 E.g. O.Corteggiani D1 (c. 150–30 BCE), see Quack 2001; 2010, 318.

159 E.g. the "Apis Embalming Ritual" of P.Vind. Kunsthistorisches Museum 3873 from Saqqara, conventionally dated to the second half of the Ptolemaic Period—although P.Zagreb 597-2 dates the archetype to the middle of the 4th century BCE (Meyrat 2014, 300–301)—, see Quack 2010, 320–323.

160 See now Love 2021a, esp. §4, with bibliography.

hieroglyphs.[161] The ritual domain, then, was fertile ground for this shift, and it is no surprise that the latest preserved manuscripts of magical texts in pre-Coptic Egyptian—the *PDM*—exhibit sections that are written in different forms/stages of the Egyptian language all rendered in demotic or a hierato-demotic hybrid. In the consideration of how certain textual traditions could have made their way into the Michigan codex, then, it must be borne in mind that the corpora of texts from the Roman Period that are best known, such as those in hieroglyphs on the walls of Ptolemaic and Roman temples, are extant in one *form*, but the context of this form is entirely detached from a context appropriate to their practicable *function*. Every text inscribed upon a temple wall was copied from a source manuscript on a portable and ephemeral medium. Not only were many of these texts kept in the "House of Books"[162]—rather than the so-called House of Life[163]—of a temple and supposed to be recopied on a regular basis, the pattern of evidence of interscript transcription suggests that they too were also in circulation not only in hieratic, but also potentially transcribed in demotic—at least in certain priestly milieux at certain sites. These considerations, which have yet to be brought to bear on the wider question of textual transmission during the early Roman Period, therefore unlock the potential routes of textual transmission among and from priestly milieux.

Prime examples for both the traditionalist and innovative scribal practices of transcription and compilation evidenced in the latter part of the early Roman Period are the *PDM*. Comprising the latest substantial manuscripts of any pre-Coptic Egyptian texts, this corpus is at once an appropriate point of comparison given the contents (magical texts), and an outlier in the pattern of extant evidence for textual culture production in the Theban region during the last quarter of the 2nd or first quarter of the 3rd century CE.[164] Within the *PDM* a distinction is to be made between P.Louvre E 3229, P.Leiden I 384, and *P.London-Leiden*, which belong to the so-called Theban Magical Library (TML),[165] and P.Brit.Mus. EA 10588, which does not, and is perhaps even slightly later. P.Louvre E 3229 (c. 151–225 CE)[166] is interspersed with hieratic signs and groups, which are not necessarily purely graphic in nature, but also relate to linguistic archaisms, and thus betray older source texts in both hieratic and dem-

[161] Hoffmann 2002, 228; Quack 2009a.

[162] See Wespi 2017, synthesized in Love 2021a, §1.2.3.3.

[163] The revisionist identification of the *pr-ʿnḫ* as the "House of the bound/rolled (i.e. Bookrolls)", rather than "House of Life", is synthesized in Love 2021a, §1.2.3.2, with bibliography there.

[164] With no substantial manuscripts in Demotic or hieratic dating securely to the 3rd century CE, the dating of the *PDM* into even the first quarter of the 3rd century CE remains problematic.

[165] A collection, or archive, of ten manuscripts of mostly magical but also alchemical texts: see Dosoo 2016a.

[166] *PDM* Suppl. = *GEMF* 18.

otic—unsurprising given the predominance of spells for sending dreams in this manuscript, and the millennia-long importance of dreams in Egyptian culture.[167] P.Leiden I 384 verso (c. 151–225 CE)[168] features one recipe in particular, an invocation to Imhotep (I*/1–29), which can most plausibly be understood as the adaptation of a hieratic source text, not least because of the likely identification of a centuries-older example thereof,[169] but also because of its disproportionate utilization of hieratic signs. *P.London-Leiden* (c. 151–225 CE)[170] features several sections which exhibit instances of hybrid hieratic and demotic writings, as well as linguistic archaisms. These include *P.London-Leiden* recto 6/1–7/4, which is among the linguistically oldest part of the compiled magical texts of the manuscript, although the ritual instructions accompanying the invocations are linguistically younger.[171] This manuscript also contains two versions of the same invocations within a vessel divination in order to see the Bark of Pre (recto 10/20–30; 27/1–12), in the latter copy of which the hieratic and hierato-demotic spellings are more prominent than in the former,[172] suggesting a compilation of two distinct source texts that themselves share a history of textual transmission. P.Brit.Mus. EA 10588 (c.176–225 CE)[173] is also interspersed with hieratic signs and groups, which are not necessarily purely graphic in nature, but also relate to linguistic archaisms, with the portion at 5/7–17 exhibiting Middle Egyptian lexical and syntactical features.[174]

In maintaining textual traditions across the boundaries of a trigraphic writing system and—even to simplify—a diglossic written language, the script communities embedded within priestly communities of practice were both traditionalist and innovative. The use of Greek in the bilingual recipes of these manuscripts has been treated in the aforementioned study by the present author,[175] but one final consideration of note here is that where the patterns of copying in the *PDM* are suggestive of later additions to phases of initial copying, these later additions feature numerous recipes in Greek, not Demotic. Take, for example, the final recipe added in the final column of P.Leiden I 384, as well as of P.Louvre E 3229, and all the recipes of the verso of P.Brit.Mus. EA 10588. These appear to be later additions, which were added into the manuscript later than their initial compilation, and so they are also suggestive of *written language shift* in the course of the use-lives of these manuscripts. The exact opposite of

167 Quack 2010, 332.
168 *PDM* xii (*GEMF* 15).
169 Quack 2010, 323.
170 P.Leiden I 383 + P.Brit.Mus. EA 10070 (*PDM* xiv; *GEMF* 16).
171 Quack 2010, 323.
172 Quack 2010, 323.
173 *PDM* lxi (*GEMF* 17).
174 Quack 2010, 322–323.
175 Love fc. c.

this process, perhaps no more than a century later, appears in the Michigan codex, which evidences first bilingual, and subsequently monolingual, phases of compilation—shifting *from* Greek *to* Coptic (Egyptian). This pattern is reflected also in the development of the TML over time, in which the initial collection of manuscripts, comprising the three aforementioned *PDM*, was augmented with the addition of several others over several generations, all of which were exclusively Greek—the only exceptions being five Egyptian-language sections in the codex *PGM* IV,[176] and a handful of Egyptian-language invocations in otherwise entirely monolingual Greek recipes in other manuscripts, discussed below. This transition, from principally Egyptian-language and some bilingual recipes to monolingual Greek-language recipes, shows that the script communities embedded within priestly *communities of practice* and their descendent milieux that maintained and transmitted these textual traditions were not limited even to the multiple scripts and forms of their written language, but also undertook translations of their textual culture into Greek.[177]

From hymns praising Isis in Greek that are comparable to compositions in Demotic attested in numerous manuscripts,[178] to the so-called Aretalogy of Imouthes in Greek also potentially preserved in at least one Demotic source text,[179] "Graeco-Egyptian" literature evidences how certain script communities broke the language barrier and facilitated the transmission of textual culture—otherwise the preserve of the priestly milieux—into distinct linguistic and thereby cultural frames.[180] Other than the quotidian domains of administrative, judicial, and technical textual culture, magical texts comprise the genre of textual culture production that saw the most pronounced shift from forms of written Egyptian to Greek. Admittedly, a precondition is the fact that those ritual texts for personal benefit did not, unlike ritual texts for the benefit of Pharaoh and the

---

[176] For these, see Love 2016.

[177] For the hypothesis that the later (4th century CE) compilers, owners, and practitioners of the TML were—based on an analysis of primary vs. literary sources for priestly milieux during the 4th century CE—not necessarily priests, but perhaps only those with a cultural or genealogical relationship to a priestly lineage, see Love 2016, §7.3. To those considerations, add the principal one here, that—even if they were "priests" (irrespective of what that would mean in the 4th century CE)—they were evidently not priests who could write Egyptian.

[178] E.g. *P.Oxy.* XI 1380 recto (c. 98–136 CE) from Oxyrhynchus, compared to *P.Carlsberg* XI 2–4 (c. 1–200 CE) from Tebtunis. P.Vind. inv. D 6927+6329+10101 recto, another Roman Period Demotic example but from Soknopaiou Nesos, is being edited by Martin Stadler: see Stadler 2017a, 70–77; 2017b; cf. Nagel 2019, 599–600. For a modelling of the relationship between Egyptian- and Greek-language hymns to Isis, see Stadler 2017a, 72–75. For *P.Oxy.* XI 1380 recto, see now Nagel 2019, 600–645; 840–852.

[179] I.e. *P.Oxy.* XI 1381 verso (2nd century CE). For reports on the Demotic source texts, see Quack 2009, 143; 2016a, 279; 2016b, 111.

[180] For an analysis of how this differed among sites during the early Roman period, see Love 2021a, §§5.1; 6.1; 7.1; 8.1.

deities of traditional Egyptian cults or the afterlife of deceased individuals, disappear with the dissolution of the priesthoods, and their *communities of practice*.

This tradition of *language shift* is notable not only because these magical texts are continually attested into the late Roman Period, but because it actually began rather early. For example, *P.Oxy*. LXV 4468,[181] dating to the second half of the 2nd century CE, a bookroll formulary of recipes for favor and erotic magic as well as a recipe to cause sleep and a phylactery, features sections both transliterated and translated from Egyptian.[182] A single *logos* at verso 2/23–25 in a phylactery features identifying statements transliterated into Greek script,[183] while a Greek hymn to the Sun with an unambiguously Egyptian background is utilized in a likely erotic recipe at recto 1/1–37. Consider also *P.Oxy*. III 433,[184] dating to the 2nd or 3rd century CE, a fragment of a formulary bookroll on papyrus preserving four recipes, one of which describes the activation of a divine image related to the Egyptian ritual of *Opening the Mouth*.[185]

Such a reengineering of ritual texts practiced otherwise in temple or funerary contexts, otherwise the preserve of priestly *script communities* and *communities of practice*, into those practiced for private benefit itself has a millennia-long tradition in Egypt. Some of the Hymns to Amun discussed in the excursus to §9 attested from the New Kingdom are found reengineered in rituals for personal benefit. A notable example is P.Harris 501, a papyrus bookroll of magical texts dating to the late 20th Dynasty.[186] Certain recipes are paralleled in, among others, the hymns to the Bas of Amun from the Temple of Amun at Hibis in the el-Khargeh Oasis, decorated during the 27th Dynasty in the reign of Darius I.[187] In such composite recipes, older hymnic sections are redacted alongside younger invocations and commands that reengineer the desired outcome of the ritual to be for personal benefit. Thus, attested already in the New Kingdom are practitioners who "have access to temple texts and were in all probability at home in

---

181 *GEMF* 6, perhaps one and the same manuscript as *GEMF* 5 (*PGM* LII; P.Lips. inv. 429).

182 Not to mention numerous other examples of transcription identified by Quack in 2013, 189–193.

183 Contrary to ed.pr., αγκ and ανκ are simply the reduced form of the 1st person singular independent pronoun, the former utilizing the Greek orthographic convention whereby γγ is vocalized νγ (κ and γ being, after all, indistinguishable for an Egyptophone). Thus, this *logos* contains a string of identifying statements on the part of the practitioner. For μν, consider also how close this is to a Demotic form, as opposed to the ɴɪᴍ that is attested in Old Coptic transliteration elsewhere, e.g. *PGM* IV.118. This is no "pre-old Coptic" (*pace* ed.pr.), see Love 2021a, §4.2; Love 2021b, §3.3–3.4, nor an isolated example from the "few examples of Egyptian transcribed in Greek", as noted in the main text.

184 *GEMF* 25.

185 See Zellmann-Rohrer 2018 and Dieleman 2005, 170–182.

186 P.Brit.Mus. EA 10042, ed.pr. Lange 1927; Leitz 1999, 31–50; with Quack 1998, 88 n. 75.

187 Quack 1998, 87–88 with references and 88 n. 75 for the date.

the temple milieu".[188] Parallels to two hymns to the Bas of Amun from the Temple of Amun at Hibis are also found in Demotic transcriptions dating to the late Ptolemaic or early Roman Period,[189] evidencing a productive textual transmission of both *intralingual translation* and *interscript transcription* during the Graeco-Roman Period that continued until the broad obsolescence of Egyptian writing during the 3rd century CE.

These examples from magical texts, alongside those other manuscripts from Oxyrhynchus that evidence the translation of Egyptian temple and ritual textual culture into Greek, can no longer be framed within outdated assumptions as to the identities of those who read and wrote Greek in Roman Egypt. Whitehorne, for example, concluded that *P.Oxy.* XI 1380 recto and 1381 verso "bespeak a profound antiquarian interest in Egyptian religious traditions on the part of the educated Greek-speaking élite of Oxyrhynchus".[190] Such an assumption cannot be maintained, not least because the Egyptian (Demotic) source texts would only have been accessible, let alone legible, to individuals trained within priesthoods—of which there were dozens at Oxyrhynchus—who must have then been responsible for translating them into Greek.[191] This is borne out by P.Brit.Mus. EA 10808, a trigraphic (Old Coptic, demotic, and Greek) and diglossic (Classical Egyptian and Demotic) Egyptian papyrus bookroll of ritual texts for personal benefit, dating to the second half of the 2nd century CE.[192] Column x+1 preserves two ritual practices,[193] both in Demotic with *voces magicae* in Greek script: the first is to acquire a supernatural πάρεδρος, an assistant in ritual practices, through invoking an "angel", while the second invokes a "ghost", most likely to be sent in a dream.[194] Column x+2 can be clearly delineated into three invocations in which a deity is invoked preceding the invocation of "Enemy of Wennefer, Enemy of Osiris, Khentyimentiu". This manuscript, then, at once evidences the translation or composition of a Greek practice in(to) Dem-

---

[188] Quack 1998, 89.

[189] O.Brit.Mus. EA 50601, ed. Smith 1977; 1999.

[190] Whitehorne 1995, 3071. Even if Whitehorne's point here were only that such "Greek-speaking élites" were interested in reading such translations, in spite of the fact that they were unable to undertake such translations themselves, that point nevertheless both divorces such textual culture from its principal milieu and fails to acknowledge the existence of that principal milieu.

[191] In hindsight, a particularly extraordinary example of this is *P.Wash.Univ.* II 71–72 + *P.Oslo* I 2, a manuscript whose content was so misunderstood that part of it was included in *PGM* XXXVII. In fact, this text comprises a Greek translation of the oath section of the Book of the Temple, the verso of which was inscribed with a Greek translation of a collection of temple rules and priestly law (Quack 2016b, 113).

[192] *GEMF* 14, ed. Osing 1976b; cf. Quack 2009, 32; 2017, 63–64; Love fc. a.

[193] Column x+1 (Dieleman 2004) was augmented by the discovery of a connecting fragment of the upper third of column x+2 by Quack (2017, 64).

[194] Dieleman 2004, 125–127; Love fc. a.

otic and the transcription into Old Coptic of a significantly older set of Classical Egyptian ritual texts reengineered to fulfill erotic intentions.[195]

Indeed, while the rate of publication of Egyptian-language sources from the Roman Period lags behind that of Greek-language sources, the Demotic parallels to the hymns to Isis already noted, among other compositions, go to show how the source texts for many Egyptian-looking Greek-language texts remain to be identified, edited, and thereby incorporated into a critical analysis of textual transmission during the early Roman Period. This transmission, however, need not be limited to Egypt. The availability of textual content transliterated and translated from written Egyptian in the GEMP also facilitated its transmission throughout the Eastern Mediterranean and to Europe. A gold lamella from Roman Period Rome, now lost, invoked Πτα νεβρ αν, i.e. *ptḥ-nfr-ʿn* "Ptah entirely beautiful", as the deity who will facilitate an exorcism,[196] while numerous etymologically Egyptian *voces magicae*—notably transliterated into Greek script with their *Egyptian* as opposed to Graecized vocalizations—which derive from Egyptian deities with funerary associations are to be found among Wünsch's "Sethian" curse-tablets from Rome.[197] These textual elements appear alongside a host of figural elements transmitted across similarly large spatial frames which have also been argued to derive from Egyptian iconographic tradition.[198] Such examples are likely the tip of the iceberg, and indicate that if the transliteration and translation of certain of types of Egyptian ritual texts into Greek script or language had already begun in the 1st century CE, much more remains to be found. This should be unsurprising given the emerging evidence for the translation of Demotic literature into Greek,[199] catalyzing the tradition of Graeco-Egyptian literature, which Quack suggests could have begun to occur as early as during the 4th or 3rd, but at the latest during the 2nd century BCE—,[200] roughly contemporary with the translation of the Septuagint into Greek, with the Pentateuch completed during the 3rd century BCE.[201]

---

[195] Quack 2009, 32; 2017, 63–64.

[196] *IG* XIV 2413 (13); *GMA* 25.

[197] E.g. βαχυχ, i.e. *bꜣ kky* "*Ba* of Darkness", σωρω, i.e. *sr* ꜥꜣ "Great Ram", ουσιρι, i.e. *wsir* "Osiris" (with a Lower Egyptian vocalization), and μνω, i.e. *mn-wr* "Mnevis", see Wünsch 1898, 23–28 no. 20; Tremel 2004, no. 70. Elsewhere, note also ουσιρι απι, i.e. *wsir-ḥp* "Osiris Apis", ουσιρι μνε, μνο as well as μνω, i.e. *wsir mn-wr* "Osiris Mnevis", and ουσιρι μνεφρι, i.e. *wsir mn-wr-pꜣ-rʿ* "Osiris Mnevis Pre" (Wünsch 1898, 121), exhibiting principally Lower Egyptian vocalizations.

[198] See Love, fc. d.

[199] Quack 2009, 6.

[200] An early example is the Dream of Nectanebo on P.Leiden I 396 (first half of the 2nd century BCE; ed. *UPZ* I 81), from the family archive of Ptolemaios found at the Serapeum at Saqqara, which describes itself as a translation from Egyptian—also attested in a Demotic copy from the Tebtunis temple library. For such Graeco-Egyptian literature, see Dieleman and Moyer 2010.

[201] Aitken 2015, 3.

In summary, the translation of texts into a written language that was not the preserve of priestly script communities and thus only in circulation within priestly communities of practice facilitated their transmission into distinct linguistic, and thereby cultural, milieux that would never otherwise have had access to this textual culture. It is in the context of this extraordinary variety of textual culture (re)production and transmission across the boundaries of script and language, and thereby generations, that the reflexes of earlier magical traditions evidenced in the recipes of the Michigan codex can be considered. First, however, it is necessary to consider the situation in the late Roman Period, during which the source texts of the Michigan codex would have been in transmission, and in the later part of which the Michigan codex was itself compiled.

III. Transcribing and Translating Textual Traditions in the Late Roman Period (3rd–4th centuries CE)

Consistent with the fact that textual culture production in Egyptian had broadly ceased and the scripts of the Egyptian writing system had thereby broadly obsolesced by the middle of the 3rd century CE, the magical texts attested from the turn of the 3rd century CE are essentially all in Greek. Thus, where collections of magical manuscripts are found—whether collections of applied, or archives of formulary texts—these are, unlike the *PGM* III archive and TML discussed further in this section, of monolingual Greek texts. For example, a scribe active at Hawara in the 2nd or 3rd century CE produced three different applied erotic recipes for three different targets in Greek,[202] while the compiler of the "Hermonthis Magical Archive" dating to the 4th century CE collected four papyrus bookroll formularies and one papyrus sheet formulary with various recipes for cursing, restraining anger, erotic intentions, as well as divination and healing.[203] Bilingual archives and manuscripts are, by comparison, rarer.

The *PGM* III archive merits consideration in some detail due to the numerous similarities shared with the compilation of the recipes copied into the Michigan codex. *PGM* III.1 and III.2[204] form a 3rd century CE bilingual archive of magical texts of unknown provenance written in Greek and Old Coptic. *PGM* III.1 verso

[202] *PGM* XXXII; XXXIIa; LXVIII.

[203] *PGM* VII; VIII; IX; X; XIa and perhaps also *P.Lips*. I 97, an account relating to the same estate as that on the recto of *PGM* XIa, re-used for copying Psalms: see Dosoo 2016a, 265–266.

[204] P.Louvre E 2391 (P.Mimaut), edited as a single text in *PGM* III but now recognized as two separate manuscripts, see Love 2017 and now Torallas Tovar, Martín Hernández, and Love fc.

4/22–6/44 comprises a manual for sunlight divination[205] consisting of sections in Egyptian (4/22–5/10; 5/11–21; 5/22–30; 5/31–6/2), which feature the invocations and commands within a hymn-like text to the Sun that bring about a theophany, alongside a longer section in Greek (6/3–44), which features instructions for the preparation of the ritual and its ritual paraphernalia. *PGM* III.2 verso 1/28–37 likewise has a divinatory aim,[206] with Greek-language ritual instructions prescribing that a set of identifying statements are to be recited before the sunrise (1/28–31), followed by a section in Egyptian specifying those identifying statements (as Thoth, etc.) (1/32–34), before further fragmentary Greek-language ritual instructions or annotations which conclude the composite recipe (1/35–37). *PGM* III.2 verso 2/10–3/4 features Greek-language ritual instructions (2/10–34) for the preparation of the ritual space and paraphernalia for this recipe to be able to read a sealed letter, while a subsequent Egyptian-language section (invoking "the ferryman" and others to "awaken") (2/35–3/4) provides the first-person invocations and commands. *PGM* III.2 verso 3/5–3/18 consists of three sections: the first in the Greek language (3/5–12) provides ritual instructions for the production of a lamella to be inscribed with Greek and Egyptian in order to bring about "memory", and—unlike the preceding examples—invocations and commands; the second in Egyptian gives the invocations to be inscribed upon the lamella and perhaps also to be recited seven times (3/13–15); the third in Greek (3/16–18) provides further ritual instructions to recite either the Egyptian, the preceding Greek, or both sets of invocations in a certain setting.

Directly comparable to the Michigan codex, this archive not only contains recipes in more than one language but was also compiled by more than one copyist. The fact that this archive comprises two manuscripts does not limit this comparison, given that the same compilation of recipes could have been compiled as one longer papyrus bookroll or several shorter papyrus bookrolls—*form* is no indicator of *function*. Copyist A copied only monolingual—Greek-language—texts onto the recto and verso of *PGM* III.1 and recto of *PGM* III.2, whereas Copyist B was responsible for filling the remainder of the verso of *PGM* III.1 and *PGM* III.2 with bilingual composite recipes in Egyptian (written in Old Coptic) and Greek. That is to say, Copyist A compiled a monolingual archive of recipes upon two manuscripts, which was acquired by Copyist B, who added bilingual recipes for similar purposes to these manuscripts. This is the opposite pattern to that found in the Michigan codex, where a first bilingual phase was supplemented by four subsequent monolingual phases—demon-

205 For this newly identified practice within the typology of divination, see Love 2016, 113 n. 1; §4.3. For a concordance of line numbers for the newly distinguished *PGM* III.1 and III.2 with the edition in *PGM*, see Love 2017, 182 fig. 1.

206 As well as fitting the typology of magical texts in this section of that manuscript by following on from the monolingual sunlight divination recipe in *PGM* III.2 verso 1/16–27.

strating the rapidity of *written language shift* in the production of magical texts during the 3rd and 4th centuries CE. Nevertheless, the *PGM* III manuscripts evidence the compilation of source texts together into "master copies" by and for bilingual and biliterate individuals. Datable only roughly to the 3rd century CE, and with an unknown provenance, the *PGM* III archive is difficult to contextualize further. Yet, given the trends in *written language shift* described above, it must be either contemporary with or slightly later than the production of the *PDM*, and thus the *PGM* III archive illustrates the wider trend of the obsolescence of the scripts of the Egyptian writing system in the magical domain and thereby how reflexes of earlier Egyptian textual culture could only be preserved in Old Coptic transliterations. These particular Old Coptic transliterations themselves in turn attest that it was possible for aspects of earlier Egyptian textual culture to survive the broad obsolescence of the Egyptian writing system. One final manuscript featuring texts transliterated into Old Coptic suggests that this was the case not only in the 3rd century—contemporary perhaps with the *PDM* and with the *PGM* III archive—but also into the 4th century—making the investigation contemporary with the production and use of the Michigan codex.

PGM IV, a bilingual (Egyptian-Greek) papyrus codex of magical texts written in Greek and Old Coptic, dating to the end of the 3rd or early 4th century CE, is ascribed to the TML and thus, while the context is distinct from the Michigan codex, is roughly contemporary with its production and initial use. The present author (Love 2016) has identified five composite bilingual recipes in this codex, for divinatory, erotic, and exorcistic purposes. The pattern of language use in all but the bilingual exorcism is typically that ritual instructions for each recipe are in Greek, whereas invocations and commands that are part of the practiced rituals are in Egyptian-Coptic rendered in different Old Coptic scripts. The complex history of textual transmission in the idioms exhibited by, and distinct Old Coptic scripts used to write, each of these composite recipes was also undertaken in that study.[207] This demonstrated that the extant bilingual recipes were compiled from a variety of source texts, some of which were in distinct idioms that show in turn that those texts were sourced from elsewhere in Egypt, and thereby transmitted along the Nile valley. While the bilingual exorcism of *PGM* IV.1227–1264 contains nothing diagnostically Egyptian in its textual content, and thereby can instead be described as an Egyptian-Greek bilingual composite recipe in which the Egyptian is written in a non-standard script, the Egyptian-language sections of the composite divinatory and erotic recipes are suggestive of a different history of textual transmission. By comparison, while the invocations and commands of the recipe for a theophany of *PGM* IV.11–25 are partially paralleled in the invocations and commands of the recipe for a the-

[207] See esp. the summary in Love 2016, §2.5.

ophany of *P.London-Leiden* 21/1–9, and thereby found in a directly comparable context,[208] parallels to the motifs found in the divine drama of the composite erotic recipe of *PGM* IV.94–153 have since been found in a much wider body of Egyptian textual culture from the Roman Period.

In *Code-switching with the Gods*, such parallel motifs, whether words or phrases, were referred to as "ritual language" because they appeared to cluster in parallels to invocations in the names or epithets of particular deities that were otherwise only attested in other magical or in funerary ritual texts.[209] Such instances were then interpreted as evidence for the transmission of textual culture not only across spheres of ritual practice, e.g. temple or funerary to magical, but also for *interscript* and *intralingual* transmission through adaptation and redaction, e.g. from hieratic (Classical Egyptian) and demotic (Demotic) source texts into Old Coptic. Further examples of this have been elaborated in a recent study,[210] which in turn were interpreted in the light of viable parallels for the transmission of motifs found across different domains of textual culture production and, importantly, scripts and media. Indeed, with a few illustrative examples, that study evidenced the transmission of textual motifs across different types of ritual texts as well as between all forms/stages of the Egyptian language and scripts of the Egyptian writing system. Nevertheless, it was argued that while it is informative to identify syntactical, lexical, and semantic parallels for their own sake, this is not necessarily informative of direct transmission. After all, shared motifs could be anything from evidence of direct textual transmission to independently written-down attestations of idioms common to spoken Egyptian. In that study, these parallels were therefore analyzed alongside evidence from the early Roman Period of *intralingual* and *interscript* transmission described above. Parallel motifs found in Demotic and Old Coptic among the papyri were therefore compared to parallel texts found in hieratic and hieroglyphs, on papyri and temple walls respectively. This in turn demonstrated how the slow but sure publication of Egyptian-language textual sources, especially those upon ephemeral media such as papyri, from the Roman Period is refocusing an understanding of Egyptian textual culture away from the temple walls upon which they were quite literally set in stone, and back into the hands of the responders (readers) and producers (writers) of these texts during that time who were thereby able to retransmit these texts horizontally within a generation or vertically across different generations of *script communities*. The written language and script communities which transcribed and translated these textual traditions were also, at least up until the first half of the 3rd century CE, embedded in priestly *communities of practice* who recited, redacted, and reified the

[208] See the discussion in Love 2016, 129–130, and the notes to the commentary there.

[209] Love 2016, §2.1.1.2.

[210] Discussed fully in Love 2018/19b.

contents of that textual culture in textual, oral, and aural form through the practice of those rituals.

Further manuscripts to be considered here, however briefly, also evidence bilingual practitioners and their script communities. *PGM* I is a bilingual papyrus bookroll dated to the second half of the 3rd century CE, ascribed by Dosoo to the TML.[211] In a "tested" recipe for invisibility (ἀμαύρωσι(ς) δοκίμη, *PGM* I.247–262), the ritual instructions at the beginning and end of the recipe are in Greek, the identifying statements in Egyptian-Coptic (with no notable difference in script), and the commands in Greek. The identifying statements read: "I am Anubis, I am Osiris-Pre, I am *Ōsōt*, *Sōrōnouier*. It is I, Osiris, he whom Seth destroyed".[212] Besides its more or less traditional Egyptian resonances, this bilingual recipe demonstrates the continued transmission of bilingual magical texts by bilingual practitioners during the 3rd century CE. Indeed, although in proportionally small quantities, Egyptian-Coptic is found elsewhere in the wider corpus of the GEMP, often hidden amongst otherwise entirely Greek-language recipes, but nevertheless betraying bilingual practitioners.[213] A later example is found in a recipe titled "door-opener" (ἄνοιξις θύρας) in *PGM* XXXVI.312–320, dating to the 4th century CE, where the ritual instructions are again in Greek, while the commands are first in Egyptian-Coptic and then repeated in a Greek version, before identifying statements and further commands are also given in Greek—within a recipe that, with the exception of certain *voces magicae*, is rather Egyptian in its content. The commands in fact repeat one another, as if the latter first served as a translation or gloss to the former: "Open for me; open for me; oh door bolt! Be opened; be opened, door bolt!".[214] Consequently, they serve as further evidence of the continued practice and transmission of bilingual magical texts by bilingual practitioners.

---

[211] *GEMF* 31; Dosoo 2016a, 270. While the editors of *GEMF* 31 note lambdacisms in ll. 145–146, implicitly suggesting that this casts doubt on the ascription of the manuscript to the TML, such dialectal features could just as easily stem from a source text, and at most evidence only the origin of a particular scribe as opposed to text or manuscript.

[212] ⲁⲛⲟⲕ ⲁⲛⲟⲩⲡ ⲁⲛⲟⲕ ⲟⲩⲥⲓⲣⲫⲣⲏ ⲁⲛⲟⲕ ⲱⲥⲱⲧ ⲥⲱⲣⲱⲛⲟⲩⲓⲉⲣ ⲁⲛⲟⲕ ⲡⲉ ⲟⲩⲥⲓⲣⲉ ⲡⲉⲛⲧⲁ ⲥⲏⲧ ⲧⲁⲕⲟ (4/20–21 = *PGM* I.251–252). Note the lexically Coptic ⲧⲁⲕⲟ, found only rarely in late Demotic as *ḏi̓.t-/ti̓.t-ʿḳ*. This is not perfect Egyptian-Coptic grammar, however, which would require a resumptive pronoun ⲧⲁⲕⲟ⸗ϥ. Yet this does not render the text incomprehensible. Although φ and β were sometimes utilized (see Love 2016, §2.3.1), the Greek alphabet does, in principle, lack a letter for Egyptian /f/, which may explain the omission of the resumptive pronoun here.

[213] Even odd and isolated examples of *voces magicae* evidence this, for example ⲑⲟⲣϫⲟⲫⲁⲛⲱ in *PGM* VII.510 featuring the Coptic letter ϫ in a manuscript otherwise written in Greek language and script.

[214] ⲁⲩⲱⲛ ⲛⲏⲓ ⲁⲩⲱⲛ ⲛⲏⲓ ⲧⲕⲉⲗⲗⲓ ἀνοίγηθι ἀνοίγηθι κλεῖστρον (*PGM* XXXVI.316–317), discussed in Love 2016, §6.5.2 (there, read κλεῖστρον in place of κλεςτρον).

Furthermore, two formulary manuscripts offer early evidence of Greek-Coptic bilingualism in the magical tradition. *PGM* LXXIX and LXXX[215] date to the late 3rd or early 4th century CE and are thus contemporaneous to *PGM* IV and perhaps also the Michigan codex. Both of these contain anger-restraining recipes (θυμοκάτοχον), where the ritual instructions to recite the text "three times" are in Greek, as are the commands to "restrain the anger and wrath of NN towards me, NN", while the identifying statements that imbue the practitioner with the efficacy to bring about this desired outcome are given in Egyptian-Coptic.[216] While written in standard Coptic,[217] even in one case including supralinear strokes, and thus evidencing bilingual and biliterate practitioners and their *script communities*, the syntax of the Coptic-Egyptian *logos* would not actually be any different if rendered in Demotic[218]—further blurring the boundaries of transliteration vs. translation across *interscript* and *intralingual* divides.

These examples bring the discussion back to the texts of the Michigan codex which exhibit reflexes of traditionally Egyptian content. There are a few lexemes in §§9 and 10 of the Michigan codex which are shown by the transliteration of the text into a hypothetical source text not to be common to Demotic (see the excurses to §§9 and 10). However, this is also the case for a few counterparts in the Egyptian (Old Coptic) texts of *PGM* IV. Nevertheless, while principally Coptic, both §§9 and 10 and the Egyptian Old Coptic texts of *PGM* IV exhibit elements of pre-Coptic grammar. These distinctions, while slight, are important. Indeed, when Greek loanwords are taken out of the equation—which are, notably, absent in §§9 and 10, and almost absent from the Egyptian (Old Coptic) texts of *PGM* IV—there is not much "not Coptic" about late Demotic, i.e. Demotic of the 2nd century CE. Through such considerations it becomes clear that if there were anything non-standard about the Coptic script used in §§9 and 10, these sections would already have been appraised as being Old Coptic through the presence of their reflexes of traditional Egyptian content.[219] An illustration of the viability of the transmission of both §§9 and 10 from pre-Coptic Egyptian (Demotic) source texts is given in the reconstructed transliteration of the two hypothetical source texts interwoven into the excurses to §§9 and 10 below. A further implication, then, is that of syntactical, lexical, and orthographic up-

---

215 *GEMF* 53 and 54.

216 ⲁⲛⲟⲕ ⲡⲉ ⲃⲁïⲛⲭⲱⲱⲭ/ⲃⲉⲛⲭⲱⲱⲱⲭ ⲁⲃⲣⲁⲥⲁⲝ ⲉⲣⲓⲛⲧ ⲙⲓⲭⲁⲏⲗ (ⲡⲉ) ⲡⲁⲣⲁⲛ ⲛ̄ⲙⲏⲧ/ⲕⲙⲏⲧ "It is I, Ba of Darkness. Abrasax is my name. Michael is my true name" (*PGM* LXXIX.2–4).

217 Utilized as opposed to "Old Coptic" to refer to the varied dialects, orthographies, and grammars depending on domain and thus register of writing that encompass the writing system and the totality of idioms of the dialects of written Coptic.

218 Compare **ỉnk pꜣy bꜣ n kk.w ꜣ-b-r-ꜥ-s-ꜥ-k-s*^{Go} *ỉw rn.ṯ⸗ỉ m-y-k-h-ꜥ-e-l*^{Go} *pꜣy pꜣy⸗ỉ rn n mꜣꜥ.t.*

219 Perhaps the same would also have been true of the Egyptian *logos* in *PGM* LXXIX and LXXX.

dating, first proposed to explain the transmission of the Old Coptic texts of *PGM* IV from their Demotic source texts.[220]

Syntactical, lexical, and orthographic updating were proposed in *Code-switching with the Gods* as scribal processes through which semantically understood—as opposed to transcribed/transliterated but semantically meaningless—textual content could be updated in line with changes to the register of written language or standardization of the writing system used, respectively. As introduced above, this has since been shown to have been in line with Egyptian scribal practices from the late Ptolemaic to early Roman Period, and indeed became increasingly prominent in the transmission of Egyptian textual culture during the 2nd century CE. At this time, Egyptian scribal culture *required* the syntactical and lexical updating of older texts through *intralingual translation* from, for example, Middle/Classical Egyptian to Demotic, and similarly orthographic updating of texts in hieratic into demotic, the predominant contemporary script. Old Coptic texts could, through the standardization of their script and, in certain cases, certain changes to their syntax, be updated enough to be legible to literates of standard Coptic who did not belong to the *script communities* and thereby linguistic and cultural milieux in which those Old Coptic texts were first transcribed from hieratic, demotic, or both. Indeed, given that reflexes of traditional Egyptian content are found in *PGM* IV, and yet it is to be placed in the context of the late 3rd or early 4th century CE, a temporal frame during which there is limited primary source evidence for priestly *communities of practice*,[221] the possibility that these texts had been transmitted into milieux that were no longer the same as the milieux in which they were originally redacted and transmitted through interscript transcription or transliteration rather requires such an interpretation.

Thus, it is clear that the 3rd century CE served, in notably limited but nonetheless secure cases, as a bridge between the pre-Coptic Egyptian textual traditions of the *PDM* and the sparse attestations of magical texts rendered in Old Coptic scripts and bilingual magical texts where the Egyptian-language sections are simply rendered in Greek script. The fact that the manuscripts treated thus far were *compiled* together in the 3rd and 4th centuries, and that their texts were therefore *copied and edited* during this time, demonstrates that they are not necessarily an end point in textual transmission. This, then, seems also to be the case for the Michigan codex, produced in the 4th century, but itself a compilation from source texts that were undoubtedly older, and which most likely themselves stretch back into the 3rd century CE, if not earlier.

---

220 Love 2016, §§2.3.5.2 and 2.4.1.

221 The dichotomy of primary vs. literacy sources for such communities is made throughout the near exhaustive treatment of the latter—often argued to be evidence for historical cults and their priesthoods—in Love 2016, §7.

IV. Composing, Redacting, and Compiling Scribes—Past, Prior, and Contemporary Practitioners

The consideration of the intergenerational transmission of magical texts was developed in *Code-switching with the Gods* through a consideration of the "priestly", "potential", and "contemporary" practitioners of the bilingual composite recipes in *PGM* IV. That is to say, by considering the history of textual transmission vertically across generations over time, the milieux in which certain texts may have been practiced and from which they would have been further transmitted can be considered. The script communities in which the source texts of the Old Coptic sections of the bilingual composite recipes in *PGM* IV were produced were those embedded within priestly *communities of practice*—"priestly", i.e. "past" practitioners and their "composing" scribes. But given the pattern of evidence of extant Old Coptic sources, this process is most likely to have occurred in the second half of the 2nd century CE, or first quarter of the 3rd century CE at the latest. In the intervening generations, then, there is a period of textual transmission accounting for this hypothesized point of origin and the extant copy of these Old Coptic texts in *PGM* IV. This period can be considered as populated by the intervening "prior" practitioners and their "redacting" scribes. By comparison, the "contemporary" practitioners are those who could have practiced the texts as extant in the late 3rd or early 4th century CE recipes in *PGM* IV—the "compiling" scribes of the extant manuscripts. In this way, while it is perfectly plausible that there was a genealogical, and thereby cultural-linguistic, relationship among all these "priestly", "potential", and "contemporary" practitioners, to suggest that the latter, those practitioners of the early 4th century CE, were from the same priestly *communities of practice*, unchanged by the significant processes of written *language shift*, *script obsolescence*, and the vanishing of primary source evidence for the majority of cults attested in the early Roman Period, is extremely problematic.[222]

Further considerations in *Code-switching with the Gods* included not only the desacralizing but also democratizing functions of transliteration into Old Coptic on the one hand, and translation into Greek on the other. Given that the original contextual milieu in which a magical text was produced or compiled and practiced, and from which it was transmitted in one generation, could subsequently have differed, the translation of an Egyptian-language magical text into the Greek language by bilingual individuals within a priestly *written language* and *script community* facilitated the transmission of that text into, or the practice of that text for clients within, a distinct and solely Grecophone milieu. That is to say, the magical texts left the sacred context of the temple priesthood and the

[222] This is developed in Love 2016, §7.7.

textual culture of its script community and entered a phase of transmission among the *demos*.

Thus, while the following section will serve to compare the respective feasibility of oral as opposed to textual transmission as the mechanisms through which texts featuring reflexes of traditional Egyptian religious content appeared in the Michigan codex, the human element must be borne in mind at all times. All of the texts copied into the Michigan codex can be robustly assumed to have been copied from source texts by "compiling" scribes who were likely also to be the "contemporary" practitioners. All of these source texts had their own "redacting" scribes and thereby their own "prior" practitioners. This history of textual transmission could have spanned generations. Each of these source texts had its own starting point, even if that point was itself a compilation from other source texts—or from oral motifs—which was produced by "composing" scribes and practiced by "past" practitioners.

Counterpoints to the overemphasis on the *script communities*—as this study would term them—embedded within monastic *communities of practice* as being the principal practitioners in Egypt of the 4th century CE and later are the considerations presented in **Context in the Practice of Medicine and Healing**. There, several parallels for the private as opposed to institutional practice of professional physicians are highlighted, and a case is made for refocusing a discussion on textual culture production from the late Roman Period onwards that has exhibited an evidentiary bias in favor of monastic contexts for the responders (readers) and producers (writers) of Coptic technical and ritual textual culture. Similarly, while priestly *written language* and *script communities* have been the focus of the preceding discussion in order to explain the presence of traditionally Egyptian content in the Michigan codex as in *PGM* IV, this recapitulation of the thesis of the desacralizing and democratizing functions of transliteration into Old Coptic on the one hand, and translation into Greek on the other, provide a counterpoint to the continued emphasis on priestly practitioners. That is to say, there is evidently a complexity of processes in the transmission of magical texts and a complexity of identities regarding their copyists and practitioners, to which a dichotomy between priestly and monastic practitioners from the 3rd to 4th century CE does not do justice. In the following section, the assumption that the Michigan codex belongs in such a Christian monastic context will be taken up further, within a wider discussion of the proposed routes of oral and textual transmission of some of its recipes, alongside a revisionist set of considerations regarding what constitutes "Christianizing" and "diagnostically Christian" in the context of the Graeco-Egyptian magical tradition.

V. Textual vs. Oral Transmission

As noted above, and in the excurses to §§9 and 10, the principle thesis concerning the "divine dramas" contained in magical texts, variously termed "*historiolae*" or "charms", extant among the CMP has been that they are the products of oral, or a mixed oral and textual, transmission. The definition and nature of such "divine dramas" in the context of Egyptian ritual tradition—spanning temple, afterlife, and magical texts—is discussed in the introduction to the excurses to §§9 and 10. Interpretations of such oral transmission have been applied principally to account for the presence of the reflexes of traditionally Egyptian content in magical texts that postdate by centuries the dissolution of priestly *written language* and *script communities* as well as priestly *communities of practice*. That is to say, they became, or had always been, part of an oral cultural repertoire. While the viability of the textual transmission of §§9 and 10 from pre-Coptic source texts has been demonstrated through an analysis of the processes of transcription, transliteration, translation, and lexical and syntactical updating presented above (II–III), as well as the reconstruction of hypothetical source texts interwoven with the excurses to §§9 and 10 below, oral transmission is also, of course, a viable explanation for the presence of these later reflexes of traditional Egyptian content in §§9 and 10.

The most important consideration from the outset, however, is that the principal corpus of divine dramas containing reflexes of traditionally Egyptian content—the so-called Horus-Isis charms[223]—are all dated much later than the Michigan codex, into the 6th, 7th, and even 8th centuries CE, and therefore none of those examples have the same direct temporal or cultural connection to the Graeco-Egyptian magical tradition as §§9 and 10 of the Michigan codex. The revision of the date of the Michigan to the 4th, not 6th, century CE thereby separates the divine dramas of §§9 and 10 and *PGM* IV from the later corpus of "Horus-Isis charms" in time, in addition to the differences in their textual content—neither concern the explicit mother-son relationship that is central to the "Horus-Isis charms"—and in questions of cultural resonances and textual transmission. That is to say, although the case has been made here for the transmission of §§9 and 10 from pre-Coptic source texts, as elsewhere for the divine drama of *PGM* IV.94–113, this does not appear viable for the "Horus-Isis charms". Those texts date later, concern only Horus and Isis, and contain very little traditional Egyptian content—sometimes simply those theonyms—compared to the divine dramas of §§9 and 10, whose deep Egyptian cosmogonic and mythological resonances are discussed at length in the excurses to §§9 and 10. Nevertheless, it will be useful to review the important discussions in scholarship

[223] The term applied to the corpus compiled and studied most recently by Blumell and Dosoo 2018, 221–256, building on the earlier study of Frankfurter 2009.

on the composition and compilation of "*historiolae*" or "charms" among both the CMP and the preceding GEMP.[224]

Frankfurter (2009) first presented and developed the thesis that the Coptic "*historiolae*", as he terms them, comprising what Blumell and Dosoo (2018) term the "Horus-Isis charms", were principally derived from myths that were most prevalent not in textual, but oral tradition. Although Frankfurter's assessment that there are not any potential intermediaries between the GEMP and CMP that could evidence textual transmission is mistaken in the case of *PGM* IV and the Michigan codex,[225] there *is* a significant temporal gap between the GEMP and the "Horus-Isis charms" proper of the 6th, 7th, and 8th century CE. While Frankfurter's reasoning, that because certain myths found in earlier Egyptian divine dramas are not paralleled in "official mythology", they principally drew from "folklore motifs",[226] could be undermined by the publication of new Egyptian texts, the divine dramas in magical, as opposed to larger temple or afterlife, ritual texts do sometimes appear to exhibit a reduced repertoire.[227] Consequently, Frankfurter sees the divine dramas of magical texts as "not a prescriptive *extension of* official cult traditions but rather a descriptive *collecting from* folk traditions".[228] Such "folklore genres", asserts Frankfurter, "would have been fundamentally the memory-store of all".[229] These two considerations are, however, rather cyclical: by asserting that these traditions belong to "folklore", Frankfurter is able to claim that they would be part of a shared cultural repertoire, which apparently explains how they are in turn derived from "folklore".[230]

---

[224] See also the introduction to the excurses to §§9 and 10.

[225] Frankfurter (2009, 236) concluded that Old Coptic could not have served as an intermediary because he thought that Old Coptic "more often translated Greek", a misunderstanding of Satzinger's conclusions (1994, 220), where he presents the—also erroneous—conclusion that the Old Coptic texts of *PGM* IV were copied by a Grecophone. Frankfurter's misunderstanding of Satzinger was also highlighted in Blumell and Dosoo 2018, 244 n. 122.

[226] Frankfurter 1995, 472; 2009, 240.

[227] This conclusion does not, however, explain why Frankfurter expects that "*historiolae*", if they were composed from textual sources redacted by priests, *would* reflect official mythology closely. After all, one is never going to find the depth and complexity of Egyptian mythological and cosmogonical associations in a brief recitation or amulet. Thus, this conclusion was reached without the question ever having been posed as to why official mythology would be reflected.

[228] Frankfurter 2009, 238, allowing that they may have been "edited to correspond to priestly or ecclesiastical tradition". Elsewhere, Frankfurter states that these "*historiolae*" "do not resemble temple prayers to these Egyptian gods, given their specific, even intimate applications" (2018, 208), but nowhere is a textual comparison provided that might evidence this assertion. As before, this does not however explain why Frankfurter *expects* that "*historiolae*" *should* resemble temple prayers—and Frankfurter never clarifies what a "temple prayer" consists of in an Egyptian context.

[229] Frankfurter 2009, 238.

[230] Again, Frankfurter sees that "this model seems still to cover texts from the Greek and Demotic magical papyri", but does not develop this consideration further (2009, 238).

Nevertheless, while this hypothesis is feasible, Frankfurter then suggested that this is not only the case for the CMP, but indeed throughout all of Egyptian history, where it was more "wise women" than priests "who would have had the authority and creativity to compose new depictions of Horus's crises and Isis's distress according to situation".[231] Given that there must have been an oral tradition of magical practice that existed throughout all of Egyptian history contemporary, and to a greater or lesser extent overlapping, with a textual tradition of magical practice, this is a crucial consideration. Frankfurter does not, however, develop this hypothesis sufficiently to test its viability, but rather builds upon this point of departure without ever establishing it.[232]

By considering Pache's (2004) work on the mythological undertones of lullabies in Ancient Greece, Frankfurter proposed that the desired outcome of sleep in certain "Horus-Isis charms", and their extension for erotic outcomes, relates to the fact that they were drawn from "an oral culture of magical song".[233] Rightly highlighting that the "Horus-Isis charms" have a "repetitive, even strophic structure", in light of Pache's work Frankfurter sees such a textual structure as "point[ing] us to the folklore genre of the *lullaby*".[234] Frankfurter contextualizes Coptic magical texts principally within the milieux of "monastic ritual experts", and thereby conceives of a combination of textual and oral activities—the reading and copying of written texts and the chanting and recollection of oral texts.[235] It is in such a context that Frankfurter then locates the origin of such "*historiolae*", "whence at some point they shifted to writing".[236] Comparable to the hypothesis of lullabies, Frankfurter sees §§9 and 10 as a "herding song or blessing",[237] compiled from "oral tradition", which—after being "lightly edited"—were copied among ritual texts exhibiting "Christian language otherwise typical

---

231 Frankfurter 2009, 238. Frankfurter's preference for illiterate oral practitioners is later contradicted in the remark that "we might imagine that the persistence of Isis cults at Menouthis and Philae—and undoubtedly elsewhere—through the 5th century would itself have grounded or legitimized a larger, popular folklore of Isis, Horus, and other gods" (2009, 241), whereby the reader is confused as to whether Frankfurter really sees these traditions as being able to persist as independent folklore traditions without (scribal) institutions or not.

232 "Such stories were not the exclusive innovations of ritual experts but came about in the quotidian oral culture *around* the ritual expert." (Frankfurter 2009, 243).

233 Frankfurter 2009, 239; 2018, 210.

234 Frankfurter 2009, 239.

235 Frankfurter 2009, 237.

236 Frankfurter 2009, 237.

237 Frankfurter 2009, 242. Indeed, in both studies Frankfurter demonstrates a misunderstanding of the desired outcome—purpose—of §§9 and 10: while first stating that §9 "pertain[s] to maternity and childbirth" (2009, 242), later this becomes a "desire for pregnancy" (2018, 208); it is first stated that §10 concerns "the fertility of cattle" (2009, 242), later that it is a "blessing of the expansion of the herd" (Frankfurter 2018, 208).

of monastic scribal culture".[238] While the dating of the Michigan codex to the 4th century CE and the absence of diagnostically Christian content (VI) undermine Frankfurter's ascription of the codex to "monastic scribal culture",[239] Frankfurter suggests that "blessing one's herd"[240] is so widespread a cross-cultural phenomenon as to make his interpretation clear. In making this statement, Frankfurter cites cattle songs from other cultures, but at no point are these examples even described, let alone discussed and developed in order to make his case.[241]

Frankfurter concludes that "the principle of continuity, of tradition" in these "*historiolae*" "was not reverence for old gods (or nostalgic archaism) but simply the efficacy of sung formulae".[242] Further mixing, rather than clarifying, the idea of oral and textual transmission, Frankfurter then states that this principle explains why the copyist did not "edit out" the archaic names, but added the "add-

---

[238] Frankfurter 2018, 208.

[239] Regardless, this was only otherwise asserted by Frankfurter (2018, 206–208). By stating that the Michigan codex was compiled by monks, Frankfurter was able to interpret its contents through the lens of his understanding of "syncretism". But nowhere was a justification given as to why the Michigan codex would have been compiled and used by monks. Given the counterpoint of private professional physicians given in **Context in the Practice of Medicine and Healing**, even if it were dated to the 6th century CE, it cannot simply be assumed that the Michigan codex is to be ascribed to monastic practitioners.

[240] Notably, Frankfurter (2018, 208 n. 90) does not provide any comparisons from Egyptian textual culture of songs or magical texts to bless one's herd. The single example cited is P.Heid. inv. Kopt. 686, ed. Kropp 1966, 16/10–12, to remove the enchantment, i.e. a curse, from a cattle pasture. This does not, however, require the recitation of songs, but the inscription of a "bird-faced power", i.e. one of the magical figures inscribed in the codex, which is then to be buried while an offering of mastic is made. (ⲕ̄= ⲟⲩⲁϩⲓ ⲛⲧⲉⲃⲛⲏⲛ= ⲧⲁⲩⲉⲗⲟⲩϩⲓⲕ ⲉⲣⲁⲕ: ⲥϩⲁⲓ= ⳨ⲧⲉⲛⲁⲙⲓⲥ= ⲛϩⲁⲛϩⲁⲗⲏⲧ·= ⲧⲁⲙⲥ: ⲉϩⲟⲩⲛ ⲉⲣⲁⲃ= ϣⲁⲃⲃⲱⲗ ⲉⲃⲁⲗ: ⲕⲁⲗⲟⲥ= ⲑ̄ⲩ̄ ⲙ̄ⲁ̄ⲥ̄⳨̄ⲭ̄ⲓ̄=). Recipes to protect or disarm the enchantment of herds are found in the earlier Egyptian magical tradition, yet these comprise divine dramas concluding with commands, rather than "songs", e.g. P.Brit.Mus. EA 10042 verso 1/1–2/1. Recitations to protect herds from crocodiles as they cross the river are also found inscribed upon the walls of Old Kingdom mastabas, but once again these are not "songs", but invocations and commands. For a summary of such "water praising" (*ḥsi.w-mw*), see now Gundacker 2019 and the substantial bibliography there.

[241] Frankfurter 2018, 208 n. 90. Van der Vliet describes these as "aptly chosen ethnographic parallels" (2018, 160) but does not elaborate as to why. In the first instance, comparisons with pastoralist societies without scribal classes and textual traditions do not appear so "apt". Although Egypt had pastoralist communities, Egypt was not a pastoralist society. Egypt was a settled agricultural society with a complex infrastructure of administration and governance, maintaining and maintained by a scribal elite class, that produced and reified textual culture and traditions, to which Frankfurter is arguing these texts do not belong. Thus, to compare cultural repertoires that have prominent oral traditions due to the absence of textual culture with proposed oral traditions in an Egyptian context is tenuous.

[242] Frankfurter 2018, 209.

itional authority of the Christian god".[243] This is, however, both a non-sequitur and a contradiction in point: (ia) if the old gods were not revered and the efficacy was through sung formulae, why were the old gods not replaced, given that Frankfurter considers the text Christianized—(ib) or why was it that songs about the old gods rather than Christian deities were sung if those old gods were insignificant and instead the efficacy was through sung formulae—(ii) if the sung formulae were considered efficacious by themselves, why did the additional authority of the Christian god need to be added?

Besides the problems with certain assumptions behind Frankfurter's thesis, one fundamental question it also leaves unanswered regarding the viability of oral transmission is when to stop the metaphorical clock. That is to say, did an oral text cease to be an oral text when it was first written down?[244] If a previously oral text was written down, did it cease being an oral text? Could not a ritual text that had always been written then enter oral tradition and thence become an oral text? None of these questions and potential issues were addressed by Frankfurter, and thus the unresolved problem can be considered as one of the conflation between the orality (production) of such texts and their aurality (responses to them)—their *textual structure*—and their origins, context of (re)production, and thereby their transmission—in textual *form*.

A potential resolution is van der Vliet's introduction of Foley's typology of a "voiced text" for written texts that are "aimed at oral performance" and for texts which are "incomplete without that performance".[245] Crucially, this does not mean that such texts are one and the same as an "oral text". While divine dramas and other rituals texts are genres that require orality (recitation), and often also aurality (reception), because "poetic qualities provide the key to [their] efficacy in performance", "oral literary strategies and formats, while they may profoundly shape a written text, are not themselves indicative of the oral origins of that text or even its oral transmission over time".[246] That is to say, "oral formats" are "geared to [a] live performance", but this does not necessarily say anything about the origins or transmission of texts with such structures. The fact that a written text "bears the stamp of orality" may come not from its being an "oral text", but rather a "voiced text"—"a written text that is aimed at oral perform-

[243] Frankfurter 2018, 209. A cyclical and ultimately contradictory statement to the same effect is that made by Hevesi (2019, 49), following Frankfurter (2009, 243): "The aim of the use of Christian and Jewish elements within the spells … could be to assimilate these native narratives to the Christian background which would, again, show that the scribes were aware of the fact that at least, these elements were not Christian at all."

[244] For this, see Bohak's consideration of a "scribalization gap" to bridge the "Jewish scribal magical tradition of late antiquity from its non-scribal predecessors" (2008, 298). That is to say, the process by which once exclusively "oral texts" became "written texts".

[245] Van der Vliet 2018, 161 with n. 48.

[246] Van der Vliet 2018, 161.

ance”.[247] Theater scripts are, for example, “voiced texts”. They are to be performed (recited), although they are nonetheless composed and transmitted in written form (inscribed). Without question, texts that were orally produced for an aural response would have had an oral transmission of production and aural transmission of reception—for example, audience members (responders) would leave a theater being able to quote (produce) due to such *oral to aural transmission*. But to extrapolate from such “oral formats” in *textual structure* an underlying thesis about *oral transmission*, when all the texts under consideration are written, and certain motifs and aspects of *textual content* are paralleled in textual culture across millennia,[248] is problematic. While the philologist focuses firstly on the written text, that is not to deny the oral transmission and aural reception of that written text: there were not only monks who recited—sung—hymns and liturgies, thereby both orally transmitting and aurally receiving otherwise written texts, there were also priestly practitioners who, for millennia, undertook the cults in Egyptian temples through hymns and liturgies. It is crucial to bear in mind that these priestly practitioners were one and the same as the priestly scribes who composed, redacted, and compiled those written—yet “voiced”—texts.[249]

A model of oral transmission has, however, been presented recently by Blumell and Dosoo (2018). Laying out their considerations that “most of the surviving magical texts derive from a mixed oral-written environment”—such as that just described—, they consider the “Horus-Isis charms” as well as other charms to “more often [have] been transmitted orally rather than through writing”.[250] In order to make this case, Blumell and Dosoo adopt Carr’s model of the formation of the Hebrew Bible, which shows that oral transmission creates distinctive textual alterations to textual transmission: while textual transmission is evidenced by closer reproduction, changes being principally graphic variants or the accidental omissions of letters, words, or lines, oral transmission is evidenced by gradual abbreviation of texts, replacement of less common terms with more familiar synonyms, rationalization of familiar material, and the loss of

[247] Van der Vliet 2018, 161.

[248] Van der Vliet (2018, 161) stresses that “magic is transmitted through a rich written record, reflecting a variety of scribal practices” which “represent a distinct literate tradition in its own right”. It is this “literate tradition”, indeed the “weight of tradition”, that van der Vliet sees as the medium through which such motifs and textual content are transmitted across millennia (2018, 162). Here, van der Vliet is close to the proposed thesis of “textual authority”, which accounts for the conceptualized efficacy of ritual texts over such vast temporal frames, see Love 2020, §§5–6, developing Love 2016, §§7.6.3–7.7.

[249] Indeed, as discussed in Love 2021a, §1.2.3.2, the *Book of the Temple* describes how one aspect of priestly training required a trainee to “learn telling (*sḏꜣḏꜣ* < *stwt*) praises (*ḥnk.w*), uttering (*wšꜣ*) praises (*ḥś(w.wt)*), (and) screeching (*diꜣ*)” (17/11).

[250] Blumell and Dosoo 2018, 251.

proper names, numbers, etc. Although it is difficult to distinguish accidental from deliberate variants, an illustrative example of how one might reason between the two is demonstrated.[251] In the "Horus-Isis charms" more specifically, Blumell and Dosoo present pairs of synonyms, ⲃⲱⲕ and ⲙⲟⲟϣⲉ and ⲡⲏⲗⲏ and ⲣⲟ respectively,[252] compared with the more "graphic" variants in two copies of a Coptic magical text.[253] These show that the "content being transmitted might be described as semantic or narrative rather than lexical", "stored in the memory as a series of narrative episodes, which would be retold with slightly different word choice and constructions in each telling".[254]

While Carr's model is certainly informative, certain questions must be raised as to the appropriateness of applying a model for the oral to textual transmission of authoritative, canonical, and scriptural textual culture to the genre of magical texts. After all, magical texts were not canonical: there was no one authoritative version of any particular text, centrally maintained, reified, and transmitted within the Coptophone world. Instead, the transmission of magical texts could instead be termed an "open" textual transmission. Copyists, compilers, and redactors were freer to copy genres of textual culture that did not have single authoritative, canonical versions. Through such "open" textual transmission, textual complexities could be rationalized, specific points of reference could be generalized, and unfamiliar textual content could be banalized. Given that the CMP and the Hebrew Bible are not at all like-for-like comparisons, then, the question must be posed how different oral transmission would indeed look from "open" textual transmission, the decentralized transmission of non-canonical texts lacking an authoritative version.

Blumell and Dosoo do not go as far as Frankfurter, however, in positing a milieu of "wise women" throughout Egyptian history who were the composers and practitioners of these "charms", but they do conclude that their study might suggest such "charms" "were not restricted to literate specialists, but were used by a wider public".[255] One difficulty of the model—the point "where this model breaks down"—was transparently presented by Blumell and Dosoo when considering the supplications that usually close such "charms".[256] While "performative phrases" such as "I invoke you" never feature, the supplications, e.g.

---

[251] Blumell and Dosoo 2018, 253 n. 147.

[252] Given the hierarchy of borrowing between languages in *contact situations*, the striking substitution of an Egyptian lexeme for a Greek loanword (πύλη) in the latter case requires further explanation. In the former case, further explanation is required to clarify why the variation between ⲃⲱⲕ and ⲙⲟⲟϣⲉ could not also represent dialectal differences, given that interdialectal translation was common in the transmission of Coptic textual culture.

[253] Blumell and Dosoo 2018, 253–254.

[254] Blumell and Dosoo 2018, 253.

[255] Blumell and Dosoo 2018, 254–255.

[256] Blumell and Dosoo 2018, 255.

"through the power of the lord god", "show no real continuity with one another, but often significant similarities with other magical material"—instead suggesting that the charms and supplications that follow "circulated separately".[257] This should then be considered alongside the fact that the "Horus-Isis charm" in O.BYU Mag. opens with a series of *voces magicae* inscribed before the divine drama begins. Although Blumell and Dosoo rightly note that these are not integrated into the charm itself,[258] according to their adopted model, where personal names are lost in oral transmission, this instead suggests that this particular "charm" was transmitted textually—bringing the discussion back to when to stop the metaphorical clock of oral to textual transmission, and whether such "charms" were definitely the product of a *unique* strand of mixed oral and textual transmission.

As noted above, there must have been an oral tradition of magical practice that existed throughout all of Egyptian history contemporary, and to a greater or lesser extent overlapping, with a textual tradition of magical practice. Blumell and Dosoo (2018) have therefore, building upon Frankfurter (2009), presented a feasible hypothesis for interrogating the difference between the written reifications of a potentially oral tradition, as thereby evidenced through a mixed oral *and* textual transmission, and the written reifications of a principally textual tradition. Before its utility can be fully evaluated, however, a consideration of an "open" textual transmission must be integrated into this discussion. Furthermore, while their synoptic treatment of the episodes exhibited in the "Horus-Isis charms" was elucidatory, the distinct lack of parallels for the vast majority of all magical texts across all of Egyptian history, quite unlike the source base utilized by Carr in his treatment of the formation of the Hebrew Bible, nevertheless makes interpretations of the nature of transmission tentative. Given that the conventional understanding of all ritual texts in the Egyptian context throughout all of Egyptian history is that they were principally "voiced texts", that is, texts that had to be recited in order for their efficacy to actualize their desired outcome, and thereby that they exhibit such "stamps of orality", it will be paramount for later studies advocating oral transmission not to conflate textual *structure* with textual *transmission*.

An important further distinction when considering the transmission of §§9 and 10 is that, unlike the considerably later "Horus-Isis charms", the Michigan codex is contemporary with the GEMP, and most importantly, the latest reflexes of traditionally Egyptian content found in the aforementioned Old Coptic texts in

[257] Blumell and Dosoo 2018, 255.

[258] Blumell and Dosoo 2018, 254; but contrary to its presentation there, the magical name in the parallel texts of P.Schmidt 1 (ed. Kropp, *AKZ* I, text A) *is* integrated into the command closing that "charm".

that corpus. While nothing comparable to the texts of *PGM* and §§9 and 10 are found among the CMP, the existence of divine dramas that may exhibit reflexes of traditionally Egyptian content in Greek translation indicates further viable routes of textual transmission—especially as these translations are significantly divorced from contemporary Egyptophone oral transmission.[259] Another crucially important distinction is that the "myths" contained within the later "Horus-Isis charms" are either not paralleled, and have no obvious resonances with, earlier Egyptian traditions, or they are entirely Christianized with Horus and Isis simply "pagan placeholders". Although a lack of parallels for the divine dramas in magical texts is also found during the Pharaonic and Graeco-Roman Period, at that time there was a substantial cultural repertoire from which to draw, which was not the case during the 6th–8th centuries. In the case of the Michigan codex, however, this cultural repertoire—albeit not the same as in the 1st–3rd centuries CE—was still in limited textual transmission, from which a reifying oral and aural reception could build.

Notwithstanding some novelties and unparalleled points of reference, the otherwise extensive mythological and cosmogonic associations and resonances discussed in the excurses to §§9 and 10 instead suggest that they were composed, redacted, copied and therefore first practiced at a time when their textual content still accorded with contemporary cultural repertoires. When the textual content of §§9 and 10 is compared with the "Horus-Isis charms" that are almost entirely stripped of any traditionally Egyptian content, the contrast is one of night and day. Indeed, while *stylistic motifs*, that is, stylized and generalized syntax, are shared among §§9–10, the divine drama of *PGM* IV.94–113, and the later "Horus-Isis charms", those later texts are lacking in the *descriptive* and *specific semantics* that are found in §§9–10 and *PGM* IV. These include, for example, aspects as simple as toponyms such as Abydos that, while being concrete place names, have only direct resonance and thereby relevance within an Egyptian as opposed to Christian cultural repertoire, or as developed as "those of the Great of Five", which would only have resonance and thereby relevance within the Egyptian cultural repertoire. Given that none of these traditional fea-

[259] Although the names of the characters in the "Horus-Isis charms" are given in their Egyptian rather than Graecized vocalizations, if those names were understood, an Egyptian-Greek bilingual could well have rendered them from a Greek translation. Thus, the so-called Philinna papyrus (*PGM* XX; *GEMF* 3) and its reflex in *Suppl.Mag*. II 88 as a potential case study for the textual transmission of these divine dramas needs to be considered further by those arguing for the oral transmission of "charms", as do the potential indices of a Greek translation or at least source texts for other "charms", see Richter 2007, 263. For studies of the "Philinna papyrus", see Ritner 1998; Faraone 2000; Zellmann-Rohrer 2020a, 44–49. The insecure foundation of Ritner's conjecture that that particular divine drama concerns Horus is presented by Zellmann-Rohrer (2020a, 46), who ultimately concurs with Faraone that the most parsimonious interpretation is that of a Near Eastern/Mesopotamian background—as is indeed described in the text's very title.

tures are found in the later "Horus-Isis charms", and that those texts are instead replete with textual content from other cultural repertoires, §§9–10 and *PGM* IV.94–113 must be interpreted as significantly different from the "Horus-Isis charms".

This difference can in turn be explained by the location of the earlier texts within the orbit of the Graeco-Egyptian magical tradition. That is to say, it should be no surprise that after the broad Christianization of Egypt by the middle of the 5th century CE, no such comparable divine dramas to those in §§9–10 and *PGM* IV.94–113 are found, whether in Old or standard Coptic.[260] Where is Amun, the south-wind, where is Thoth, the Great of Five? Where are the mythological and cosmogonic associations of Abydos and Thinis resonant and thereby relevant within an Egyptian cultural repertoire? The reification by modern scholars of the isolated persistence of incredibly limited aspects of the traditionally Egyptian cultural repertoire in magical texts during the late Roman Period onwards, without a contextualized analysis of the sheer scale of how much was, by comparison, lost, risks falsifying the reality of the contemporary individuals who interacted with these aspects of the cultural repertoire.[261] The contraction of the cultural repertoire of traditionally Egyptian content that occurred during the 3rd and 4th centuries CE, itself partly a consequence of the broad obsolescence of Egyptian writing during the 3rd century CE and the dissolution of priestly *communities of practice*, resulted in its gradual replacement with a new cultural repertoire that otherwise dominated the CMP, and it is how this transition is reflected in the Michigan codex which concerns the following, final section.

[260] Indeed, other than those few divine dramas, the presence of traditionally Egyptian content is seen in just a few theonyms and what I have previously called "mythical allusions" (Love 2016, 154 with n. 22)—see now the table in Blumell and Dosoo 2018, 257–259.

[261] Indeed, this in turn risks a slip of the scholarly discourse away from the lived experience of those contemporary individuals and into the realms of reifying—even lionizing—survivals in cultural repertoires at the expense of the predominant cultural complexes contemporary to those survivals by assuming that such survivals were as meaningful to contemporary individuals as they are to modern scholars. After all, the persistence of any aspect of a cultural repertoire is only meaningful in that temporal frame when it is actually contextualized among the contemporary cultural repertoires of which it was part, not when it is placed in an etic temporal frame of transmission of which contemporary individuals would not have been conscious, and for whom it may have been entirely irrelevant.

VI. Syncretism in the Other Direction

One of the principal concerns of Frankfurter's most recent study of "syncretism" in late Roman and Byzantine Egypt (2018), is what was Egyptian about the Christianity in Egypt; that is to say, which local cultural practices persisted there under the weight—prestige, authority, and institutional influence—of Christianity. Given that all prior commentators on §§9 and 10 have considered them to have been Christianized through later additions, without examining whether these later additions are truly diagnostically Christian in the context of the 3rd and 4th centuries CE,[262] the nature of the syncretism that existed in the magical texts of Graeco-Roman Egypt must be examined.

Significant absences from the recipes of the Michigan codex should first be considered. No compiler or practitioner introduced into, or would find within the Michigan codex any direct references to Jesus and/or Christ, the use of trinitarian language for the superordinate deity "God" that—unlike a monotheistic "God"—is unique to Christianity, evidence of the cult of saints, unambiguous Christian symbols,[263] *nomina sacra*, or citations from Christian scripture—whether canonical or apocryphal. In the supplications at the end of §§9 and 10, however, reference is made to the "lord god" and "Iao Sabaoth". While these formulations are instantly recognizable in the later CMP, they are not diagnostically Christian epithets or theonyms, nor are they therefore unambiguous evidence of Christianization. Indeed, given the host of Jewish elements in pre- and non-Christian magical texts from the GEMP that were evidently redacted and practiced by non-Christians, the conclusion that the "lord god" and "Iao Sabaoth" are evidence of Christianization is in fact rather tenuous. After all, as noted above and discussed further below, although the Michigan codex was produced during the 4th century CE, it was itself a compilation from source texts, most if not all of which, given their direct resonance with the GEMP, must date back at least to the 3rd century CE, if not earlier.

In the ritual for "petitioning god" (*pḥ-nṯr*) of *P.London-Leiden* recto 5/3–33 (*PDM* xiv.117–149), "God" (*pꜣ nṯr*) is commanded to reveal himself to the practitioner "in the fashion of your revelation to Moses (*m-w-s-e-s*[Go]) which you enacted upon the mountain, before whom you, yourself, created the darkness (and) the light".[264] This is, then, an undoubtedly Jewish addition to a traditionally Egyptian ritual practice that otherwise invokes a god to give answer without falsehood because the practitioner will glorify him in Abydos (5/15–16), i.e.

---

[262] Frankfurter 2009, 242; 2018, 208; van der Vliet 2018, 159; Dosoo 2021.

[263] The chi-rho symbols among the magical signs on p. 2 and a rho-headed cross in the stele-amulet for demoniacs on p. 11 can both be explained through other derivations (see commentary).

[264] *wnḥ=k r-ỉrỉ̯=y ty n pꜣ(-h)rw mw-ky pꜣ ky n wnḥ=k r m-w-s-e-s*[Go] *ntỉ-r(ỉw) ỉ:ỉrỉ̯ =k r-r=f ḥr pꜣ tw ntỉ-ỉw ḥr=k tỉ.t ḫpr pꜣ kke pꜣ wyn nꜣe-ḥr=f* (*P.London-Leiden* 5/13–14).

Osiris' paramount cult center. Such a feature is not, however, considered evidence of the Judaization, let alone Christianization of that recipe, even though it is evidently the Judaeo-Christian "God" who is commanded to appear. Presumably, this later addition was conceptualized as an efficacious motif in contemporary non- and preceding pre-Christian milieux, drawn from a distinct cultural repertoire—albeit one, in the case of Judaism, which had been present in Egypt for centuries.

Moses figures again as an addition to traditional Egyptian content in a string of mythical allusions regarding the state of the practitioner in the erotic recipe of *P.London-Leiden* verso 12/1–13/12 (*PDM* xiv.1026–1045). There, the practitioner declares that his heart feels "the longing that God, the son of Sirius (?), felt for Moses while he was going to the hill of Ninaretos to offer water to [h]is god, his lord, his Iaō Sabaō(th)".[265] Of particular note is that Iao Sabaoth is glossed in Old Coptic, which—following the revisionist study of Dieleman[266]—indicates that the scribe was retaining the integrity of a source text.[267] A comparable phenomenon is the appearance of an "angel" in the aforementioned diglossic and trigraphic P.Brit.Mus. EA 10808, where the supernatural assistant (*parhedros*) to be acquired is named, in Demotic, *ʿ-n-g-y-l-w-s*[Sl-Go].[268] These two examples are further evidence of the utilization of motifs from distinct cultural repertoires that were conceptualized as efficacious, but would never be considered by modern scholars as evidence for the Judaization or Christianization of those recipes in contemporary non- and preceding pre-Christian milieux.

Within the aforementioned bilingual *PGM* III archive, two further bilingual recipes are relevant. In the bilingual memory recipe of *PGM* III.2 verso 3/5–3/18, introduced above, one of the Egyptian-language sections contains the identifying statement "I am Jesus, the great god",[269] utilizing a novel and unambiguously Christian theonym alongside a traditionally Egyptian epithet several millennia older. This interpolation of diagnostically Christian content would not, however, be considered by modern scholars as a conscious attempt to Christian-

[265] *⸌pꜣ wḫꜣ⸍ nti-ỉw pꜣ nṯr sꜣ spd* (?) *ỉyi̯.yṯ=f r m-w-s.t-s*[Go] *ỉw=f ỉni̯-nꜥ.k r tꜣ sbt.t n n-y-n-ꜣ-r-e-tꜣ-s*[Or] *r wꜣḥ mw n [p]ꜣe=f nṯr pꜣe=f ḥrye pꜣe=f y-ꜥ-h-ꜥꜣ*[Go] (glossed ⲓⲁⲱ) *s-ꜥ-b-ꜣ-h-ꜥꜣ*[Go] (glossed ⲥⲁⲃⲁⲱ) (*P.London-Leiden* verso 12/6–7).

[266] Dieleman 2005, 73–77; 125–130; 2006, 77–81. See also Quack 2004, 430–432, discussed in Love 2016, §2.4.4.4.

[267] Although it would be easier to assume that this source text would have been in Greek, the Old Coptic gloss to Sabaoth (ⲥⲁⲃⲁⲱ) is highly suggestive of an Egyptian substrate text due to the absence of the final consonant ⲑ. Such renderings are in fact common to Egyptian-language transcriptions and transliterations, consider *s-ꜥ-b-ꜥ-h-ꜥꜣ*[Go] (*P.London-Leiden* 19/39; 21/6) and *s-ꜥ-b-ꜣ-h-w*[Go] (*P.London-Leiden* verso 12/10).

[268] Discussed in Love 2016, 20 n. 28; since then I have been able to correct the reading, with thanks to Joachim Quack.

[269] ⲁⲛⲅ ⲓ̈ⲏⲥⲟⲩⲥ ⲡⲛⲉⲧⲟ (*PGM* III.2 verso 3/13–15).

ize the recipe, even though this identifying statement means that it is Jesus who is providing the authority and thereby efficacy through which the desired outcome could be actualized. In this case, perhaps one divine name was replaced with another because Jesus was conceptualized within contemporary milieux as an efficacious deity to invoke. In the bilingual sunlight divination of *PGM* III.1 verso 4/22–6/44, also introduced above, a mix of traditionally Egyptian content, such as "It is you who are Prē, Coming forth is your [true] name"[270] is found alongside the Judaeo-Christian divine names and epithets "Sabao[th] Adōnai".[271] This mixture, while entirely unremarkable in the GEMP, specifically shows that—just as with the Demotic examples presented above—biliterate bilinguals, whose first language was in all likelihood Egyptian, were invested in utilizing—appropriating—material from distinct cultural repertoires, presumably because they were conceptualized as providing certain efficacy. Nevertheless, this appropriation would not be considered by modern scholars as evidence of the Christianization of these recipes among contemporary non- and preceding pre-Christian milieux.

In the bilingual recipe for a direct vision of *PGM* IV.5–51,[272] introduced above, which features nondescript *voces magicae* (5–10) preceding Egyptian-language invocations for that direct-vision (11–25) and Greek-language ritual instructions for preparations and practice (26–51), traditionally Egyptian content is found alongside that of Jewish, or perhaps Judaeo-Christian, origins. While the opening line of invocations in Egyptian reads: "Hail Osiris, King of the Underworld, Lord of Mummification",[273] this is followed shortly by, "Hail Althabot (i.e. Ialdabaoth), bring Sabaoth in to me"[274] and "Hail Althonai (i.e. Adonai)",[275] before concluding "Bring Michael in to me, this mighty one of angels who is with God".[276] Given that the opening lines of this Egyptian-language section in Old Coptic are paralleled in Demotic in *P.London-Leiden*,[277] where no such Jewish or Judaeo-Christian features are found, would this too be considered evidence of the Judaization or Christianization of that recipe?

In a prior treatment of these parallels, I argued that such "unambiguous interpolations of the Old Testament God, and Moses, attest a similar phenomenon of incorporating religious elements from the milieu of the client rather than the

[270] [ⲛ]ⲧ̣ⲟ̣ⲕ̣ ⲡⲉ ⲡⲓⲣⲉ ⲡⲉⲣ̣ⲉ ⲉⲣⲓⲛⲕ̣ ⲛ̄[ⲙⲏⲧ] (*PGM* III.1 verso 4/23–24).
[271] ⲥⲁⲃⲁⲱ[ⲑ] ⲁⲇⲱⲛⲁⲓ (*PGM* III.1 verso 5/5).
[272] Love 2016, §1.2; §4.1.
[273] ⲉⲟⲩⲱ́ⲧϥ ⲟⲩⲥⲓ́ⲣⲉ· ⲡⲉⲣⲟⲛ̄ⲧⲏ́ ⲡⲛⲏ́ⲃ ⲛ̄ⲧⲕⲁⲏ́ⲥⲉ· (*PGM* IV.11).
[274] ⲉⲩⲱ́ⲧϥ ⲁⲗⲑⲁⲃⲱ́ⲧ · ⲉⲛⲓ ⲥⲁⲃⲁⲱ́ⲑ ⲛⲁⲓ̈ ⲉⳍⲟⲩⲛ (*PGM* IV.14–15).
[275] ⲉⲩⲱ́ⲧϥ ⲁⲗⲑⲱⲛⲁⲓ (*PGM* IV.15).
[276] ⲁⲛⲓ ⲙⲓⲭⲁⲏ́ⲗ ⲛⲁⲓ̈ ⲉⳍⲟⲩⲛ ⲡⲓϭⲁ́ϥ ⲛ̄ⲁⲅⲅⲉⲗⲟⲓ ⲉⲧⲟⲓ̈ ⲛ̄ⲧⲉⲙ ⲡⲛⲟ́ⲩⲧⲉ (*PGM* IV.16–17).
[277] Discussed in the commentary to the edition of *PGM* IV.11–25 in Love 2016, §1.2.

milieu of the practitioner".[278] That is to say, the prominence of Jewish or Judaeo-Christian motifs in the wider mixed cultural repertoires of Graeco-Roman Egypt meant that, during the second half of the 2nd century CE, they found their way into the repertoire of the practitioners of the GEMP. A refinement to that point may be made, however: even in the absence of such "market forces", redactors and compilers were clearly interested in utilizing—appropriating—motifs from different cultural repertoires in order to enhance the efficacy of their own recipes. A final example of a comparable phenomenon in *PGM* IV is the presence of a bilingual exorcism (1227–1264) which is either a Christianized version of an earlier Jewish liturgical exorcism or a directly Christian redaction.[279] This manuscript was compiled and practiced by non-Christians, as were its source texts, but these were individuals who evidently had an interest in redacting and compiling magical texts from Jewish or Judaeo-Christian cultural repertoires. A further example may be mentioned, which will not be treated in detail here, of the "Stele of Jeu the hieroglyphist"[280] (*PGM* V.96–145), in which the practitioner identifies himself with "Moses your prophet to whom you have transmitted your mysteries" (109–111) as well as the "messenger" (ἄγγελος) of "the king Osiris-Wennefer" (Φαπρω Οσοροννωφρις, 114) who knows "your true name which has been transmitted to the prophets of Israel" (114–117).

Even in the CMP, there are examples in which texts of later centuries have not been unambiguously Christianized and can—if investigating scholars do not begin with the assumption that everything that could resonate with Christianity is, from the 4th century CE onwards, diagnostic of a Christian(ized) text—instead be interpreted as descendants of the GEMP. Consider, for example, the third text (p. 4/1–6/2) in the miniature papyrus codex formulary of the 6th century CE, P.Mil.Vogl. Copt. 16.[281] This erotic recipe invokes both the traditional Egyptian deities Petbe and the triad of "three gods" Apis, Isis, and Osiris as well as the—in the Graeco-Egyptian magical tradition—pan-cultural Abrasax, Typhon-Seth (through his epithets in the so-called Typhonic *Logos*), and Iao Sabaoth. Although the entire recipe concludes with the phrase "Seize NN, bring her to the feet of NN by <the> power of Iao Sabaoth!", [282] Iao Sabaoth is so common throughout the GEMP in Demotic and Greek magical texts as to not be diagnostic of Christianization or Christianity. Thus, even into the 6th century

[278] Love 2016, 219. In the case of a divinatory recipe, the practitioner would have been commissioned to acquire foreknowledge on behalf of the client, who may have observed the ritual or—even if not—have been encouraged by the invocation and commanding of a deity that exhibited particular resonances with an individual cultural repertoire.

[279] As discussed in Love 2016, §6.5.1.

[280] Also discussed in Love 2016, §6.4.1.

[281] Ed. Pernigotti 1979; 1993. For the multilingual archive of magical texts to which this manuscript belongs, see Love fc. c.

[282] ϩⲁⲣⲡⲁ[ⲥ]ⲥⲉ ⲛⲇ̣ⲇ̣ ⲁⲛⲓⲧ̣ⲥ̣ ⲉⲣⲁⲧϥ ⲇ̣ⲇ̣ ϩⲛ ϭⲟⲙ ⲓⲁⲱ ⲥⲁⲃⲁⲱⲑ (p. 6/1–2).

CE, there were magical texts of evident antiquity in circulation in an unambiguously Christianized society that had themselves not been unambiguously Christianized. Indeed, of all the "Horus-Isis charms" studied by Blumell and Dosoo that do not contain unambiguously Christianized content, only one closes with an unambiguously Christian invocation,[283] and this is an example from the 8th century CE,[284] which may include Horus and Isis as named deities, but otherwise features characters from the Christian cultural repertoire.

This phenomenon, then, should be considered alongside a directly comparable one attested towards the end of the tradition of Coptic magical texts. That is, comparable to the late Roman Period in which *written language* and *script shift* were also indices of changing cultural repertoires, a curse on a sheet of paper from the Cairo Genizah of the 9th–11th century CE (Cambridge, University Library T.-S. 12.207)[285] is informative of analogous trends during the shift from Coptic to Arabic in an increasingly Arabized and Islamized Egypt. This manuscript contains a bilingual (Arabic-Coptic) text inscribed in a monographic redaction, where the first six lines contain the Basmala/Bismillāh,[286] followed by an Arabic-language text in Coptic script: "May the tongue of the resentful Gharib bin Sit al-Kul[287] be bound, so that the speaker is not able to speak", "May his tongue be bound on behalf of Thijar bint Siti,[288] through the power of these

---

[283] Blumell and Dosoo 2018, 235–237. By contrast, Blumell and Dosoo state that the invocation "by the power of Iaō Sabaōth" that ends the "charm" of O.BYU Mag. "suggests an attempt to integrate a non-Christian charm into a Christian framework" (2018, 238). Given that Iao Sabaoth is found in pre- and non-Christian magical texts, however, the dating of this ostracon to a period in which the superordinate cultural and religious community is Christian does not render this invocation diagnostically Christian. Later Christians could have reinterpreted this supplication through a Christian lens, and thereby perceived no need to Christianize it, meaning that a source text from centuries earlier, that is, of pre-Christian date, would in fact look the same.

[284] At the end of a recipe for healing stomach-ache in P.Berl. inv. 8313 (ed. *BKU* I 1) 2/1–verso/8, Isis provides her suffering son Horus with commands that conclude: "Every sickness and every suffering and every pain which is in the belly of NN, the son of NN, let it cease! It is I who calls, it is the Lord Jesus who grants healing" (ϣⲟⲛⲉ ⲛⲓⲙ ϩⲓ ϩⲓⲥⲉ ⲛⲓⲙ ϩⲓ ⲧⲓⲧⲕⲁⲥ ⲛⲓⲙ ⲉⲧϩⲛ ϩⲏⲧϥ ⲉ-ⲛⲓⲙ ⲡϣⲛ ⲛⲓⲙ ⲙⲁⲣⲉϥ ⲗⲟ ⲛⲧⲉⲩⲛⲟⲩ ⲁⲛⲟⲕ ⲉⲧⲙⲟⲩⲧⲉ ⲡϫⲟⲉⲓⲥ ⲓ̅ⲥ̅ ⲡⲉⲧⲧⲓ ⲛⲡⲧⲁⲗϭⲟ, verso/6–8), and the copy closes with a rho-headed staurogram (⳨).

[285] Ed. Crum 1902; see further the German translation in Kropp, *AKZ* II, 242–243 and the English translation in Meyer and Smith 1994, 197–199 no. 94, and for an image, https://cudl.lib.cam.ac.uk/view/MS-TS-00012-00207/1.

[286] ⲡⲉⲥⲙⲉⲗⲗⲉ ⲉⲗⲣⲁϩⲙⲉⲛ ⲉⲗⲣⲁϩⲓⲙ (بسم الله الرحمن الرحيم) (l. 1).

[287] As noted in Love fc. c, it could be that these names are in fact pseudonymous, as they could be read "strange-man, son of the woman-of-everything". As there, Jack Clift is thanked for his contribution to reading this text.

[288] As noted in Love fc. c and the preceding footnote, it could be that these names are in fact pseudonymous, as they could be read "thick-one daughter of my-mistress".

names here. Amen".[289] The opening Arabic-language invocation and command, then, are framed in a format that would be characteristic of a prayer, applying epithets evidently from the Islamic tradition. The second section is clearly delineated from the first by three lines of *charaktēres*, featuring an exclusively Coptic-language invocation in Coptic script to God (ⲫⲛⲟⲩⲧⲓ), "the one who bound heaven and earth" and "the voice which was uttered at the top of the wood (i.e. the Cross)"[290] —, among other diagnostically Christian motifs.

Richter considers that the initial element of the invocation, "In the name of God", was in fact "unmarked by confession", that is, a monotheistic formula which related not only to the beginning of the Basmala/Bismillāh, but also to Christian formulae.[291] This is thereby a case in which the cultural repertoire of a distinct religious tradition was adopted, resulting in stylistic changes in language that occurred relatively rapidly in comparison to the structural changes exerted by Arabization on Coptic texts.[292] Indeed, examples of this opening invocation are found in multiple genres of texts, whether magical as the present text, medical,[293] or financial,[294] or other documents.[295] A remarkable linguistic feature of the rendering of the Basmala/Bismillāh in the present text is the lack of phonetic assimilation of the definite article, which suggests that the copyist knew the orthographic form of the formula in written Arabic, and thus that he was not reliant on an aural version.[296] The presence of a feature that stems from the Arabic and/or Islamic cultural repertoire and, indeed, has not even been translated into the linguistic frame of the wider recipe is not, therefore, diagnostic of the Islamization of the recipe into which it has been added. It is in light of this later development that the utilization—appropriation—of theonyms, invocations, and supplications from other cultural repertoires by practitioners of the late Roman Period that are assumed to be evidence of Christianization should be reconsidered.

[289] ⲡⲉⲥⲙⲉⲗⲗⲉ ⲉⲗⲣⲁϩⲙⲉⲛ ⲉⲗⲣⲁϩⲓⲙ ϩⲁⲕⲁⲧ ⲗⲓⲥⲏⲛ ⲛⲁⲕⲓⲙ̣ ϧⲁⲣⲓⲡ ⲡⲉⲛ ⲥⲓⲧ ⲉⲗⲭⲟⲩⲗ ⲗⲏ ⲓⲏⲥⲧⲁ̣ⲧⲓϩ ⲓⲏⲧⲓⲏⲭⲏⲗⲗⲉⲙ ⲉⲗⲭⲏⲗⲉⲙ ϩⲁⲕⲁⲧ ⲗⲓⲥⲉⲛⲟⲩ ϩⲁⲛ ⲑⲓϫⲁⲣ ⲡⲉⲛⲧ ⲥⲉⲧⲉ ⲡⲉϩⲁⲕ ϩⲏⲧⲓ ⲗⲉⲥⲙⲏ ϩⲁⲩⲗⲏⲓ ⲏⲙⲓⲛ (ll. 1–6).

[290] ⲫⲏ ⲉⲧⲁϥⲙⲟⲩⲣ ⲧⲫⲉ ⲁ̣ϥⲙⲟⲩⲣ ⲡⲕⲁ̣ϩⲓ (ll. 7–8); †ⲥⲙⲏ ⲉⲧ̣ⲁⲩⲧⲏⲓⲥ̣ ⲥⲁⲡϣⲱⲓ ⲙ̀ⲡⲓϣⲉ (ll. 24–25).

[291] Richter 2003, 216.

[292] Legendre 2014, 340.

[293] E.g. *P.Ryl.Copt*. 106.

[294] E.g. *P.Stras.Copt*. 67.

[295] E.g. *P.Lond.Copt*. I 487, with Richter 2003, 214–223. Bagnall and Worp (2004, 99–100) do not directly treat Greek renderings of the Basmalla/Bismillah, but rather "invocation formulae" in Greek-language texts produced under Islamic governance that they considered to include examples clearly "influenced by the Bismillah".

[296] I.e. ⲉⲣⲣⲁϩⲙⲉⲛ and ⲉⲣⲣⲁϩⲓⲙ could instead be expected.

An important further consideration is that, unlike the previous example, which is preceded by the hundreds of manuscripts comprising the corpus of the CMP and among which this distinct later development can be contextualized, there is—essentially—no non-Christian, or at least no non-monotheistic, Coptic textual culture other than the magical texts treated here. Notwithstanding those few Old Coptic exceptions, the break between the textual culture of the early Roman Period, in demotic, hieratic, and hieroglyphs, and Coptic textual culture is all but absolute. As a result, an understandable assumption—nevertheless to be resisted—has come about among modern scholars that the motifs prominent in Christian texts of the 4th century CE and later are diagnostic of processes of Christianization in other, earlier texts. Indeed, the sparseness of sources for the late Roman Period permits no direct comparison. This study has, however, instead shown that indirect comparisons can be made, between Jewish and/or Judaeo-Christian motifs in Demotic and Old Coptic magical texts, which were embedded in contemporary and preceding pre- and/or non-Christian milieux, as well as that these indirect comparisons provide both a counterpoint to such assumptions and a note of caution when considering what constitutes diagnostically Christian in the late Roman Period. Christianity is not the only monotheistic tradition from which motifs regarding "God" could be drawn during the late Roman Period, and the use of the Basmala/Bismillāh in a non-confessional way, even in a monotheistic society, indicates that formulae stemming from certain cultural repertoires are not necessarily diagnostic of influence exerted by that repertoire on another, but rather of adoption from that repertoire into another.

While the Iao Sabaoth appearing in §10 is sufficiently pan-cultural and attested throughout the GEMP to not be considered diagnostically Christian, even the supplication to "lord god" in §9 which is ubiquitous in Christian Egypt can be called into question as evidence of Christianization in the 4th century CE. In Jewish tradition, the Greek version of the Hebrew bible contains renderings of the name of the supreme deity as κύριος "lord" (including in combination with Σαβαώθ in the *trishagion* of Isaiah 6:3), while in Egyptian tradition, Greek-language oracle tickets contain supplications to both κύριος and θεός "god",[297] relating closely to petitioning practices in which Roman officials can be referred to as both κύριος and θεός,[298] practices descending in turn from how the deified Pharaohs of the Ptolemaic Period were addressed. Of even greater significance is a letter of the 1st century BCE from the Fayum town of Tebtunis referring to the traditional Egyptian deity Seknebtunis directly as ὁ κύριος θεός "the lord god".[299] In the excursus to §9, the Egyptian conceptualization of the divine as a

[297] E.g. *SB* XVIII 13853 and 14043 (2nd century CE).
[298] E.g. *BGU* IV 1197 (7–4 BCE).
[299] *P.Tebt.* II 284.5–6.

unity of pluralities, in particular regarding the role of the superordinate deity—often Amun—as primordial creator, was discussed. This conceptualization of the divine in which one name or epithet would stand for that superordinate deity and the unity of pluralities that they represent not only persists but is even transferred into the pantheistic, henotheistic, or megatheistic trends of the Roman Period, in which one particular deity, e.g. Sarapis, Isis, or Helios, is revered as the superordinate deity, of which all others are either manifestations or derivatives. In such contexts, epithets connoting supremacy, such as κύριος as well as δεσπότης "master" and *nṯr-ꜥꜣ* "great god", are often found.[300]

In the excursus to §9, it will be demonstrated that P.Saqqara inv. F.17.10,[301] exhibiting a partial parallel to the mythological scene setting in §9, does not exhibit any diagnostic features of Christianization. While the divine names featured in the text could have been comfortably reinterpreted through a Christian lens, the fact that the text, dating perhaps to the second half of the 10th or 11th century CE, would have been just as much at home among the GEMP, i.e. in pre- and non-Christian milieux, demonstrates that arbitrary and etic formulations by modern scholars of what comprises a Christian(ized) text based exclusively on the temporal frame of their attestations are erroneous.[302] Furthermore, when a frame of interpretation that does not assume Christianization based on the presence of textual content that would also be at home in other religious traditions, whether Jewish or Graeco-Egyptian, is applied, this leads to a rather fascinating result: among the CMP there is a significant corpus of magical texts that were not overtly Christianized,[303] and are therefore highly suggestive of having been transmitted more or less unchanged from the late Roman to Islamic Period. Thus, the "textual authority" of such compositions becomes evident.[304]

While it is perfectly possible that Christian(ized) practitioners could have later (re)interpreted a prayer to Gabriel (§6), supplication to the "lord god" (§9), or reference to "Iao Sabaoth" (§10) through a Christian lens, this does not require their conceptualization as such in the context of the compilation of the Michigan codex. Indeed, although ancient Christian exegetes had an impressive capacity to read Christianity into Jewish and even Graeco-Roman texts where they wished to, this does not indicate whether the source texts of the Michigan codex were Christian(ized). It is crucial to bear in mind, especially given the sections on **The**

---

[300] Consider "Jesus, the great god", noted above.

[301] Re-edited here in the appendix.

[302] For example, van der Vliet (2018, 159–160) notes that "the original evocation of a snake-shaped healing power" is "at odds" with "names of the biblical God", and yet if the text had been Christianized—as van der Vliet maintains—, this apparent problem has rather been resolved by the very co-existence of these entities in a Christian(ized) text.

[303] Consider also the example of the third text from the c. 6th century CE P.Mil.Vogl. Copt. 16, discussed above, and the example of P.Donadoni, cited below.

[304] For this thesis, see Love 2020, §§5–6, developing Love 2016, §§7.6.3–7.7.

Compilation of Michigan Ms. 136 and **Linguistic and Orthographic Features**, that the texts of the Michigan codex were redacted from source texts. These source texts, then, were almost certainly in circulation during the 3rd century CE, a period in which Christians were in a decided minority. Even connecting the alleged Christian(zing) additions with the steady Christianization of Egypt during the 4th century CE fails to remove the objection that these supplications are not diagnostically Christian because—as demonstrated—they appear in pre- and non-Christian magical texts compiled by pre- and non-Christian practitioners. Christian(ized) magical texts in turn do not become dominant until the 5th century CE, while magical texts without diagnostically Christian content are attested still much later than that.[305]

One final consideration in the comparison of §§9 and 10 with the "Horus-Isis charms", in addition to how Christian(ized) they are, is how traditionally Egyptian they remain. The most recently published witness, a group of ostraca dating to the 7th or 8th century CE (O.BYU Mag.), was argued by its editors to be a composition that "draws extensively upon the earlier cosmology of Pharaonic Egypt".[306] Yet, they in fact concluded that the text at most "reflect[s] a memory of a particular late myth, now lost to us, of Horus finding his wife or wives in the underworld".[307] While the motifs of that composition are found elsewhere, and while Horus had a wife and wives in earlier traditions, nothing of any semantic substance has been retained—most likely because those earlier motifs had no resonance in the contemporary cultural repertoire of a Christian(ized) society. Nevertheless, the only superficial Christianization of this text is found in the closing supplication "by the power of Iao Sabaoth", which—especially when

[305] Consider in particular P.Donadoni, ed. Donadoni 1965–1966, one of the "Horus-Isis charms" which, despite being dated to the 7th century CE and therefore having been copied in a decidedly Christian(ized) Egypt, contains no diagnostically Christian features in the text whatsoever, the only such feature present at all being the chi-rho monogram (⳨) that precedes the text: "I went to the door of Hell, I found a beauty, white with black eyes sitting upon a well of stone, a wallet (?) beside her, drawing water with a bronze bucket, ... of iron. I said to her, "O beauty, give me a kiss!" She said to me … to the door of Hell. I ran away from her. I was in pain, I cried, I groaned. Isis said to me, "Why do you cry, why do you groan?" (I) said, "It is not my fault that I cry. I found a beautiful woman whom I wanted to kiss, but she did not return (?) my heart." She said to me, "Even if you did not find me, if you did not find my name, if you did not find the name of these three angels, Kirie, Kirie, prostrate (?) … you (pl.) shall bring NN daughter of NN to my feet, that I might be with her, that I might cast my desire at her, and she ... into her womb, to (?) the seventy nerves which surround it! Quickly, quickly!" (Collaborative translation from a re-edition of the text from a photograph of the original by Korshi Dosoo, Markéta Preininger Svobodová, and Edward O. D. Love for the *Kyprianos* database). Of course, angels could subsequently be (re)interpreted through a Christian lens, but they also appear throughout the GEMP, having already entered the magical tradition before Christianity even came into existence.

[306] Blumell and Dosoo 2018, 202.

[307] Blumell and Dosoo 2018, 255.

taken alongside the *voces magicae* which precede that text's divine drama—could be as much at home among the GEMP as the CMP.[308]

Likewise, the aforementioned "Horus-Isis charm" of P.Schmidt 1 (ed. Kropp, *AKZ* I, text A) retains, other than the obvious theonyms, only one toponym ϩⲁⲃⲓⲛ, the temple of which Isis is said to be within, which might be derived from *Ḫbn.w* (Hebenu), and yet the divine drama itself is otherwise based around the apocryphal Judaeo-Christian motif of Abimelech. The "Horus-Isis charm" of P.Schmidt 2 (ed. Kropp, *AKZ* I, text B), by comparison, retains nothing traditionally Egyptian in terms of semantic content, but also exhibits no Christianization. Comparable to P.Schmidt 1 is the aforementioned "Horus-Isis charm" of P.Berl. inv. 8313, which exhibits Christian motifs with the possible exception of the toponym ⲟⲛ "Heliopolis", but this actually had contemporary cultural relevance because it appears in the Bible (e.g. ⲱⲛ in Ge 41:45). While the "Horus-Isis charm" of P.Berl. inv. 5565 (ed. *BKU* I 22) may preserve a reference to the "Primaeval Ocean" (*nwn*), this term could just as easily render the "Abyss" of Judaeo-Christian cosmogony and eschatology, given the presence of other Gnostic and Judaeo-Christian features. It is also notable that the "Horus-Isis charms" are, with the exception of that in P.Berl. inv. 8313, principally applied for erotic aims, whereas §§9 and 10 concern healing, like their predecessors in earlier Egyptian.

Indeed, in surveying and summarizing the motifs common to the divine dramas of the Egyptian magical texts that they term "Horus-Isis charms", Blumell and Dosoo demonstrate the extraordinary contraction of a complex and productive tradition into a stripped-back and reductive one.[309] These authors also stress that the decline of the temples and therefore, within the framework of this study, the dissolution of the priestly *communities of practice* and their *written language* and *script communities*, "led to the almost total disappearance of explicitly 'Egyptian' or even 'Graeco-Egyptian' material culture from the fourth century onwards".[310] Where characters are subsequently added to divine dramas, these are drawn from the Christian cultural repertoire.[311] The significance, let alone identity, ascribed to the theonyms "Isis" and "Horus" during this period is,

[308] In the temporal context in which the text was inscribed, however, the editors take this as "an attempt to integrate a non-Christian charm into a Christian framework" (Blumell and Dosoo 2018, 238).

[309] Blumell and Dosoo 2018, 241–244. Their analogy is that "the Coptic charms represent the last surviving branch of a tree that was once much larger" (2018, 243), but an analogy to the desiccated root of a dead stump might be more appropriate.

[310] Blumell and Dosoo 2018, 245.

[311] Blumell and Dosoo 2018, 250.

then, incredibly hard to discern.[312] Of note, finally, is that among the nine episodes in the typology of the divine dramas constructed by Blumell and Dosoo from their comprehensive study of the "Horus-Isis charms", the divine dramas of §9 and *PGM* IV.94–113 accord with only one. Therefore, alongside the significantly different textual *content* in §§9–10 and *PGM* IV.94–113 compared with the "Horus-Isis charms", the textual *structure* also differs significantly.

The studies of Clarysse and Depauw (2013; 2015), which built upon Bagnall's formative (1982) and refined (1987) study, of onomastics to trace Christianization in Egypt have analyzed compelling evidence to suggest that Christians were a "sizeable minority of 20 to 30% when Constantine converted in 313", and "when Theodosios proclaimed Christianity as the official state religion in 380, probably already more than two-thirds of the new born came from Christian families. Around 450, to take the council of Chalkedon as a symbolic date, probably not many pagans were left in Egypt."[313] This perhaps surprisingly rapid Christianization during the 4th century CE is crucial for understanding the changing cultural context in which the Michigan codex was produced. Nevertheless, by that same evidence Egypt was not comprehensively Christian(ized) until the second half of the 5th century.[314] Consequently, the considerations laid out above as well as the case studies of motifs that could be read through a Christian(izing) lens evidently appearing in pre- and non-Christian magical texts—among others—, suggest that the copyists of the Michigan codex need not have been Christian, and still less the redactors of the source texts. Even if the Michigan codex was produced during the second half of the 4th century CE, a significant proportion of the population were still not Christian. Indeed, the growing number of Christians may present one reason for the utilization—appropriation—of motifs from a Judaeo-Christian cultural repertoire in §§9 and 10. It does not, however, have to be taken as an index for the Christian(ized) identity of the copyists and practitioners of the Michigan codex.

This point, then, brings the discussion back to the central consideration of "Syncretism in the Other Direction". That is to say, a syncretism that has been overlooked in favor of a model of cultural replacement of indigenous Egyptian by imported Christian tradition. This imbalance manifests in the study of ancient magic principally as a lack of consideration as to whether the same borrowing

---

[312] For modern scholars interested in such phenomena, of which the present author is one, it is all too easy to reify the phenomenon under investigation and project significance from the contemporary into the past context.

[313] Clarysse and Depauw 2013, 434.

[314] By naming his study "Isis in Christian Egypt", Dosoo (2021) rather presupposes that this was also the case a century earlier, an assumption which is seen in his reading of these aforementioned motifs as diagnostic of an at least nominally Christian practitioner who Christianized certain texts when compiling them into the codex.

could instead demonstrate that the cultural repertoire of the GEMP was the principal tradition—at home in, emic to Egypt—, into which etic motifs—imported into, foreign to, Egypt—were borrowed, without fundamentally changing or undermining the Graeco-Egyptian magical tradition. As proposed throughout this section, then, an important counterpoint to the assumptions made and conclusions reached by prior commentators about the alleged Christianization of §§9 and 10 is that the Graeco-Egyptian magical tradition, to which the texts of the Michigan codex belong, is fundamentally a syncretic one. Although aspects of the Graeco-Egyptian cultural repertoire were syncretized into Christianity, and magical texts were undoubtedly Christianized, or (re)interpreted through a Christian lens, there was a time during the late Roman Period in which Jewish and Judaeo-Christian motifs were syncretized into the Graeco-Egyptian cultural repertoire. Given, then, the temporal frame in which the Michigan codex was produced, and the preceding generation(s) in which its source texts were undoubtedly in circulation, the most parsimonious contextualization of the Michigan codex is not among the Christian(ized) CMP, but the pan-cultural GEMP of the early to late Roman Period.

Context in the Practice of Medicine and Healing (MZR)

The medicinal portions of the Michigan codex may be divided roughly between the properly pharmacological, in which simple or compound drugs and preparations are prescribed on their own, and healing methods that include ritual means, such as incantations, textual amulets, and strictures for the gathering and application of substances. This healing ritual category, iatromagical by a recently proposed categorization, is abundantly attested in contemporary and later Greek texts and continues to some extent in Coptic, though a systematic collection and study remains to be made.[315] Pharmacological medical texts, the majority being simple recipes or collections thereof, make up only a small fraction of surviving Coptic manuscripts, outnumbered even by magical texts. The situation is roughly comparable for Greek medical papyri, which have on the whole been better served by editions and studies.[316] The available Coptic witnesses were studied in detail by Walter C. Till in his monograph of 1951, already mentioned, in which the Michigan codex claimed a place. Till laid the foundations of an inventory of the medical ingredients and pathologies referenced by the surviving textual witnesses, a corpus usefully surveyed and supplemented recently by Tonio Sebastian Richter, who has also published three important, additional witnesses that allow such texts to be traced back as early as the third or fourth century CE.[317]

Before the contribution of the Michigan codex to the history of Coptic medicine can be assessed, the character of its witness should be briefly surveyed. The codex in full addresses 21 distinct pathologies (see also the section **Outline**

---

[315] Greek: for the definition and a checklist of texts, see De Haro Sanchez 2004 and 2012; add now *P.Oxy.* LXXX 5245 with the introduction; P.Mich. inv. 4451a, ed. Zellmann-Rohrer 2015b, 177–183; P.Harr. inv. 303a front, ed. Zellmann-Rohrer 2016; and P.Utrecht Copt. Ms. B3.8, ed. van den Broek 2017. Coptic: beyond finished products (amulets) and isolated recipes, some more substantial collections are, e.g., *P.Borg.Copt.* 278 and *P.Ryl.Copt.* 104; of particular interest as a witness to continued bilingualism in this genre is *SB Kopt.* I 1, a fragment of a parchment codex combining medical recipes with the Greek version of Psalm 150.

[316] See recently *P.Oxy.* LXXX for a representative selection of texts from the city of Oxyrhynchus, with introductory discussions and references to further literature, and the two volumes of *GMP* already published (a third is forthcoming) and the companion volume of studies, Reggiani (ed.) 2019.

[317] For checklists of texts, see Till 1951a, 110–112; Richter 2014, 189–191. Add now a codex fragment dated to the 9th or 10th century from the Monastery of St. Anthony on the Red Sea (cat. no. 137 [98:Ms4]), ed. H. Lundhaug ap. Blid et al. 2016, 191–193.

of Contents and Phases), in no readily perceptible order beyond the occasional pairing of recipes for the same indication. The field of gynecology covers five of the recipes, more specifically for uterine disorders (§§3, 16–17) and problems with fertility and birth (§§9–10), a unique concentration among surviving medical or iatromagical comparanda, and dysuria in either sex and possibly a disorder of the male testicles are the subjects of one each (§§14, 22). The broad category of internal medicine is the best represented, by recipes against head- and stomach-ache (§13), splenitis (§4), constipation (§27), sciatica (§31), sores "in the posterior" perhaps to be identified more specifically as hemorrhoids or anal fissures (§24), and a general-purpose pediatric remedy targeting discomfort resulting in crying (§28), to which are closely allied others against earache (§26), teething and toothache (§§7, 25), rheum in the eyes (§23), and gout (§2, and possibly §1). Swellings and skin conditions receive three recipes (§§8, 20–21), and excessive or abnormal eyelash growth one (§5). External trauma in the form of wounds is addressed, possibly, only once (§30, a poultice or dressing), while the bleeding targeted in §11 is described in the most general terms. Fever and mental illness, the latter conceived in turn as the result of demonic possession, round out the collection (§§6, 18).

The choice between the two categories, pharmacological and ritual or iatromagical, which are somewhat porous in themselves, is strongly correlated to the phase of copying, with the later phases preferring the former category. The compilers may have been motivated purely by opportunity and the availability of existing recipes for copying. The same indication, the treatment of uterine disorders, may be sought by recipes of both kinds (§§3, 16–17). Further nuance may still emerge from a closer analysis of the two groups. The properly pharmacological methods (§§4, 7–8, 16–17, 20–28, 30; similarly, the pest-control methods §§19 and 29) are restricted to the application, be it topical or oral, of various medicinal substances, both organic and inorganic, and compounds thereof. A preference for such procedures in the case of the more specific, and readily apparent and outwardly perceptible pathologies might be identified.

The ritual or iatromagical methods are fewer but more diverse, centered on the power attributed to words, whether uttered aloud or inscribed as textual amulets, and ritual actions analogizing the desired resolution of the healing scenario. Those purely verbal are textual amulets on silver and tin against gout and head- and stomach-aches (§§2, 13), on a calcareous "stone" from the human womb against mental illness arising from demonic possession (§18), and invocations of divine powers or direct incantatory addresses to aid fertility and birth (§§9–10) and to staunch bleeding (§11). Incantation and invocation are combined with ritual action, for example, the tying of knots in a cure for fever (§6). There may be some, but only slight correlation between less specific and visible, more internal and amorphous conditions—such as general-purpose remedies for bleeding, and mental illness—and prescription of methods of this type. Cases in which an incantation or amulet is combined with the administration of medicinal substances, against gout (§1?) and uterine disorders (§3), or a medicinal potion is accompanied by a healing ritual or related observances, against excessive hair growth (§5: the application is timed with the waning moon), dysuria (§14: the patient is to wallow in a horse-wallow), and sciatica (§31: strictures for gathering of medicinal substances, use of right or left hand, avoidance of speech), are further indications of the permeability of the two categories.

With the newly proposed dating—fourth century for the majority, and no later than the fifth for the final portion (§§30–31)—the medical portions of the Michigan codex take their place among the earliest surviving Coptic medical recipes. Based on the 2014 survey of Richter, where they were placed in the fifth or sixth century or later, the Michigan recipes are the earliest attested on parchment, and of the 38 texts listed in total, only three among the papyri could be earlier: from the third or fourth century, the small fragment P.Heid. inv. G 698c (ed. Richter 2014, 164–165 no. 2; and no. 9 in Richter's checklist), and from the fourth or fifth, P.Berl. inv. 22164 (ed. *BKU* III 396; no. 8 in Richter's checklist) and P.TT 157-470, the only other document with secure provenance (Thebes) (ed. Richter 2014, 156–164 no. 1; and no. 1 in Richter's checklist), the latter two somewhat more substantial but attesting no more than nine recipes between them.

As Richter has noted for other early witnesses, in particular P.TT 157-470, this stage of Coptic medicine is marked by heavy dependence on Greek. Richter's Theban papyrus shows both the wholesale translation of Graeco-Roman recipes into Coptic and the further reliance on the Greek language for technical terms in the form of loanwords. Both are also illustrated by the Michigan codex. Examples of more or less direct translation are §§5, 22, 25, and 29–31, the dynamics of which are discussed in the commentary. Loanwords are also frequent, with two instances of direct transliteration from a Greek oblique case as would have been found in the exemplar, rather than the lexical form usually used in loanwords (pp. 11/11 ⲥⲁⲧ[ⲏ]\`ⲩ´ⲣⲁⲕⲏⲥ, Greek σανδαράκης and 13/15 ⲡⲥⲓⲙⲓⲑⲓⲟⲩ, Greek ψιμυθίου; and partially at p. 12/5–6, ⲗⲓⲃⲁⲛⲟⲥ ⲛ̄ⲝⲉⲛⲓⲕⲟⲛ, Greek λίβανον ξενικόν), on record also in Richter's Theban papyrus (e.g. ⲯⲓⲙⲓⲑⲓⲟⲩ at 1/5 and 1/11). For metrology the Coptic texts are particularly dependent on Greek, of which the system in the Michigan codex is an unusually complex reflection. Six Graeco-Roman terms are in use—the stater (pp. 12/2 and 13/15), the pint (sextarius, p. 13/12, 13), the litra (pound or liter, p. 13/14), the ounce (p. 14/2–4), and the gram (p. 14/5)—alongside the generic ϣⲓ "measure" (p. 9/2–5), ⲁⲡⲟⲧ and ⲟⲧ̄ⲍ̄ "cup" (pp. 9/8, 14/4), and ϭⲟⲡⲉ "vessel" (pp. 10/17, 12/18–19), and the obscure ⲁⲙⲟⲅ ("mouthful"? see p. 9/13 with the commentary). The Theban papyrus for its part uses only the drachm.

The debt to the Graeco-Roman tradition illustrated by the Michigan codex overall, which contrasts with the traditional Egyptian background of the motifs of §§9–10, consists not only in the recipes found in learned authors such as Galen but also in more popular traditions (see especially §§5, 14, 23, 31). These are best reflected in the roughly contemporary Latin collection, drawing heavily on Greek sources, of the so-called Marcellus Empiricus. This Marcellus is probably to be identified with the Marcellus attached to the court of Theodosius I and serving as *magister officiorum* circa 394–395, possibly a native of Gaul and if not a practicing physician, certainly a well-read layman with a keen interest in the subject.[318] He is responsible for a collection of medical recipes and healing advice, organized roughly from head to foot, compiled after 408, in part from literary sources, but also including practices observed by the author in contemporary use. The epistolary prologue openly acknowledges collection of proven remedies from rural and popular sources, that is, healers operating outside of the elite, learned tradition of Galenic medicine. The collection of Marcellus, which like the Michigan codex may be termed iatromagical, shows a comparable interest in gathering pre-Christian healing lore, adapting and augmenting it, and allowing it to continue in a form attractive or at least unoffensive to Christian practitioners. Three further, anonymous Latin collections, adduced at points here in the commentary, continue this tradition into the early medieval period.[319]

On the Greek side a comparison can be drawn with the *Kyranides*, a compendium on the occult natural properties of animal, vegetable and mineral products with late ancient roots and a wide circulation in Byzantium.[320] Advice in the Michigan codex on the occult properties of the green lizard has close parallels in this corpus (2.14: see §23 with the commentary), and more broadly the arrangement of indications for body parts of the bull follows a similar style (§§26–28 with the commentary). These parallels constitute new evidence for the tradition of the *Kyranides* in Coptic; an antecedent in a Greek collection of prescriptions for the use of the dung of various animals has recently come to light, copied on the back of a magical formulary on a papyrus from Roman Oxyrhynchus (*P.Oxy.* LXXXII 5315). A later Coptic witness from the Islamic period can also be iden-

---

[318] On Marcellus and his career, see Ewers 2009. Among his sources Marcellus mentions the Jewish patriarch of Constantinople, Gamaliel, as author of a remedy for splenitis (*De medicamentis* 23.77, ed. Niedermann 1916), which, in addition to illustrating the range of his contacts, also provides a chronological datum: Gamaliel is attested in office in 415 (see most recently Matthews 2010, 339–340).

[319] Found in a sixth-century manuscript, Leiden, Universiteitsbibliotheek cod. VLQ 9, ed. Piechotta 1887; the ninth-century Glasgow, University Library Ms. Hunter 96 (T.4.13), ff. 137r–177r, ed. Sigerist 1923, 99–160; and in some interpolations in the *Euporiston* of Theodore Priscianus, ed. Rose 1894.

[320] Edited by Kaimakis 1976; see recently Bain 2006. A version may already have been known in the time of Lucian: see the commentary to 2/11–12 below.

tified in the paper codex fragment P.Berl. inv. 8116+8117 (ed. *BKU* I 26), with sequences of prescriptions for amuletic and healing purposes involving parts of the hoopoe (P.Berl. 8116a, 12–29), the cockerel (P.Berl. 8117, 5–19), the bat (ibid., 20–22), and another bird whose name is lost (P.Berl. 8116b, 20–40). The presence of Arabic loanwords alongside Greek might suggest a translation from the former language rather than a continuous local tradition.

Comparable patterns of borrowing can also be found in the advice for household management. The prescription for ridding a home of pests in §19 in particular bears a close relation to recipes for pest control in a Byzantine agricultural encyclopedia, the *Geoponica* (13.9.3), which in turn depends on late ancient sources.[321] A Greek papyrological witness to the same tradition from Byzantine Egypt has been identified, and Syriac translation of one of its late ancient predecessors is known, in fact from a codex brought to the Syrian monastery in the Egyptian Wadi el-Natrun in the medieval period,[322] but the Michigan codex offers new evidence for a Coptic phase of its tradition. Such home-economic compendia are otherwise not much in evidence in Coptic, but the survival of two almanacs,[323] combining methods for meteorological prognostication and crop forecasts with miscellaneous ritual healing advice, may be noted. A fragmentary ninth-century papyrus pairs a treatise on agriculturally-focused divination based on the weekday on which the first of the month falls (calendologium), on the front, with instructions, on the back, for a ritual to overcome insomnia by inscribing an incantation.[324] The more extensive remains of a parchment codex of the ninth or tenth century combine prognoses on harvests, based on thunder, earthquakes, and calendar-divination, and a table of recommendations for auspicious times for the management of agricultural estates based on the course of the moon, with instructions for a ritual to gain a revelation on crop forecasts, featuring a prayer (ⲡⲣⲟⲥⲉⲩⲭⲏ) that opens with two verses from the Psalms (90:2–3).[325] A colophon identifies the copyist, the deacon Chaēl, as the son of a priest Geōrge.

As Richter concludes for medical texts, based also on the replacement of Greek technical terms with Arabic ones in later witnesses, there was little contribution of contemporary Coptic-language medical scholarship or theory, and little solid evidence of continuity from ancient Egyptian medical traditions. Alongside the obvious borrowings, however, signs of what may best be considered local

---

[321] See Guignard 2009.

[322] Greek: P.Vind. inv. G 40302, ed. Papathomas 2000 (cf. *Geoponica* 17.8, 22). Syriac: London, British Library Add. Ms. 14662, ed. Lagarde 1860, with Guignard 2014.

[323] On the almanacs, see in general Wilfong 1999, 224–234.

[324] *SB Kopt.* I 4; see further the commentary of ed.pr., Till 1943, 329–334.

[325] P.Vind. inv. K 1112+4858+9885–9899, ed. Till 1936; cf. Till 1943, 328–332; on the calendologium, see also Browne 1979, 45–63.

color, or adaptations to maximize utility and appeal in the context of use, may be noted: the feathers of the once sacred ibis are pressed into service as ointment applicators (§§20–21), and fresh palm leaves have crept into a recipe otherwise probably derived from a northern Mediterranean context (§31; cf. also §30).

What can be said of the context of use of the Michigan codex and the identity of its users? It would be tempting, in view of the combined emphasis in recent scholarship on monks and monasteries as repositories and practitioners of both medical and magical knowledge in the Coptic tradition,[326] to look to such a context. While the surviving iatromagical texts more often than not lack a secure provenance, the parchment codex fragment *P.Med.Bouriant*, which will have belonged to a manuscript of no fewer than 215 pages, is known to come from the White Monastery (Sohag), and the iatromagical *P.Borg.Copt.* 278, fragments from a parchment codex of similar format and at least an original 244 pages, has a good chance of belonging to a similar context, perhaps even the same original manuscript.[327] In a study of the Theban area of the seventh and eighth centuries, Richter has focused on monasteries as centers for the production of medical books and on monks as providers of medical care, and most recently, Frankfurter has inscribed some of the recipes of the Michigan codex within "monastic scribal culture."[328]

This situation, however, need not have pertained in the earlier, fourth-century context of the production of the Michigan codex or its later re-use. After the removal of ⲫ̄ϯ̄ (p. 3/10), wrongly read by ed.pr., there remain no unambiguous marks of Christian context. Some chi-rho symbols among the magical signs on p. 2 and a rho-headed cross in the stele-amulet for demoniacs on p. 11 can both be explained through other derivations (see the commentary), while invocations with a Jewish background can more positively be identified, of the angels Gabriel and Michael (pp. 4, 7), of a supreme "lord god" and Ia(ō) Sabaōth (p. 7), but without requiring a religious affiliation, as such elements had been circulating in Egypt for centuries by this time. Several pre-Christian divinities, in turn, including Isis, Amun, Thoth, and Damnameneus, are plainly referenced.

Beyond the practical objection that the attention to pediatrics (§7) and fertility and birthing (§§9–10) would have been of little use to a monastic community unless it accepted outside patients, to say nothing of the recipes for ridding apparently private houses of pests (§§19, 29), contemporary data suggest a more diverse world of healing practice. It was in the later part of this same century that the distinctive late ancient institution of the private hospital (ξεν(ε)ών) came onto the scene in Egypt: independent of state and ecclesiastical impetus, these centers of treatment were established by the private initiative of wealthy donors.

[326] For a cautionary example, however, see Zellmann-Rohrer 2020e.
[327] So Richter 2014, 191, under no. 27.
[328] Richter 2017, with mention of the Michigan codex at 155; Frankfurter 2017, 208.

In turn private, professional physicians worked in the hospitals and even came to establish and own hospitals in their own right. A document of prime importance is the will of one such physician, the ἀρχιατρός Flavius Phoebammon drafted in 570 CE: Phoebammon took after his father Euprepius both in professional title and ownership of a hospital in the Middle Egyptian city of Antinoupolis, and while he frames its administration as a pious act, and dispenses charity to monastic institutions among his other bequests, he takes care to keep the hospital in the family by bequeathing it to his brother.[329] We also know of lay medical personnel entrusted with state functions in Roman Egypt, the performance of forensic examinations in juridical contexts by individuals sometimes titled "public doctor" (δημόσιος ἰατρός).[330]

Beyond the *archiatroi*, who could draw public salaries and enjoy other privileges as civic officials in towns and cities already in the Roman period,[331] the provision of iatromagical services offered a profitable sideline for literate people to monetize their skills by putting written formulary recipes into practice for a broader clientele. A notebook in the form of a papyrus codex owned by a minor official responsible for tax collection in the Middle Egyptian city of Hermopolis Magna in the second half of the fourth century, one Aurelius Philammon,[332] bears witness to this practice. After purchasing a premade, blank codex, Philammon progressively filled up the pages with documents from his public and private dealings, as well as ritual recipes. The latter include healing and broader personal advancement, in the form of requests for favor (*charitesion*, p. 23) comparable to one found in the Michigan codex (§12 with the excursus), and divinatory vision (εἰς ὀπτ̣[ασί]α̣ν), victory (νικητικόν), the "muzzling" of enemies and restraint of anger, and erotic attraction (φίλτρον, p. 9).

The accounts entered in the codex also show that Philammon did business with a physician (ἰατρός), and it is possible that the healing incantations at least were intended for use in the same context.[333] That the healing in particular had paying clients in view is suggested by a gathering of medical applications of Homeric verses, inscribed as amulets or uttered out loud (pp. 22–23), paralleled in general in the Michigan codex (§6 with the excursus). Portions of at least

---

[329] *P.Cair.Masp.* II 67151 with van Minnen 1995. For the development of monastic hospitals as a parallel system, wholly replacing the civic antecedents, see Crislip 2005.

[330] See in general Amundsen and Ferngren 1978, and for the resulting reports in the papyrological record, recently *P.Oxy.* LXXX 5254–5257 and Reggiani 2018.

[331] On the office, Nutton 1977; for its later Egyptian instantiations, *CPR* XXV 1.1 n. and *P.Oxy.* LXXXIII 5392.4 n.

[332] P.Berl. inv. 9873, (ed. *P.Philammon*; some excerpts also in *PGM* P XXIIa); on the juristic texts included in the codex see recently Kanavou 2020.

[333] Three payments in cash to the physician Theodosios are recorded at p. 25.8–10, of which the amounts are unclear (one is at least 15,000 drachmas); this same man is also paid in rations (eight pounds of meat, p. 28.18).

eight recipes of this kind survive; where indications can be determined, they cover headache, fever, hemorrhage, pain in the breasts and uterus, and contraception, and the recipe addressing hemorrhage provides for the case of non-payment, allowing the affliction to be re-inflicted on an ungrateful patient by further manipulation of the medicinal substance used in the healing.

The later witness of *P.Med.Chassinat*, a long papyrus roll from the ninth century in which the ingredients are partly concealed by cryptography, belongs very much to private practice, purporting to be written by a physician, himself the son of a physician, for the benefit of his son who would succeed him in the profession. The intersection of bureaucracy and magical healing continued in this later period too, when a recently-published Coptic business letter from the Fayum shows Christians seeking healing not from monasteries but, in this case, from an anonymous copyist in the service of the Muslim Caliph Al-Walīd, said to have cured no fewer than 100 sick men and women by writing "book-rolls" (ϫωⲙⲉ) for them.[334] This wider medical world contemporary with and succeeding the Michigan codex suggests that the evidentiary bias in favor of monastic contexts for Coptic technical literature should be approached with caution.

Before concluding this discussion of medical context, one further piece of evidence for transmission of ritual texts more broadly considered in non-institutional contexts may be adduced. This unique document, a private letter from a Manichaean context in fourth-century Kellis (P.Kell.Copt. 35),[335] concerns aggressive as opposed to the healing magic at the center of the Michigan manuscript. It nevertheless attests the same interest and capacity of bilingual, and to all appearances private individuals—as opposed to priests and monks—to collect and transmit magical texts. The sender, a man with the Roman name Ouales (Valens), writes in effect a Coptic cover-letter to his correspondent Psai in Kellis for a copy of a formulary for a bilingual Greek-Coptic incantation to cause the separation of two other individuals. After the copy a personal message is appended that suggests that Psai had requested and Ouales actively sought out a particular source-text, for which he substituted the best alternative to hand, probably from his own papers, after failing to find it.

Nowhere in this correspondence are third-party experts mentioned, priestly or otherwise, such that the exchange is best contextualized in the collecting activity of curious individuals who may also, like Aurelius Philammon, have intended to put the material to use for their own benefit or that of paying clients. Bilingualism among personnel involved in tax collection, the same class of literate but non-priestly individuals, mediating between Egyptian-speaking taxpayers and Greek-language administration, are on record more broadly in documentary

334 P.Vind. inv. K 55, ed. Garel 2016.

335 Ed. *P.Kell.Copt.* V 35; see recently Love 2016, 273–276; Zellmann-Rohrer 2020b, 177; Love fc. c.

papyri. One such text is a tax-register from the Hermopolite nome of the mid-6th century CE (*P.Lond.Herm.*). The records are primarily Greek, but there are occasional hints of a Coptophone background. One entry, for example, concerns a man with a Greek version of an originally Roman name, further identified by a Coptic professional title: Τατιανοῦ ⲙⲁⲧⲟⲓ̈ "from Tatianus, soldier" (f. 3r/17).[336]

[336] See in general Bagnall 2017, esp. 22–23.

The Compilation of Michigan Ms. 136 (EL)

Following the considerations of the previous sections, a brief sketch of the history of compilation and use of Michigan Ms. 136 can be provided. The treatment of the palaeographic, linguistic, and orthographic features suggests that three hands copied the extant contents of the manuscript into the pre-made codex over the course of an unknown number of years. While the palaeography of all three of these hands suggests near contemporary activity, and no more than a century of chronological distance, this century encompasses approximately four generations, and it cannot be established when in that century the five phases of compilation were undertaken by the three different copyists. As established in the preceding section, all three of these copyists were interested in treatments for the healing of patients; both those conventionally termed pharmacological, in which simple or compound drugs and preparations are prescribed on their own, and those conventionally termed ritual, in which the recitation of incantations and the production of textual and figural amulets were prescribed. Although entirely conjectural, it is conceivable that the codex was handed down over generations, and thus a compilation of the content of the codex as now extant occurred over three generations, but it is also conceivable that it was passed between colleagues over a shorter time. A relatively safe assumption is that all three copyists were bilingual, with the copyist of Hand 1 inscribing the only Greek-language texts in the codex, and the copyists of Hand 2 and 3 presumably also making use of these Greek-language texts, although only adding Coptic-language texts to the codex themselves. The analysis of the textual content of the codex suggests that a core bilingual compilation of texts, directly comparable to the multilingual Roman-period ritual handbooks but more medicinal in scope, was copied by Hand 1 and progressively supplemented with Coptic-language recipes by Hands 2 and 3. None of the text has been removed or replaced, suggesting that the entire contents of the codex were valued by these genealogically or socially related users—physicians—over its use life. From such a master copy, or "formulary", the owners of the codex would have been able to copy and send the recipes in the codex when practicing them on clients or sharing them with colleagues.[337] Finally, given the robustness of the codex itself, it should be borne in mind that the fourth century palaeographic dating is only a terminus post quem

[337] For a treatment of selected historical primary sources for the sharing of magical texts among practitioners in 3rd and 4th century CE Egypt, see Love 2016, §7.6.

for copies made from it, and does not rule out that the codex was in circulation for generations beyond the lifespan of its three copyists.

Although the assumption that the textual content of the codex is an incomplete translation from Greek-language source texts, as stated by ed.pr. and maintained by subsequent commentators,[338] cannot be maintained, it is possible to propose a delineation of the five phases of compilation into hypothetical source texts from which the codex was compiled, some of which were Greek. Phase 1 comprises the only properly bilingual phase of compilation, but it can itself be delineated into at three phases of prior compilation. That is not to say, however, that the copyist of Hand 1 copied these three source texts as Phase 1. Phase 1 could have been copied from a source text with exactly the same layout, and this hypothetical compilation could have occurred much earlier in Phase 1's hypothetical history of textual transmission.

Block A of Phase 1 comprises §§1–8, the entirety of pages 2, 3, and 4, and also the lost preceding page 1, which are internally coherent in their textual content. No space is left between these sections, unlike between the end of §8 and §9, which suggests that they were copied as a continuous whole, divided by paragraphoi. As treated in the section on linguistic and orthographic features, above, there are no significant inconsistencies within the Sahidic of §§1–8, with §4 and §8 exhibiting phonetic features which are suggestive of southern dialects, although the magical words (*voces magicae*) of Egyptian etymology in §3 instead are suggestive of northern vocalizations (see the commentary). Evidently, at some point in the history of textual transmission these texts were brought together from difference source manuscripts—and perhaps even from different parts of Egypt. Conceivably all of the Coptic recipes were translated from Greek at some point in this history of textual transmission,[339] but their current form instead suggests that they were already established in a source manuscript before being copied into the codex as Block A of Phase 1. Further delineations within Block A appear possible between: (i) §§1–2, two recipes for the production of textual amulets against gout, the former in Coptic, the latter in Greek; (ii) §3, Greek-language invocation of Isis against uterine disorder with magical words derived from Egyptian; (iii) §§4–5, two medical recipes, the first bilingual, the second in Coptic; (iv) §6 a Greek-language incantation and prayer to Gabriel; (v) §§7–8, two Coptic-language medical recipes. When and where these are to be located in their hypothetical history of textual transmission is, however, a matter of conjecture.

---

[338] "The original was, in part at least, Greek; and some of the text has been taken over, untranslated" (Worrell 1935, 17); "At least a portion of the document has been translated from Greek, and some of the present text ... has been left, untranslated, in Greek" (Meyer in *ACM* p. 83).

[339] §5 is certainly a more or less direct translation from Greek: see the commentary.

Block B of Phase 1 comprises §§9–10, pages 5, 6, and the beginning of page 7. These texts, titled here "The Voice of Amun" and "The Cow of Amun", respectively, are also internally coherent in their textual content, concerning fertility, childbirth, and lactation, but exhibit linguistic and orthographic features suggestive of a distinct history of textual transmission.[340] While both were written in Sahidic, several linguistic and orthographic features discussed above suggest that §9 originated in a source text that expressed Mesokemic tendencies,[341] as well as a few orthographies and orthographic conventions ascribable to southern dialects.[342] By comparison, §10 exhibits none of those Mesokemic tendencies, and only a few orthographic conventions consistent with southern dialects[343] alongside a few suggestive of Fayumic.[344] The discontinuities of the orthographies between §§9–10, and between these sections and the others copied in Hand 1, suggest that these orthographic conventions have been carried over from their source texts, with the discontinuities between the two further suggesting that they were once separate source texts, i.e. (i) and (ii), compiled together as Block B of Phase 2. For a discussion of the hypothetical prehistory of the textual transmission of §§9–10, see the discussion of **Transmitting Textual Traditions**, above.

Block C of Phase 1 comprises §§11–13, copied directly below §10, filling the remainder of page 7 and most of page 8—leaving a small space empty at the bottom of that page that was never filled with text. This is again a bilingual block, containing two Greek-language texts for healing (§11 and §13), but the first comprises simply an invocation whereas the second requires the production of a textual amulet. Between them was copied a Coptic-language invocation for favor (§12), which features numerous loanwords from Greek, is indeed titled in Greek, and therefore was most likely also translated from Greek at some point in its textual history. Furthermore, given that §§11–13 present more miscellaneous prescriptions and purposes than those of Block A (§§1–8), they were perhaps directly copied from separate source manuscripts, i.e. (i), (ii), and (iii), into the codex as Block C of Phase 3, instead of being precompiled in a source manuscript.

---

[340] Simple orthographic distinctions include ⲡⲉϊ- (p. 5/3; 5/4) and ⲡⲁϊ- (p. 5/6) in §9 but ⲡⲓ- (p. 6/10) and ⲡⲁϊ- (p. 7/7) in §10.

[341] In particular, (ⲟ)ⲟⲩ, ⲱ for ⲟⲟ, ⲱ for ⲱⲱ, ⲟ for ⲱ, and ⲟ for ⲟⲟ.

[342] In particular, ϩⲟϊⲙⲉ and ⲧⲙⲁⲥϊⲟ alongside the adjustment of southern ⲉ- to S ⲁ-.

[343] E.g. free variation between ϭ and ⲕ in ⲧⲏϭ+ (p. 6/18) and ⲧⲏⲕ+ (p. 7/1) and S ⲙⲉ⸗ (p. 6/13; 6/14) alongside A ⲙⲁ⸗ (p. 6/15).

[344] In particular, compare F ⲕⲉⲙ (p. 6/18) in contrast to S ⲕⲁⲙ (p. 7/2) and the penchant for ⲃ over ϥ in certain orthographies.

Bookrolls and codices as compilations of pharmacological and especially of magical texts are the exception in the historical record rather than the rule.[345] Loose-leaf compendia of manuscripts that were collected or copied from source manuscripts acquired, or borrowed, by the individual copyist would have been the most affordable and flexible way to go about compiling like texts.[346] Thus, it seems the most parsimonious assumption that the copyist of Hand 1 had already compiled a collection of source manuscripts, upon which were inscribed the first 13 separate texts that he wished to copy, or have copied, into one "master copy" handbook. The proposal of at least three blocks comprising Phase 1, here, thereby highlights that several source manuscripts, already collected and sorted by type, were brought together to fill out the majority of this codex.

Phase 2 comprises §15. This section appears to have been copied at a later date by Hand 1, whose copyist, after leaving page 9 blank (perhaps having something else already in mind for it), copied this short invocation for general assistance from a distinct source manuscript to the preceding Phase 1, in some cases, along with the distinct orthographic conventions of the source text.[347]

Phase 3 comprises §14 and appears also to belong to later copying by Hand 1,[348] who added a recipe against dysuria upon the blank page 9, and—running out of space—under §15 on page 10. While lacking diagnostic differences in the morphology of graphemes or orthographic and linguistic features that would suggest they were the work of different hands, the differences in the handwriting of Phases 1, 2, and 3 do suggest that Hand 1 copied these on different occasions, perhaps returning after weeks or even years having acquired or borrowed other source texts to be copied into this "master copy" handbook.

At a later point in the history of Michigan Ms. 136, the codex passed into the possession of another individual, either one and the same as Hand 2, or the individual who commissioned the addition of a series of 12 Coptic-language medicinal and household recipes and rituals in that hand. §§18–29 are thereby consistent with the broader theme of the textual content of the codex and are sug-

---

[345] This deduction can now be supplemented by the statistics of *Kyprianos*, a database of Coptic magical texts (see the **Preface**): of the 521 manuscripts that contain texts conventionally characterized as "magical", 302 (58%) are in "sheet", 47 (9%) in "codex", 38 (7.3%) in "rotulus", and 6 (0.01%) in "roll" form, while 61 (11.7%) are on ostraca (as of May 2020). The remainder are upon unidentified fragments, or rare media such as bone, inscribed objects and architecture.

[346] A recent treatment has made the case that the transmission of magical texts was most likely through such loose-leaf manuscripts rather than in compiled bookroll or codex form, see Love 2016, §7.6.3.

[347] Compare ⲛⲓⲙ ⲡϣⲉ ⲛⲓⲙ (p. 10/5–6) where §12 has ϯϯ (p. 8/3).

[348] Not least because the page begins with the distinctive paragraphos and waved dividing line found in the earlier pages of the codex.

gestive of an individual who had broadly the same interests as the preceding owner(s) and user(s) of the texts copied by Hand 1.[349]

The hypothetical history of the textual transmission of Phase 4 is harder to discern, with shorter recipes leaving less opportunity for orthographic or linguistic variation. While §21, §23, and §27 exhibit a consistent orthographic convention diagnostic of a middle or southern dialect,[350] this is interspersed with those suggestive of a northern dialect—Fayumic in §16, §19, and §20[351] and Bohairic in §16, §22, and §28[352]—, alongside a unique orthographic convention that seems to be suggestive of the copyist's idiolect or similar source texts because it appears in both §19 and §29,[353] the two household recipes against pests. These orthographic and/or linguistic features are otherwise embedded within short texts that are comfortably characterized in the main as Sahidic. Two distinctive orthographies for the same word in §16 compared with §24 and §26 suggest that the copyist was carrying over the orthographic conventions of source texts,[354] but when in the hypothetical history of textual transmission this occurred is a matter of conjecture.

Nevertheless, given the coherence of the textual content of §§16–17, against uterine disorder, and the aforementioned orthographic and linguistic features, these two recipes, which complete page 10, seem contenders for a Block A of Phase 4. Block B of Phase 4 could comprise simply §18,[355] a healing ritual against mental illness (framed as demonic possession) involving the production of a textual amulet. Distinct from the textual content of the preceding and following recipes, this text appears to have been added onto the end of those for uterine disorder at some point in its history of textual transmission. Added to this at some point in their history of textual transmission were §§19–29, where §§20–28 comprise an internally coherent block of medical recipes against a variety of ailments, preceded (§19) and followed (§29) by two household recipes against pests. Perhaps, then, §19 and §29 were added to this list of recipes from separate source texts and each comprise a block, or perhaps there is nothing significant in their framing the list of otherwise medical recipes.[356] When begin-

[349] There is no reason to rule out, after all, that there were other owners and users of the codex who simply did not copy any further texts into the codex.

[350] ϫϩ over ⲕϩ.

[351] ⲃ for ϥ in the first two instances, ⲁⲛⲏϣ (p. 12/2) in the latter.

[352] ϭⲓⲱⲟⲩ (p. 10/13), ⲗⲁⲗⲉ- (p. 12/12), and ⲁⲧⲕⲁⲥ (p. 13/7), respectively.

[353] ⲛⲟⲩϫ̅ⲧ̅⸗ (p. 11/15) and ⲛⲟϫⲧ̅⸗ (p. 13/9), respectively.

[354] ϯ-ⲧⲕⲁⲥ (p. 10/17) in the first instance; ⲧⲓ-ⲧⲕⲁⲥ (pp. 12/18; 13/1) in the latter two.

[355] Exhibiting either the orthographic conventions of the source text, or the copyist's idiolect in the variation between ϣⲱⲛⲉ (p. 11/1) and ⲡⲉⲧϫⲱⲛⲉ (p. 11/6).

[356] The aforementioned consistency of the unique orthographic convention ⲛⲟⲩϫ̅ⲧ̅⸗ (p. 11/15) and ⲛⲟϫⲧ̅⸗ (p. 13/9), however, is suggestive of their standardization either by the copyist or by a copyist in their history of textual transmission.

ning and ending on the same line, these recipes were separated from one another by the scribal annotation ⸗, although horizontal dividing lines and some paragraphoi are used for recipes starting on their own line. The orthographic and linguistic features that creep through a dialect that can otherwise be comfortably characterized in the main as Sahidic suggest that the copyist, or the copyists of the source texts, were expressing their regional language variety—one that finds expression in orthographies characteristic of middle and northern dialects. The most parsimonious deduction, then, seems to be to locate the penultimate phase of copying, and the source texts of Phase 4, in the Fayum, where the manuscript was acquired.

Similarly, Phase 5, copied by Hand 3 and completing pages 13 and 14 of the codex, also seems to exhibit orthographic conventions suggestive of a northern dialect[357] as well as those of a, or the, copyist's idiolect[358] and/or source texts.[359] Both §30 and §31, comprising Phase 5, are medical recipes and so maintain the internal coherence of the codex, and the few orthographic and linguistic features which are expressed in these otherwise Sahidic texts also, as (the blocks of) Phase 4, seem to locate the last phase of copying, and the source texts of Phase 5, again in the Fayum.

---

[357] Compare especially F ⲧⲁⲗⲁ⸗ (p. 14/11) with S ⲧⲁⲗⲟ⸗ by Hand 2 (p. 11/12) and ⲓ (p. 14/17) with S ⲉⲓ by Hands 1 and 2 (5/14; 6/8; 6/15; 10/9; 11/9; 13/17).

[358] Consider the reduction of the initial consonant cluster in the second person singular masculine conjunctive; inconsistent reduction of the final consonant cluster in ϣⲁⲧ̄⸗ (p. 13/17) yet ϣⲁⲛⲧ̄⸗ (p. 14/12) compared with ϣⲁⲛⲧ̄⸗ (p. 4/18–19) and ϣⲁⲛⲧⲉ⸗ (p. 7/6–7) by Hand 1, and ϣⲁⲛⲧ⸗ (p. 11/14) by Hand 2; the reduced writing of the negative perfect in ⲙⲡ⸗ (pp. 14/7; 14/17), ⲙ̄ⲡ⸗ (pp. 14/8; 14/17), and ⲙⲡ̄⸗ (pp. 14/15) compared with ⲙ̄ⲡⲉ⸗ (pp. 5/18 [twice]; 5/19) and ⲛⲡⲉ⸗ (p. 4/14) by Hand 1.

[359] Compare ⲡⲥⲓⲙⲓⲑⲓⲟⲩ from ψιμύθιον (p. 13/15) with ⲥⲓⲙⲓⲑⲓⲟⲛ (p. 13/8–9) by Hand 2.

Edition

Michigan Ms. 136: Text and Translation

At the center of the new edition is a fresh text after autopsy, accompanied by translation, line-commentary, and longer excurses.[360] The line-commentary focuses on philological questions, while the excurses contain further discussion on the traditional background of and contemporary parallels for the rituals and their texts. In contrast to ed.pr., who set the entire text in Coptic characters, the linguistic distinction between Greek and Coptic is marked here by typography, with separate typefaces for each language. The punctuation and abbreviations in the edition reproduce those in the codex as far as possible (with v to mark punctuation by vacat), except in the Greek portions where, in keeping with papyrological practice, abbreviations are expanded and middle points that function simply as word separators are omitted, but both are noted in the apparatus. This apparatus also offers orthographic normalization for Greek but not Coptic and notes divergences from ed.pr., excepting minor points of punctuation and superlineation. As the codex in fact predates "standard" Sahidic Coptic, the point of reference for the normalizations that are increasingly being given in editions of Coptic texts, such references would be anachronistic; difficult forms or variants of linguistic interest are instead discussed in the line-commentary. For convenience the line-numbering of ed.pr., which runs continuously across pages, is noted in parentheses at the first line of each page and given in a concordance in the appendix. In the translation, magical words (*logoi*) are rendered in italics.

---

[360] The text was checked on the original by Zellmann-Rohrer on 8 May 2017; he thanks Pablo Alvarez and Kate Hutchens of the University of Michigan Library for assistance.

[p. 1]

p. 2

β̄

§1 ⲁⲩⲱ ⲉϫⲛ̄ ⲟⲩⲛⲉϩ ⲛ̄ⲕⲧⲁϩⲥ̄ϥ̄ ⲕⲟⲩⲓ̈
ⲛⲁⲓ̈ ⲛⲉ ⲛ̄ⲣⲁⲛ ⲉⲧⲕ̄ⲛⲁϫⲟⲟⲩ ⲉϫⲙ̄
ⲡⲛⲉϩ ⲙ̄ⲛ̄ ⲡⲉⲧⲁⲗⲗⲟⲛ· ⲁⲛⲁⲝ· ⲥⲁ-
ⲃⲣⲏⲝ· ⲁⲡⲏⲙⲉⲛⲱⲛ· ⲃⲟⲣⲁⲩ· ⲡⲉⲣⲓ·
ⲧⲣⲁⲣⲁ· ⲛⲟⲩⲁⲛⲛⲱⲱⲛⲟⲥ: ⲡⲉⲧⲁⲛⲁ-
ⲕⲉⲛⲟⲛ· ⲟⲛⲏⲥⲓⲛ ⲛⲉϣⲁⲕⲥⲁϩⲟⲩ {ⲉ}
ⲉⲡⲡⲉⲇⲁⲗⲗⲟⲛ ⲛⲁⲓ̈ ⲛⲉ· ⲥϩⲁⲓ̈ ⲛ̄ⲛ̄-
ⲕⲉⲣⲁⲛ ⲙ̄ⲛ̄ ⲛⲉⲭⲁⲣⲁⲕⲧⲏⲣ· 
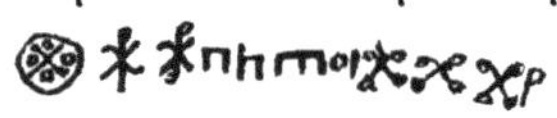 ≈>>>

---

§2 πρὸς ποδάγραν δόγιμον· 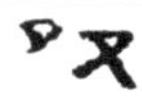
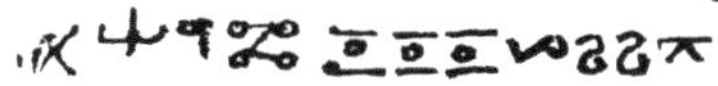 αρδαβαι
α̣μακουμ· γρ(άφε) εἰ ἀργυρᾶν σε`λή´νη
ληγούσης καὶ θαλάσσης χλι-
αρᾳ̣ καταντλῶν ἐπίλεγε
τὸ ὄνομα· λείαν ἐνεργές.
ποίησον τοῦτο ἕως μ̅δ̅ʹ ἡμέ-
§3 ρας· / ⟨...⟩ ἐπικαλοῦμαί σε τὴν μεγίσ-
την ʾΙσιν τὴν βασιλεύουσ̣α̣ν ἐν
τῷ̣ τελείῳ̣ μέλανι· ἡ δέσποινα̣

2/4 ⲡⲉⲣ̣ⲓ ed.pr. **5** ⲡⲉⲧⲁⲗⲁ ed.pr. **7** ⲥ̣ϩⲁⲓ̈ ed.pr. **8** ⲭⲁⲣ̣ⲁⲕⲧⲏⲣ ed.pr. **11** ⲁⲣⲇ̣ⲁⲃ̣ⲁ̣ⲓ ed.pr. **12** ⲙⲁ-ⲕⲟⲩⲙ ed.pr. γρ cod. ⲉⲓⲁⲣⲅⲩⲣⲓⲁⲛ ed.pr., l. εἰς ἀργυρᾶν -νη· cod., l. σελήνης **13** ληγουσης· cod. l. θαλάσσῃ χλ̣ι̣- ed.pr. **14** καταντλων· cod. **15** ονομα·, ενεργες· cod. ⲉⲛⲉⲣⲅ̣ ⲥ̣ⲟ – ed.pr. **16** τοῦτο: υ corr. from ο (?) εωσ̣ ed.pr. **17** ⲥ̣ⲉ ed.pr. ⲙ̣ⲉⲅⲓⲥ- ed.pr. **18** ϊσιν cod. ⲃⲁⲥⲓⲗⲉⲩ-ⲟⲩ[ⲥⲁ]ⲛ ed.pr. **19** μελανι· cod. : ⲙⲉⲇⲁⲛⲓ ed.pr. ⲇⲉⲥⲡⲟⲓⲛ[ⲁ] ed.pr.

§1 (*Coptic*)
[...] and over oil, and anoint him (or, it) a little. These are the names that you will speak over the oil and (the) leaf (of metal): "*Anax sabrēx apēmenōn borau peri trara nouannōōnos petanakenon onēsin*." The ones that you write on the leaf are these: write these further names and the signs: *signs*.

§2 (*Greek*)
For gout, a proven (remedy): *Signs ardabai amakoum*—write on a silver (sheet) when the moon is waning, and while rinsing with warm salt-water utter the name: (it is) very effective. Do this until 44 days (have passed).

§3 (*Greek*)
<...> "I invoke you, greatest Isis, the one who rules in the perfect black, the mistress

p. 3

ⲅ̄
θεῶν, οὐρανοῦ γένεσι· ⲁⲑⲉⲣⲛⲉ-
ⲕⲗⲏⲥⲓⲁ· ⲁⲑⲉⲣⲛⲉⲃⲟⲩⲛⲓ· ⲗⲁⲃⲓⲥⲁ-
ⲭⲑⲓ· ⲭⲱⲙⲟⲭⲟⲱⲭⲓ· ⲓⲥⲓ· ⲥⲟⲩⲥⲏ· ⲙⲟⲩⲛ-
ⲧⲏ· ⲧⲛ̄ⲧⲱⲣⲉⲱ· ϊⲱⲃⲁⲥⲧ: ⲃⲁⲥⲧⲁϊ·
ⲣⲓⲃⲁⲧ: ⲭⲣⲓⲃⲁⲧ· ⲑⲉⲣⲏⲥⲓⲃⲁⲧ· ⲭⲁ-
ⲙⲁⲣⲉⲓ· ⲭⲩⲣⲓⲑⲓⲃⲁⲑ· ⲥⲟⲩⲉⲣⲏ· ⲑⲁⲣⲑⲁ-
ⲑⲁⲃⲁⲁⲑⲑⲁ· ⲑⲁⲑ· ⲃⲁⲑⲁⲑ· ⲗⲁⲑⲁϊ·
ⲁⲭⲣⲁ· ⲁⲃⲁⲑⲁϊ· ⲁⲏ· ποίησον τὴν
μήγραν τῆς δεῖ(νος) ἣν ἔτεκαν ἡ δεῖ(να)
εἰς τὸ κατὰ φύ(σιν) γενέσθαι καὶ
ἀφλέγμαντον εἶναι, ἀκίνδυν{ω}-
ων ’βασανίστως ἤδη β̄ ταχὺ
β̄ / βάψον μαλλὸν ἐρίδη λευκοῦ,
βάλε ὑποκάτω αὐτῆς καὶ εὐθέως
§4 θεράπευσον : >>>– πρὸς σπλην(ῖτιν)
—
δόκιμον ἔμπλαστρον ἀπὸ πρωΐ-
ας ἕως ὅ(ρας) ϛ τῆς ἡρέρας· ⲛⲟϊⲧ ⲛ̄ⲉⲓ-
ⲱⲧ: ϩⲓ ⲟⲝⲩⲅⲅⲓⲛ ⲛ̄ⲣⲓⲣ: ϩⲓ ϩ̄ⲙ̄ϫ ⲉϥ-
§5 ϫⲏϥ ⲧⲟⲛⲟⲩ· ϩⲙⲟⲩ ⸗ >>>– ⲉⲧⲃⲉ ϩⲉⲛ-
—
ⲃⲟⲩϩⲉ ϫⲉ ⲛ̄ⲛⲉⲩⲣⲱⲧ ⲥⲛⲟϥ ⲛ̄ϭ[ⲓ]-
ϭⲗⲱ· ϩⲓ ⲥⲛⲟϥ ⲛ̄ⲕⲟⲩⲣⲓⲥ: ⲉⲣⲉⲡⲟⲟϩ ϭⲱ̣ϫ̄ϥ̄ ⸗

3/1 γενεσι· cod. : l. γένεσιν (?) ed.pr. **5** ⲟ̣ⲉⲣⲏⲥⲓⲃⲁⲧ ed.pr. **9** μήγραν: l. μήτραν : ⲙⲏⲧⲣⲁⲛ ed.pr. ⲇ cod. (bis) **10** ⲉ̣ⲓⲥ ed.pr. κατα φυ γενεσθαι· cod. : ⲕⲁⲧⲁⲫ† ⲉⲛⲉⲥⲑⲁⲓ ed.pr. **11** ⲁⲫⲗⲉⲅⲙⲁⲛⲧⲟ̣ⲛ ed.pr. ειναι· cod. **11–12** l. ἀκίνδυνον ⲁⲕⲓⲛⲇⲩⲛⲓ· ⲁ̣ⲉⲓ ⲛⲃⲁⲥⲁⲛⲓⲥⲧⲱⲥ ed.pr. **12** l. ἀβασανίστως ἤδη cod. **13** l. ἐριδίου **14** ὕπο- cod. **15** σπλην̄ cod. : ⲥ̣ⲡⲗⲏⲛ ed.pr. **16** πρωϊ cod. **17** ο ϛ cod., l. ὥρας ηρερας: cod., l. ἡμέρας ⲛⲟϊⲧ̣ ed.pr. **19** ϩⲙ̣ⲟⲩ ed.pr. **21** ϭⲱ̣ϫ̄ϥ̄ ⸗: -ϫ̄ϥ̄ ⸗ fitted in below line : ϭ[ⲱ]ϫϥ ed.pr.

(p. 3) of the gods, origin of heaven, (*Coptic*) *Atherneklēsia athernebouni labisachthi chōmochoōchi isi sousē mountē tentōreō iōbast bastai* *ribat chribat therēsibat chamarei churithibath souerē tharthathabaaththa thath bathath lathai achra abathai aē*, (*Greek*) make the womb of her, N, whom she, N, bore return to its natural state and be without inflammation, without peril, without torment, now", twice, "quickly", twice. Wet a flock of white wool, place it beneath her, and cure (her) at once.

§4 (*Greek*) For splenitis, a proven plaster, (applied) from morning until the sixth hour of the day: (*Coptic*) barley flour and pork lard and very sharp vinegar, salt.

§5 (*Coptic*)
For eyelashes, that they not grow: bat blood and bedbug blood, when the moon is waning.

p. 4

ⲁ̅

§6 (41) πρὸς ῥῖγος· ὅς δ' ὅτε τίς τε δράκοντα
ἰσῶν παλίνορσ̣ος ἀνέντη οὔρεος
ἐν βήσσῃς ὑπό τε τρόμος ἔλλαβε
γυῖα· ἄψ τε ἀνεχώρησσεν· κ(αὶ) τρίτε·
Γαβριὴλ θεράπευσον τὸ ⲇⲇ ἤδη
β̅ ταχὺ ταχύ. ὅταν οὖν ποιεῖς ζ̅
χορδὰς ἢ στήμονος ἢ κρόκης
δήσας ποίησον ζ̅ ἅμμα καὶ εἰς
τὶν ἀνατολὴ βλέψας εἰπὲ γ̅·
κύριε Γαβριήλ· κύριε Γαβριήλ·
κύριε Γαβριήλ· θεράπευσον τὸν
πάσχοντα ⸗ >>>——————

§7 ⲉⲧⲃⲉ ⲟⲩⲕⲟⲩⲓ̈ ⲛ̅ⲕⲉⲕⲉ ⲉⲧⲣⲉⲛⲉϥⲛⲁ-
ϫⲉ ⲣⲱⲧ ⲉⲛⲡⲉϥϩⲓⲥⲉ † ⲥϩⲃⲏⲏⲧⲉ ⲛ̅-
ⲙⲟⲩⲗⲁϩ ⲉⲛⲉϥⲛϥⲧⲉ ⸗ >>>————

§8 ⲉⲧⲃⲉ ⲟⲩⲣⲱⲙⲉ ⲉϥϣⲁϥⲃⲉ ϩⲙⲟⲩ ⲛ̣̅ⲟⲩ-
ⲛⲟⲩⲃ ⲡⲏ ⲉϣⲁⲩⲱϣ̅ⲙ̅ ⲩ ⲛⲟⲩⲃ ⲛ̅ϩⲏⲧϥ̅
ⲧ̅ⲛ̅ⲛⲟϥ ϩⲓ ⲛⲉϩ ⲧⲱϩ̅ⲥ̅ ⲉⲣⲟϥ ϣⲁⲛ-
ⲧ̅ϥ̅ⲗⲟ ⸗ >>>——————

4/1 ριγος· cod. [ο]ⲥ ⲇ̣ⲟⲧⲉ ed.pr. l. ὡς **2** ϊσων cod., l. ἰδὼν παλίνορσ̣ος: σ corr. from χ (?) : ⲡⲁⲗⲓⲛⲟⲣ[ⲥ]ⲟⲥ ed.pr. ανεντη· cod., l. ἀνέστη **3** ϋπο cod. **4** γυια· cod. l. ἀνεχώρησεν ϗ τριτε· cod. : ⲕⲧⲣⲓⲧⲉ ed.pr. **5** γαβριηλ· cod. l. τὸν ⲇⲇ: l. τοῦ δεῖ(να τῆς) δεῖ(νος) or τοῦ δεῖ(να ὃν ἔτεκεν ἡ) δεῖ(να) ἡδη cod. **6** β̅· cod. ταχυ· ταχυ· cod. l. ποιῇς **7** στημονος· cod. κροκης· cod. **8** αμμα· cod., l. ἅμματα ⲕⲁ̣ⲓ ed.pr. **9** l. τὴν ανατολη· cod., l. ἀνατολήν γ̅· cod. : ⲅ ed.pr. **10–11** γαβριηλ· cod. (ter) **14** ⲣⲱⲧⲉ ed.pr. † ⲥϩⲃⲏⲏ†ⲉ̣ⲡ̣ ed.pr. **17** ⲙ̣̅ⲛ̣̅ⲟⲩⲃ ed.pr. ⲛ̣̅ϩⲏⲧ̅ϥ̅ ed.pr. **18** ϣⲁⲛ̣- ed.pr.

§6 (*Greek*)

For fever. “As when one, having seen a snake in mountain glades, straightens up and draws back, and trembling takes hold of his limbs, and he retreats”, and three times, “Gabriēl, cure him, N, son of her, N, now”, twice, “quickly, quickly”. When you do (it), tie seven strings, either of warp or of woof, and make seven knots, and looking to the east say thrice, “Lord Gabriēl, lord Gabriēl, lord Gabriēl, cure the patient.”

§7 (*Coptic*)

For a small child, to make its teeth grow without it feeling pain: put foam of wax on its swellings.

§8 (*Coptic*)

For a person who has swellings: salt of gold, that with which gold is quenched, crush it in oil, anoint him until he gets relief.

p. 5

ⲉ̄

§**9** (60) ϩⲣⲟⲩ ⲛ̄ⲧⲏ̣ⲟⲩ ⲉⲙ̄ⲛ̄ⲧⲏ[ⲟⲩ] ϩⲣⲟⲟⲩ ⲛ̄ϩⲟⲓ̈ⲙⲉ
ⲉⲙ̄ⲛ̄ϩⲟⲓ̈ⲙⲉ· ϩⲣ´ⲟ`ⲟⲩ ⲛ̄ⲁⲙⲟⲩⲛ ⲡϣ̄ⲙ̄ⲛ̄ⲧ-
ⲛ̄ⲧⲏⲣ· ⲁⲙⲟⲩⲛ ⲉⲕⲛⲏⲩ ⲧⲱⲛ ⲙ̄ⲡⲉⲓ̈-
ⲥⲙⲟⲧ ⲙ̄ⲡⲉⲓ̈ⲣⲏⲣⲉ· ⲉⲓ̈ⲛⲏⲩ ⲙ̄ⲡⲧⲟⲩⲣⲏⲥ
ⲉϩⲏⲧ ⲟⲩⲧⲉ ⲕⲁϣ· ⲟⲩⲧⲉ ⲕⲁⲙ· ⲟⲩⲧⲉ
ⲧⲓⲛⲁⲉⲃⲱⲧ· ⲟⲩⲧⲉ ⲡⲁⲓ̈ⲧⲟⲟⲩ ⲥⲛⲁⲩ·
ⲛ̄ⲧⲉ ⲧⲉⲓ̈ⲥⲓⲃⲓⲧ ⲥ̄ⲛ̄ⲧⲉ· ⲉⲓ̈ⲧⲁⲗⲏⲩ
ⲉϩⲧⲟ ϩⲁⲧ: ϩⲧⲟ ⲕⲁⲙ ⲉⲛⲉϥϩⲁⲣⲟⲓ̈·
ⲉⲣⲉⲛ̄ⲭⲱⲱⲙⲉ ⲛ̄ⲑⲟⲟⲩⲧ ⲛ̄ⲧⲟⲧ:
ⲛⲁⲡⲟⲣϯⲟⲩ ϩ̄ⲛ̄ ⲛⲁϭⲓⲭ· ⲉⲓ̈ⲧⲙⲁ-
ⲥⲓ̈ⲟ ⲛ̄ⲛⲉⲧⲉⲉⲧ ⲉⲓ̈ⲱ̄ⲧ̄ⲡ̄ ⲛ̄ⲛⲉⲧ-
ϣⲓⲧ: ⲉⲓ̈ⲧⲣⲉⲥⲟⲟⲩϩⲉ ⲛⲓⲙ ⲣ̄ϣⲁⲩ· ϣⲁ-
ⲧ̄ⲛ̄ⲥⲟⲟⲩϩⲉ ⲛ̄ⲁϭⲣⲏⲛ· ⲁⲩⲟⲩⲱ̄ⲧ̄ϥ̄
ⲑⲟⲟⲩⲧ ⲁϥⲉⲓ ⲉⲃⲟⲗ ϩⲏⲧ: ⲁⲙⲟⲩⲛ
ⲉⲕⲛⲏⲩ ⲧⲱⲛ· ⲡϣⲟ̄ⲙ̄ⲛ̄ⲧ ⲛ̄ⲏ̄ⲥ̄ⲉ:
ⲡⲟⲟⲩ ⲉⲥϯⲛⲁⲁⲕⲉ· ϥⲧⲟⲟⲩ ⲛ̄ⲥⲟⲩ
ⲏⲣ ⲙⲉⲛ ⲟⲩ’ ⲧⲉ ϥⲡⲟ̄ⲗ̄ϭ̄ ⲉⲛⲧⲱⲃⲉ
ⲉⲙⲓⲥⲉ ⲉⲥⲧⲱ ⲙ̄ⲡⲉⲕϭ̄ⲛ̄ⲧ ⲙ̄ⲡⲉⲕ-
ϭⲓⲛⲉ ⲙ̄ⲡⲁⲣⲁⲛ· ⲙ̄ⲡⲉⲕϭⲓⲛⲉ ⲛ̄-
ⲟⲩϣⲏⲙ ⲛ̄ⲛⲉϩ ⲛ̄ⲉⲓⲛⲉ ⲉⲃⲟⲗ ϩ̄ⲙ̄

5/1 ⲛ̄ⲧ[ⲏ]ⲟ̣ⲩ ed.pr. ⲉⲙ̄ⲛ̄ⲛ̄ⲧⲏ[ⲩ] ed.pr. **2** ⲛ̄ⲁⲙ̣ⲟⲩⲛ ed.pr. **3** ⲛ̄ⲧⲏⲣ ed.pr. **4** ⲙ̄ⲡⲉⲓⲣⲏⲣⲉ ed.pr.
6 ⲧ̣ⲓ̣ⲛⲁⲉⲃⲱⲧ ed.pr. **7** ⲉⲓⲧⲁⲗⲏⲩ ed.pr. **15** ⲛ̄ⲏ̣ⲥⲉ ed.pr.

§9 (*Coptic*)

Voice (or, sound) of wind (or, breath), when there is no wind.
Voice (or, sound) of wave (or, flood), when there is no wave.
Voice of Amun, the three gods.
Amun, where is it that you are going in this form, in this manner?
It is with the south-wind that I am going, (5) northwards between reed and rush, {between} I am going to Abydos between these two mountains of these two hills.
What I am mounted on is a white horse, a black horse was before me, while the books of Thoth are with me, (10) those of the Great-of-Five in my hands.
What I cause to give birth are the ones who are pregnant.
What I close up are those who miscarry.
What I cause to be fertile is every egg, except the infertile eggs.
He was sent, Thoth. He came out before me.
"Amun, (15) where is it that you are going?"
"The Three of Isis (or, the three Isises), today, it is for four times that she is suffering (in labor). It is so-and-so many times that he releases the birth bricks".
"If you have not found me, have not found my name, have not found (20) a little oil for bringing out of <...>

p. 6

ϛ̄

(80) ⲛ̄ⲅ̄ⲧⲁⲁϥ ⲟⲩⲧⲉ̣ ⲡⲗⲉⲃⲉⲛ ⲛ̄ⲧⲉⲥϫⲓⲥⲉ
ⲉⲡⲉⲥⲏⲧ ⲛ̄ⲕ̄ϫⲟⲟⲥ ϫⲉ ⲁⲗⲟ ⲁⲗⲟ ⲙ̄ⲙⲁⲩ
ⲥⲙ̄ⲛ̄ⲧⲉ· ⲥⲙ̄ⲛ̄ⲧⲟⲩⲟⲟⲧⲉ· ϣⲙ̄ϣⲉ ⲙ̄-
ⲡⲟⲩⲙⲁⲥ ⲣ̄ⲉⲣⲱⲧⲉ ⲛ̄ϩⲱⲣ ⲡⲟⲩϣⲏⲣⲉ
ϩ̄ⲛ̄ ⲧϭⲟⲙ ⲙ̄ⲡϫⲟⲉⲓⲥ ⲡⲛⲟⲩⲧⲉ· >——
— ~~~~~~~~~~~~~~~~~~~~~~~~~~

§10 ⲧⲉϩⲉ ⲧⲉϩⲉ ⲛ̄ⲁⲙⲟⲩⲛ· ⲧⲙⲁⲁⲩ̈ ⲛ̄-
ⲛ̄ⲧ̄ⲃⲛⲟⲟⲩⲉ ⲁⲩϩⲱⲛ ⲉⲧⲟⲟⲧⲉ ϩⲧⲣⲟⲩ ⲉ-
ⲣⲁⲉⲓ ⲉⲃⲟⲗ ⲉⲙⲟⲟⲛⲉ· ⲁⲩϩⲱⲛ ⲉⲧⲟⲟ-
ⲧⲉ ϩⲓ ⲣⲟⲩϩⲉ ⲉⲣⲁⲃⲱⲕ ⲉϩⲟⲩⲛ ⲉⲧⲣⲥ̣ⲱ
ϫⲉ ϩⲁⲣⲉϩ ⲉⲣⲟ ⲉⲡⲓ ⲍ̄ ⲛ̄ⲃⲱⲛ ⲉⲡⲕⲁ-
ϩⲱⲣ· ⲡⲕⲁⲓ̈ϩ· ⲡⲃⲟⲩϩⲉ· ⲡⲃⲛ̄ⲧ ⲛ̄ⲡϣⲱ̣-
ⲡⲉ ⲉⲙⲡⲁⲧⲉϥⲡⲱⲣ̄ϣ̄ ⲡⲓⲱⲧ ⲉⲙⲡⲁ-
ⲧ̄ϥ̄ⲣ̄ ⲥⲏⲃⲉ· ⲛ̄ⲧⲏϭⲙⲉ ⲡⲁⲓ ⲉⲙⲉϥⲣ ⲕⲉ-
ⲗⲉⲗⲉ ⲛ̄ϣⲱⲥ· ⲙⲉϥⲣ̄ ϣⲃⲱⲧ ⲛ̄ⲉⲗⲟⲓ̈ϩ
ⲙⲁϥⲣ̄ ϫⲟⲟⲕⲉϥ ⲛ̄ⲉⲙⲉ· ⲁⲩⲉⲓ ⲉϫⲱⲓ̈ ⲡⲁ-
ϣⲱⲥ ⲡⲁⲉⲗⲟⲓ̈ϩ· ⲡⲁⲁⲙⲉ ⲛⲉⲩϩⲟⲓ̈ⲧⲉ
ⲡⲏϩ ⲉⲣⲁⲩ ϩⲁ ϫⲓϩ ϩⲏ̄ⲧ̄ϥ̄ ⲙ̄ⲡⲉⲩⲧⲟⲟⲩⲉ
ⲉϥⲧⲏϭ ⲛ̄ⲗⲁϩⲙⲉϥ ⲛ̄ⲕⲉⲙ· ⲁϩⲣⲟⲕ ⲉⲕ-
ⲡⲏⲧ: ⲉⲕⲓ̈ⲏⲥ ⲡⲁϣⲱⲥ ⲡⲁⲉⲗⲟⲓ̈ϩ· ⲡⲁⲁ-
ⲙ̄ⲉ ⲉ̄ⲣⲉⲛⲉⲕϩⲟⲓ̈ⲧⲉ ⲡⲏϩ· ⲁϩⲣⲟⲕ

6/1 ⲟⲩⲧ[ⲉ] ed.pr **2** ⲛ̄ⲕ̄ϫⲟⲟⲥ: -ϫⲟ- corr. from - ϫⲉ- **7** ⲉⲧⲟ̣ⲟⲧⲉ ed.pr. **11** ⲕⲁⲓ̈ϩ: corr. from ⲕⲁϩ : ⲕⲁ̣ⲓ̈ϩ ed.pr. **11–12** ⲛ̄ⲡⲟ̣ϣ̣ⲡⲉ̣ ed.pr. **12** ⲉⲙⲡ̣ⲁ̣- ed.pr. **15** ⲉϫⲱⲓ̣ ⲡ̣ⲁ̣- ed.pr. **19** ⲡⲁⲁ̣- ed.pr.

and you should put it along the ridge of her back downwards, saying: “Cease! Cease there! Prepare yourself! Prepare your womb! Serve your offspring! Produce milk for Horus your son through the power of the lord god!”

§10 (*Coptic*)
“O cow, o cow of Amun, o mother of the cattle.
They have commanded you at dawn; you should come out to pasture.
They have commanded you at evening; you should go into the fold:
Guard yourself (f.) from these seven evils against the producing of milk: the membrane-of-the-eye, the eyelid, the worm of the cucumber before it has spread, the barley before it has sprouted, the genuine (or, precious) plants, this one that never provides a crook for shepherds, never makes a staff for cowherds, never makes a goad for herdsmen.”
“They have come upon me, my shepherd, my cowherd, my herdsman.
Their garments are torn, while their mouths are drooling on the front of their shoes, being fastened with black *lahmef*.
Why are you running and hastening, my shepherd, my cowherd, my herdsman, with your garments torn? Why are you

p. 7

ⲍ̅

ϩⲁ ϫⲓϩ· ϩⲏⲧ̅ϥ̅ ⲙ̅ⲡⲉⲕⲧⲟⲟⲩⲉ ⲧⲏⲕ ⲛ̅ⲗⲁⲥ
ⲛ̅ⲕⲁⲙ· ⲍ̅· ⲛ̅ⲉⲥⲟⲩ ϩⲏⲣ· ⲍ̅ ⲛ̅ⲉⲥⲟⲩ ⲕⲁ-
ⲙⲉ· ⲍ̅ ⲛ̅ⲃⲁϩⲥⲉ· ϣⲏⲙ· ⲍ̅ ⲛ̅ϩⲉⲱ́· ⲙⲁ-
ⲣⲉ· ⲉϩⲉ ⲛⲓⲙ· ϩⲓ ⲧ̅ⲃ̅ⲛⲏ ⲛⲓⲙ ϫⲓ ⲡⲉϥ-
ϣⲏⲣⲉ ϫⲉ ⲡⲉϫⲉ ⲓⲁⲱ· ⲥⲁⲃⲁⲱⲑ· ⲣ̅
ⲡⲉⲙϩⲓⲧ ⲛ̅ⲁⲃⲱⲧ ⲣ̅ ⲡⲣⲏⲥ ⲧⲓⲛ· ϣⲁⲛ-
ⲧⲉⲕϭ̅ⲛ̅ ⲡⲁϊⲥⲟⲛ ⲥⲛⲁⲩ ⲉⲩⲱϣ ⲉⲩⲡⲏⲧ
ϭⲁϩⲏⲧ ⲉⲡⲏⲧ ⲛ̅ⲥⲱⲟⲩ ⲉⲩⲡⲏⲧ ⲥⲁⲣⲏⲥ
ⲛ̅ⲕ̅ϫⲟⲟⲥ ϫⲉ ⲃⲱⲕ ⲛ̅ⲙ̅ⲙⲉⲩⲉ ⲙ̅ⲡⲉ-
ⲧ̅ⲛ̅ϩⲏⲧ ⲉⲃⲟⲗ· ϫⲉⲕⲁⲁⲥ ⲉⲣⲉ ⲧ̅ⲃⲛⲏ
§11 ⲛⲓⲙ ⲛⲁϫⲓ ⲡⲉϥϣⲏⲣⲉ: vac. Ανουσφ.

—
ανουσφ. ανουσφ· ανουσφ. ανου`σ´φ.
ανουσφ. ανουσφιβιαχ· κάτεχε
τὸ αἷμα ἐν ποιῷ μέλει τοῦ ⲇⲇ τὶ
κελεύει σοι Δαμναμενεύς ⸗
§12 — _____ ⲭⲁⲣⲓⲧ/_______________
ⲭⲁⲓⲣⲉ· ⲡⲣⲏ· ⲭⲁⲓⲣⲉ ⲛⲉⲧⲛ̅ⲙ̅ⲙⲁⲕ
ⲭⲁⲓⲣⲉ ⲡⲉⲧⲉⲡⲱϥ ⲡⲉ ⲡⲉⲭⲁⲓⲣⲉ: ⲭⲁⲓ-
ⲣⲉ ⲙⲓⲭⲁⲏⲗ· ⲭⲁⲓⲣⲉ ⲅⲁⲃⲣⲓⲏⲗ· ⲭⲁⲓ-
ⲣⲉ ⲥⲉⲙⲉⲥⲓⲗⲁⲙⲯ. ⲙⲁϯ ⲛⲁϊ ⲛ̅ⲧϭⲟⲙ

7/2 ⲕ̣ⲁ- ed.pr. **3** ⲛϩⲉⲱ̅ ed.pr. **6** ⲧ̣ⲓ̣ⲛ̣ ed.pr. **8** ⲡⲏⲧ: ⲏ corr. from ⲱ (?) **13** ⲁⲛⲟⲩⲥⲫ · ⲓⲃⲓⲁⲭ ed.pr. **14** ⲇⲇ: l. τοῦ δεῖ(νος τῆς) δεῖ(νος) or τοῦ δεῖ(νος ὃν ἔτεκεν ἡ) δεῖ(να) l. ὅτι : ṭι ed.pr. **15** ⲕⲉⲗⲉⲩⲉⲓⲥ ⲟⲓⲇⲁ ⲙⲛⲁⲙⲉⲛⲉⲩⲥ ed.pr. **16** ⲭⲁⲣⲓⲧ/: i.e. χαριτί(σιον), l. χαριτήσιον : ⲭⲁⲣⲓⲥ ed.pr. **20** ⲛ̅ⲧϭ̣ⲟⲙ ed.pr.

drooling on the front of your shoes, being fastened with a reed-needle (or, black flax)?
Seven white sheep, seven black sheep,
seven small (or, young) calves, seven large (or, mature) cattle
—let every cow and every beast receive its offspring,
because Iaō Sabaōth has said,
“Make (for) the north of Abydos, make (for) the south (of) Thinis,
until you (m.) find these two brothers as they call out and flee northwards,
so as to chase them as they flee southwards, so that you (m.) can say:
‘Send forth the thoughts of your (pl.) hearts so that every beast will receive its offspring.’”

§11 (*Greek*)
“*Anousph anousph anousph anousph anousph anousph anousphibiak*, restrain the blood in such-and-such limb of him, N, son of her, N, for Damnameneus commands you.”

§12 (*Coptic*)
Favor-procedure (*charitesion*): “Hail, Sun. Hail, those who are with you. Hail, the one to whom ‘hail’ belongs. Hail, Michaēl. Hail, Gabriēl. Hail, Semesilamps. Give to me the power

p. 8

ⲏ̄

ⲛ̄ⲓ̄ⲁ̄ⲱ̄· ⲡⲧⲁⲭⲣⲟ ⲛ̄ⲁⲃⲣⲁⲥⲁⲝ· ⲧⲉ-
ⲭⲁⲣⲓⲥ ⲛ̄ⲥⲁⲃⲁⲱⲑ· ⲛ̄ϩⲣ̄ⲛ̄ ⲣⲱⲙⲉ ⲛⲓⲙ
ⲕⲟⲓ̸ ⲙⲁⲗⲓⲥⲧⲁ ⲛⲁϩⲣ̄ⲛ̄ ⲇⲇ· ⲡⲉⲩϩⲟ
ⲛ̄ⲥⲁ ⲡⲁϩⲟ· ⲏ̇ⲇⲏ ⲃ̄· ⲏ ⲧⲁⲭⲩ ⲃ ⸗

—~~~~~~~~~~~~~~~~~~~~~~~~~~~~

§13 φυλακτήρ(ιον) πρ(ὸς) στόμαχον καὶ
καφαλλαλγίαν· εἰς κασσίτερ(ον)
γρ(άφε)

αεηιουω
αεηιου
αεηιο
αεηι
αεη
αε
α

ωυοιηεα
ωυοιηε
ωυοιη
ωυοι
ωυο
ωυ
ω

---

vacat

8/3 κοι̸: i.e. κοινά **4** ⲃ̄ ed.pr. **5** φυλακτηρ cod. ⲡͦ cod. **6** l. κεφαλαλγίαν κασσιτερ· cod. **7** γρ cod.

of Iaō, the strength of Abrasax, the favor of Sabaōth, before every person"—the particulars—"especially before N, child of her, N, their face facing mine. Now", twice, "quickly", twice.

§13 (*Greek*)
(5) An amulet for stomach(-ache) and headache: write on tin,

a e ē i o u ō	design	*ō u o i ē e a*
a e ē i o u	design	*ō u o i ē e*
a e ē i o	design	*ō u o i ē*
a e ē i	design	*ō u o i*
a e ē	design	*ō u o*
a e	design	*ō u*
a	design	*ō*

p. 9

— ~ ——— ~ ———— ~ ————
——— ———— ———

§14 ⲉⲧⲃⲉ ⲡϣⲱ ⲛⲟⲩⲙⲏ ⸗
(134) ⲟⲩϣⲓ ⲙ̅ⲫⲓⲗⲁⲛⲓⲥ ⸗ ϣⲟⲙ̅ⲛ̅ⲧ̅
ⲛ̅ϣⲓ ⲛ̅ⲉⲃⲣⲓⲗⲁⲙ ⸗ ϣⲟⲙ̅ⲛ̅ⲧ̅
ⲛ̅ϣⲓ ⲛ̅ⲉⲃⲣⲓⲥⲉⲗⲓⲛⲏ ⸗ ϣⲟⲙ̅ⲛ̅ⲧ̅
ⲛ̅ϣⲓ ⲛ̅ⲉⲃⲣⲓⲉⲙⲓⲥⲉ ⸗ ⲛ̅ⲅ̅ϯ
ⲉⲃⲓⲱ ⲛ̅ⲥⲱⲟⲩ ⲛ̅ⲅ̅ⲧⲣⲓⲃⲉ ⲙ̅ⲙⲟⲟⲩ
ⲙ̅ⲛ̅ ⲛⲉⲩⲉⲣⲏⲩ ⲛ̅ⲕ̅ⲧⲁⲁⲩ {ⲉⲟⲩ}
ⲉⲩⲁⲡⲟⲧ ⲛ̅ϩ̅ⲛ̅ⲕⲉ ⲙ̅ⲛ̅ ⲟⲩⲁⲡⲟⲧ
ⲛ̅ⲏ̅ⲣ̅ⲡ ⲛ̅ϭ̅ⲱⲛ ⲛ̅ⲅ̅ⲧⲣⲓⲃⲉ ⲙ̅ⲙⲟⲟⲩ
ⲕⲁⲗⲱⲥ ⲙ̅ⲛ̅ʼ ⲛⲉⲩⲉⲣⲏⲟⲩ· ⲛ̅ⲅ̅ⲁⲁϥ
ⲛ̅ϣⲟⲙ̅ⲛ̅ⲧ̅ ⲛ̅ⲟⲩⲱⲛ ⲛ̅ⲅ̅ϫⲓ ⲟⲩⲱⲛ
ⲛ̅ⲙ̅ⲙⲁⲕ ⲙ̅ⲏⲛⲉ ⲛ̅ϣⲟⲙ̅ⲛ̅ⲧ̅ ⲛ̅ϩⲟⲟⲩ ⲛ̅ⲅ̅-
ⲥⲉ ⲥⲁϣ̅ϥ ⲛ̅ⲁⲙⲟⲅ ϩ̅ⲛ̅ ⲧⲕⲉⲗⲓⲥⲧⲣⲁ
ⲛ̅ⲅ̅ⲡⲁϩⲧⲕ ⲉϫ̅ⲛ̅ ϩⲏⲧⲕ ⲛ̅ⲥⲉϭ̅ⲡ̅ ⲛⲉⲕ-
ⲟⲩⲉⲣⲏⲧⲉ ⲛ̅ⲥ̣ⲉ̣ⲡⲁϩⲟⲩ ⲉϫ̅ⲛ̅ ⲡⲉⲕⲣⲁ-
ⲧϥ̅ ⲛ̅ⲥⲉϫⲓ ⲥⲁ̣ϣϥⲉ ⲛ̅ⲕⲟⲧⲥ ⲛ̅ⲙ̅ⲙⲁⲕ·
ⲙ̅ⲛ̅ⲛ̅ⲥⲱⲥ ⲛ̅ⲕⲃⲱⲕ ⲉϩⲣⲁⲓ̈ ⲉⲧϩ̅ⲙ̅ⲙⲉ
~

9/8 ⲛ̅ϩ̣̅ⲛ̣̅ⲕⲉ ed.pr. **9** ⲛ̅[.]ⲥ̣ⲁ̣ⲛ̣ⲓ ed.pr. **12** ⲛ̅ⲙ̣̅ⲙⲁⲕ ed.pr. **13** ⲛ̅ⲁⲙ̣ⲟⲅ ed.pr. **14** ⲉ̣ϫ̅ⲛ̅ ed.pr. **16** ⲛⲥⲉϫⲓ ed.pr. ⲥ̣ⲁ̣ϣ̅ϥⲉ ed.pr.

§14 (*Coptic*)

For kidney-stone: (take) a measure of anise-leaf (?), three measures of carom-seed, three measures of celery-seed, three measures of dill-seed, and you put honey in with them and grind them together and put them in a cup of beer with a cup of mild wine and grind them well together, and divide it in three parts, and take one part daily for three days and drink seven mouthfuls (?) in the horse-wallow and prostrate yourself upon your belly, and your feet are to be taken and stretched out over you as you recline (?), and seven circuits are to be made with you; and then go to the hot (bath)—

p. 10

———~———~———~———

§15 ⲟ̣ⲥ̣ⲫⲏ· ⲟⲥⲫⲏ· ⲟⲥⲫⲏ· ϊⲟⲥⲫⲏ· ϊⲟⲥⲫⲏ· ϊⲟⲥⲫⲏ·
(151) ⲃⲓⲃⲓⲟⲩ· ⲃⲓⲃⲓⲟⲩ· ⲃⲓⲃⲓⲟⲩ· ϊ̅ⲁ̅ⲥ̅ⲁ̅ⲃ̅ⲁ̅ⲱ̅ⲑ̅·
ⲁⲇⲱⲛⲁⲓ· ⲡⲉⲧⲁⲙⲁϩⲧⲉ ⲉϩⲣⲁϊ ⲉ-
ϫ̅ⲛ̅ ⲡⲉϥⲧⲟⲟⲩ ⲛ̅ⲕⲟⲟϩ ⲙ̅ⲡⲕⲟⲥⲙⲟⲥ·
ϩ̅ⲛ̅ ϩⲱⲃ ⲛⲓⲙ ⲉⲉⲓⲟⲩⲁϣ̅ϥ̅· ⲁⲛⲟⲕ ⲛⲓⲙ·
ⲡϣⲉ ⲛⲓⲙ ⲏⲇⲏ ⲏⲇⲏ ⲧⲁⲭⲩ ⲧⲁⲭⲩ:

———~———~———~———~———

§14 ~ ⲛ̅ⲅ̅ⲥⲉ ⲕⲉⲥⲁϣ̅ϥ̅ ⲛ̅ⲁⲙⲟⲕ ⲛ̅ⲅ̅ⲃⲱⲕ ⲉⲧ-
ⲕⲟⲗⲟⲙⲏⲑⲣⲁ ⲙ̅ⲙⲟⲩϩ̅ⲙ̅ⲙⲉ ⲛ̅ⲅ̅ⲥⲉ ⲕⲉⲥⲁ-
ϣ̅ϥ̅ ⲛ̅ⲁⲙⲟⲅ· ⲛ̅ⲅ̅ⲉⲓ ⲉϩⲣⲁϊ ⲛ̅ⲅ̅ⲥⲉ ⲕⲉⲥⲁ-
ϣ̅ϥ̅ ⲛ̅ⲁⲙⲟⲅ· ⲛ̅ⲅ̅ⲣ̅ ϣⲟⲙ̅ⲛ̅ⲧ ⲛ̅ϩⲟⲟⲩ ⲉⲕ-
ⲉⲓⲣⲉ ⲙ̅ⲡⲁϊ ⲙ̅ⲙⲏⲛⲉ ⲉⲕⲥⲉ ϭⲱⲛ >>—

———————————

<m2> §16 ⲉⲧⲃⲉ ⲟⲩⲥϩⲓⲙⲉ ⲉϣⲁⲣⲉⲧⲉⲥⲟⲟⲧⲉ ⲙⲕⲁϩ
ϫⲓ ⲛⲁⲕ ⲛ̅ⲟⲩⲛⲉϩ ⲛ̅ϭⲓⲱⲟⲩ ϩ̣[ⲛ̣̅]`ⲙ̣´ ⲡ̣ⲟ̣ⲩⲁϩⲉ ⲙⲛ̅ ⲟⲩ-
ϣⲏⲙ ⲛ̅ⲃⲱ ⲛ̅ϩⲉⲗⲱ ⲧⲁⲁⲩ ⲉϩⲣⲁϊ ⲉϫ̅ⲛ̅ ϩⲛ̅ϫ̅ⲃ̅ⲥ
ⲛ̅ⲛ̅ϣⲉ ⲛ̅ⲛⲟⲩϩⲉ ⲙⲁⲣⲉⲥϩⲙ̅ⲟⲟⲥ ϩⲓϫ̅ⲛ̅ ⲡⲉⲩ-
§17 ⲕⲁⲡⲛⲟⲥ ⲥ̅ⲛⲁⲗⲟ ⸗ ⲉϣⲱⲡⲉ ⲟⲩⲥϩⲓⲙⲉ

—
ⲧⲉ ⲉⲁⲥⲱ̅ⲥ̅ⲕ̅ ⲉⲥϯ ⲧⲕⲁⲥ ⲟⲩϭⲟⲡⲉ ⲛ̅ⲉⲣⲱ-
ⲧⲉ `ⲛⲉ´ϣⲁⲩ ⲧⲁⲁϥ ⲉⲟⲩϣⲏⲙ ⲛ̅ⲏⲣⲡ ⲉϥϩⲟ̅ⲗ̅ϭ̅ ⲙⲁ-
ⲣⲉⲥⲥⲟⲟϥ ⲥⲛⲁⲗⲟ >>> – – >> – >>>>> – – – –
—— ~ —— ~ ——

10/1 [ⲟⲥ]ⲫⲏ ed.pr. **11** ⲙ̅ⲙⲏⲛⲏ ed.pr. ⲉⲕⲥⲉϭⲱⲛ̣ ed.pr. **13** ⲛ̅ϭⲓⲱⲟⲩⲓⲛ̣ⲡ̣ⲟ̣ⲩⲁϩⲉ ed.pr. ϩ̣[ⲛ̣̅]`ⲙ̣´ⲡ̣ⲟ̣ⲩⲁϩⲉ: ⲟ corr. from ⲩ (?) **14** ⲧⲁ̣ⲁⲩ· ed.pr. ϫ̣̅ⲃ̅ⲥ̣̅ ed.pr. **17** ⲉⲧϯⲧ̅ⲕ̣ⲁ̣ⲥ ed.pr.

§15 (*Coptic*)
"*Osphē osphē osphē iosphē iosphē iosphē bibiou bibiou bibiou iasabaōth adōnai*, the one who has hold of (or, rules) the four corners of the universe, (assist me?) in every matter that I wish, I so-and-so, the son of so-and-so, now, now, quickly, quickly."

§14, continued
—and drink another seven mouthfuls (?) and go to the hot-water pool and drink another seven mouthfuls (?), and descend (into the pool) and drink another seven mouthfuls (?), and continue doing this daily for three days, drinking mild wine.

§16 (*Coptic*)
For a woman whose womb is in pain: take rich (?) oil from the Oasis (?) and a little hair from an old woman. Put them over coals of sycamore wood. Let her sit over their smoke. She will get relief.

§17 (*Coptic*)
If it is a woman who has been in pain constantly: a vessel of sow's milk, put it in a little sweet wine. Let her drink it. She will get relief.

p. 11

§18 ⲉⲧⲃⲉ ⲛⲉⲧⲛⲁϣⲱⲛⲉ ⲉⲡⲉⲩϩⲏⲧʼ ⲣ̄ϣⲁⲛ ⲡⲉⲩϩⲏⲧ
(170) ⲑⲗⲓⲃⲉ ⲉⲣⲟⲟⲩ ⲉⲩⲟ ⲛ̄ⲇⲁⲓⲙⲟⲛⲓⲟⲛ ϣⲁⲣⲉⲧⲉⲓ̈-
ⲥⲧⲏⲗⲏ ⲧⲣⲉⲟⲩⲗⲟ

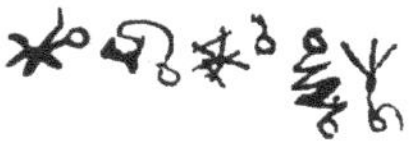

ⲭⲟⲩⲃⲁⲣⲟⲩⲭ

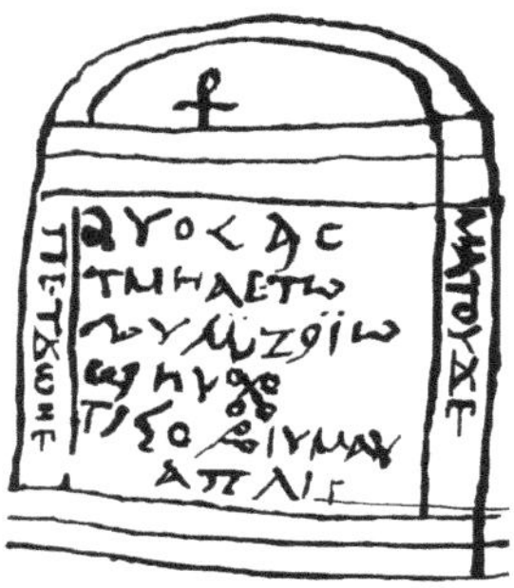

(*within stele: left border*) ⲡⲉⲧⲭⲱⲛⲉ (*right border*) ⲙⲁ ⲧⲟⲩⲭⲉ
ⲥⲁϩ̄ϥ ⲉⲟⲩⲱⲛⲉ ⲛ̄ⲟⲟⲧⲉ

§19 ⲉⲧⲃⲉ ϫⲁⲧⲃⲉ ⲛⲓⲙ ⲉⲕⲟⲩⲱϣ ⲉⲧⲣⲉⲩⲉⲓ ⲉⲃⲟⲗ
ϩⲙ̄ ⲡⲉⲕⲏⲉⲓ ⲟ̄ⲩϣⲏⲙ ⲛ̄ⲭⲁⲗⲃⲁⲛⲏ ⲟⲩ-
ϣⲏⲙ ⲛ̄ⲥⲁⲧ[ⲏ]`ⲩ´ⲣⲁⲕⲏⲥ ⲟⲩϣⲏⲙ ⲛ̄ⲕⲛ̄ⲛⲉ
ⲙ̄ⲃⲁⲁⲙⲡⲉ ⲧⲁⲗⲟϥ ⲉϩⲣⲁⲓ̈ ⲉϫⲛ̄ ⲟⲩϫ̄ⲃ̄ⲥ
ⲛ̄ⲑⲉ ⲛ̄ⲟⲩϩⲙ̣ⲙ̣ⲉ̣ ⲟ̣ⲩⲕⲗⲁⲇⲟⲥ ⲛ̄ⲕⲁⲕⲟⲇⲁ-
ⲫⲛⲏ ⲕⲁⲁϥ ϩⲙ̄ ⲡⲙⲟⲟⲩ ϣⲁⲛⲧϥ̄ⲃⲱⲕ
ⲛ̄ⲕⲛⲟⲩϫ̄ⲧ̄ ⲙ̄ⲡⲏⲉⲓ >>>> – >>>> – –

11/1 ⲡⲉⲩϩⲏⲧ̣ ed.pr. **2** ϣⲁⲣⲉⲧⲉϥ- ed.pr. **5** ⲭⲟ̣ⲩⲃⲁⲣⲱⲭ ed.pr. **7** ⲛ̄ⲉⲧⲭⲱⲛⲉ ed.pr. **8** ⲉ̣ⲟⲩⲱⲛⲉ ed.pr. **10** ⲡⲉⲕⲏⲓ ed.pr. ⲛ̄ⲭⲁⲗ̣ⲃⲁⲛⲏ ed.pr. **11** ⲥⲁⲧⲏⲣⲁⲕⲉⲓⲥ ed.pr. ⲛ̄ⲕⲛ̣̄ⲛⲉ ed.pr. **13** ⲛ̄ⲟⲩϩⲛ [. . . . .]ⲕⲗ̣ⲁⲙⲉ ed.pr. **14** ϣⲁⲛⲧϥ̄ⲃⲱⲕ̣ ed.pr. **15** ⲙ̄ⲡⲏ̣ⲉⲓ ed.pr.

§18 (*Coptic*)

For those who fall sick in their mind, if their mind distresses them and they are possessed by a demon, this stele-amulet brings them relief:

signs

Choubarouch

(*stele, left border:*) the one who is sick (?), (*right border:*) give salvation.

Write it on a uterine stone.

§19 (*Coptic*)

For any reptile that you want to make leave your house: a little galbanum, a little realgar, a little goat fat—place it over a coal like (in) a hot(-water bath); a branch of laurel, put it in water until it dissolves and sprinkle the house.

p. 12

§20 ⲉⲧⲃⲉ ⲧⲡⲁⲉⲓϣⲉ ⲉⲧⲕⲁ ⲕⲟⲩⲕⲉ v ⲟⲩⲕⲗⲁⲇⲟⲥ
(184) ⲛ̄ⲁⲛⲏϣ ⲙ̄ⲡⲣⲏ ϥⲧⲟ ⲥⲁⲧⲉⲉⲣⲉ ⲛ̄ϩⲟⲥ̄ⲙ̄ ⲛ̄ⲁⲣ-
ⲥⲉⲛⲓⲕⲟⲛ ⲧⲛⲟⲟⲩ ⲙⲛ̄ ⲛⲉⲩⲉⲣⲏⲩ ⲡⲉⲣⲓⲭⲣⲓⲁ ⲙ̄-
§21 ⲙ̄ⲟⲟⲩ ⲛ̄ⲟⲩⲙⲏϩⲉ ⲛ̄ϩⲓⲃⲱⲓ̈ >>> – ⲉⲧⲃⲉ ⲟⲩⲡⲁ-
ⲉⲓϣⲉ ⲉⲥϩⲙ̄ ⲫⲟ ⲙ̄ⲡⲣⲱⲙⲉ ⲟⲩⲗⲓⲃⲁⲛⲟⲥ
ⲛ̄ⲝⲉⲛⲓⲕⲟⲛ ⲥⲁϣϥ̄ ⲛ̄ϭⲁⲡⲁⲧ ϩⲓ ⲟⲩⲥⲟⲟⲩ ⲛ̄-
ⲕⲁⲙⲉ ⲟⲩⲧⲁⲡ ⲛ̄ⲛⲉⲥⲟⲟⲩ ⲉϥⲣⲟⲭ̄ϩ̄ ⲟⲩ-
ⲙⲏⲙⲟⲟⲩ ⲛⲕⲟⲩⲓ̈ ⲁⲫⲑⲁⲣⲧⲟⲥ ⲟⲩⲗⲟⲕ ⲛ̄-
ϩⲙ̄ⲭ̄ ⲉϥⲭⲏϥ ⲧⲁⲁⲩ ⲉⲟⲩⲗ̣ⲟⲟⲕⲉ ⲛ̄ⲃⲣ̄ⲣⲉ ⲉⲥ-
ⲭⲏⲣ ⲡⲁⲥⲧⲟⲩ ⲙⲛ̄ ⲛⲉⲩⲉⲣⲏⲩ ⲡⲉⲣⲓⲭⲣⲓⲁ ⲙ̄-
ⲙⲟⲟⲩ ⲛ̄ⲟⲩⲙⲏϩⲉ ⲛ̄ϩⲓⲃ̣ⲱⲓ̈· >>>– >>>– >>>>–>>>>–
—
§22 ⲉϣⲱⲡⲉ ⲟⲩⲁⲗ̣ ⲡⲉ ⲉϥⲟ ⲛ̣ . . . . ⲁ . ⲏ̣ ⲗⲁⲗⲉ
§23 ⲡ̣ⲉϥⲙⲟⲧⲉ ⲛ̄ⲥⲓϣⲉ ⲙ̄ⲙⲁⲥⲉ ⸗ ⲟⲩϩⲁⲃ[ⲗ]ⲉⲉⲗⲉⲓ̣ –
ⲛ̄ⲧⲉⲓ̈ϩⲉ ⲉⲥⲟⲩⲉⲧ̄ⲧ̄ⲟⲩⲱⲧ ⲣⲟⲭ̄ϩ̄ⲥ̄ ⲧⲛⲟⲥ ϩⲓ ϩ̄ⲙ̄ⲭ̄
ⲧⲁⲁⲥ ϩⲓ̈ ⲗⲓⲃⲁⲛⲟⲥ ✝ ⲉϩⲛ̄ⲃⲁⲗ ⲉⲩ`ϩ´ⲣⲉⲩⲙⲁⲧⲓ̈-
§24 ⲥⲉ ⲥⲉⲛⲁⲗⲟ ⸗ ⲟⲩϣⲏⲙ ⲛ̄ⲕⲛ̄ⲛⲉ ⲛⲉϣⲱ ⲉϥⲟⲩ-
ⲱⲧ ⲧⲛⲟϥ ✝ ⲉϩⲛ̄ⲥⲁϣ ⲉⲩⲁϣⲱⲡⲉ `ϩⲓ ⲡⲙⲁⲛⲉϩⲙⲟⲟⲥ´ ϩⲓ ⲉⲃⲓⲱ
§25 ⲙ̄ⲙⲉ ⸗ ⲉⲧⲃⲉ ϩⲛ̄ⲛⲁⲁⲭⲉ ⲉⲩⲧⲓ ⲧⲕⲁⲥ v ⲉⲩϭⲟ-
—
ⲡⲉ ⲛ̄ⲉⲣⲱⲧⲉ ⲛ̄ⲉⲱ ⲉⲥϩⲏ̣ⲙ ⲉⲓⲁ ⲣⲱⲕ ⲉⲃⲟⲗ
ⲙ̄ⲙⲟⲥ ⲁⲩⲱ ⲥⲛⲁⲗⲟ ⸗ >– >>>>– – ~~~
– –

12/6 ϩⲓ`ⲁ̣´ⲟⲩⲥⲟⲟⲩ ed.pr. **7** ⲛ̄ⲡ̣ⲉⲥⲟⲟⲩ ed.pr. **9** ⲉⲟⲩ̣ⲟⲟⲕⲉ ed.pr. **11** ⲛ̄ϩⲓ̣ⲃ̣ⲱ̣ⲓ̈ ed.pr. **12** ⲟⲩⲁⲁ ed.pr. ⲉϥⲟ [ ]ⲁⲛⲏ̣ ed.pr. **13** [ⲛ]ⲉϥⲙⲟ̣ⲧⲉ ed.pr. ⲟⲩϩⲁⲃ[ⲗ]ⲉⲉⲗⲉ ⲟ – ed.pr. **17** ϩⲓ ⲡⲙ̣ⲁⲛⲉϩⲙⲟⲟⲥ ed.pr. **19** ⲉⲥϩ[ⲏ]ⲙ̣ ed.pr.

§20 (*Coptic*)
For skin-sores that leave mange: a branch of garland-of-the-sun (plant), four staters of arsenic-natron, grind them with each other, smear them on with an ibis-feather.

§21 (*Coptic*)
For skin-sores that are on the face of a person: imported frankincense, seven shoulder blades (?) from a black sheep (?), a burnt ram's horn, a little urine from a virgin child, a cup of sharp vinegar, put them in a new cup that is black, cook them together, smear them on with an ibis-feather.

§22 (*Coptic*)
If there is a testicle (?) that is [...]: smear his neck with bull's gall.

§23 (*Coptic*)
A lizard is (useful) in the following way, if it is green: burn it, pound it with vinegar, put it with frankincense. Apply it to eyes that are rheumy. They will be relieved.

§24 (*Coptic*)
A little fresh pig's fat, crush it, apply it to sores that arise particularly on the backside (or, anus), in genuine honey.

§25 (*Coptic*)
For teeth that ache: a vessel of warm donkey's milk, rinse out your mouth with it, and there will be relief.

p. 13

§26 ⲉⲧⲃⲉ ϩⲛ̅ⲙⲁⲁϫⲉ ⲉⲩⲧⲓ ⲧⲕⲁⲥ ⲩ ⲟⲩϣⲏⲙ ⲛ̅ⲥⲓϣⲉ
(204) ⲙ̅ⲙⲁⲥⲉ ⲧⲁⲁϥ ⲉϩⲟⲩⲛ ⲉⲡⲉϥⲙⲁⲁϫⲉ ⲁⲩⲱ
§27 ϩⲁ ⲛⲉϥⲟⲃϩⲉ ⲁⲩⲱ ⲥⲉⲛⲁⲗⲟ ⸗ ⲟⲩⲣⲱⲙⲉ ⲉϥ-
ⲙⲟϫϩ ⲉⲉⲣ ⲙⲏⲟⲉⲓⲕ ⲗⲁⲗⲉ ϩⲏⲧ̅ϥ̅ ⲛ̅ⲁⲛ-
§28 ⲧⲏⲗ̅ⲙ̅ ⲛ̅ⲙⲁⲥⲉ ⲁⲩⲱ ϥⲛⲁⲗⲟ ⸗ ⲉϣⲱⲡⲉ ⲟⲩ-
ⲕⲟⲩⲓ̈ ⲛ̅ⲕⲉⲕⲉ ⲡⲉ ⲉϥⲣⲓⲙⲉ ⲗⲁⲗⲉ ⲡⲉϥ-
ⲁⲛⲧⲏⲗ̅ⲙ̅ ⲛ̅ⲁⲧⲕⲁⲥ ⲙ̅ⲙⲁⲥⲉ ⲏ ⲁ`ⲛ´ⲅⲕⲉⲫⲁ-
§29 ⲗⲟⲥ ⲙ̅ⲙⲁⲥⲉ ⸗ ⲟⲩⲕⲉⲓ ⲉϥⲟ ⲙ̅ⲡⲏⲉⲓ ⲟⲩⲥⲓ-
ⲙⲓⲑⲓⲟⲛ ⲛⲟϫ̅ϥ̅ ⲉⲟⲩⲙⲟⲩ ⲛ̅ϩⲙⲟⲩ ⲛⲟϫ̅ⲧ̅ϥ̅
<m3> **§30** ϩ̅ⲙ̅ ⲡⲏⲉⲓ ⸗ ⸗ [⸗ ⸗] ⸗ *vac.* ⲉⲧⲃⲉ ⲧⲉⲥ-

ⲕⲉ[ⲟ]ⲩⲏ ⲛ̅ⲧ̣ⲉ̣ ⲟ̣ⲩⲥ̣ⲡ̣ⲗ̣ⲉⲗⲓⲛ ⲛ̅ⲕⲁⲙⲏ
ⲟⲩⳅⲉⲥⲧ̣ⲏ̣ⲥ̣ ⲛ̅ⲛⲉϩ ⲙⲉ ⸗ ⲟⲩ-
ⳅⲉⲥⲧⲏⲥ ⲛ̅ϩ̣ⲙ̅ϫ̅ⲁⲥ ⸗ ⲟⲩⲗⲓⲧⲣⲁ
ⲛ̅ϩⲉⲗⲕⲓⲉⲙⲁ ⸗ ϣⲟⲙⲧⲉ ⲛ̅-
ⲥⲁⲧⲉⲉⲣⲉ ⲙⲡⲥⲓⲙⲓⲑⲓⲟⲩ ⸗ ⲛ̅ⲅ̅-
ⲧⲁⲁⲩ ⲉⲩⲗ̣ⲓ̣ⲕ̣ ⲛ̅ⲗⲟⲟⲕⲉ ⲛ̅ⲥⲁϩ-
ⲧⲉ ϩⲁⲣⲟⲟⲩ̣ ϣⲁⲧ̅ⲥ̅ⲉⲓ ⲉϩⲟⲩⲛ
ⲉⲕⲧⲱϩ ⲙ̅ⲙ̣ⲟ̣ⲟⲩ ⲛ̅ϩⲉⲛⲃⲁ ⲉⲩⲟⲩϣ̣ⲧ̣

— — — —

13/5 ⲙ̅ⲙⲁⲥⲉ ed.pr. **8** ⲟⲩⲕ̣ⲉ̣ⲓ ed.pr. **9** ⲙⲓⲑ̣ⲓⲟⲛ ed.pr. **10–11** ⲧⲉⲥⲕⲉ[.]ⲩ ⲏ ed.pr. **11** ⲛ̅[ϩⲁϥ]ⲗⲉⲗⲓ ⲛⲛ̅ⲕⲁⲙⲏ ed.pr. **12** ⲟⲩⳅⲉⲥ̣ⲧ̣[ⲏⲥ] ed.pr. **13** ⲛ̅ϩ̣ⲙ̣̅ϫ̅ⲁⲥ ed.pr. **14** ϩⲉⲗⲕⲓⲉⲣ̣ⲁ ed.pr. **15** ⲙ̣ⲡⲥⲓⲙⲓⲑⲓⲟⲩ ed.pr. **16** ⲉ̣ⲣ̣ⲛ [ϩ]ⲛ̅ⲗⲟⲟⲕ ⲉ- ed.pr. **18** ⲙ̅ⲙ[ⲟ]ⲟⲩ ed.pr. ⲉⲩⲟⲩϣ̣ⲧ ed.pr.

§26 (*Coptic*)
For ears that ache: a little bull's gall, put it in his ear and at the base of his teeth, and they will be relieved.

§27 (*Coptic*)
A person who has trouble defecating: smear his chest with a bull's head, and he will be relieved.

§28 (*Coptic*)
If there is a small child that is crying: smear its head with bull's marrow, or bull's brain.

§29 (*Coptic*)
A *kei* that is in the house: white lead, put it in salt water, sprinkle it in the house.

§30 (*Coptic*)
For the preparation of a black poultice: (take) a pint of genuine (i.e. olive) oil, a pint of old vinegar, a *litra* of *helkiema*, three staters of white lead, and you put them in a fresh (?) pot and kindle a fire under them until (the mixture) comes together, while you stir them with fresh palm-fronds.

p. 14

§31 [ⲉ̅]ⲧⲃⲉ ⲡⲉⲥⲭⲓⲟⲛ: ⲧⲟⲕⲓⲙⲟⲛ ⸗

(222) ⲟⲩⲟⲛⲅⲓⲁ ⲙ̅ⲙⲟⲩⲗⲁϩ
ⲟⲩⲟⲛⲅⲓⲁ ⲛ̅ϩⲙ̅ⲭ̅ⲁⲥ
ⲟⲩⲟⲧ̅ϩ̅ ⲛ̅ⲛⲉϩ ⲛ̅ⲥⲓⲙ ⲉϥ-
ⲙⲟⲕⲉ ⸗ ⲅⲣⲁⲙⲁ ⲥⲛⲁⲩ
ⲛ̅ⲗⲁⲗⲱⲏ ⸗ ⲟ̣ⲩ̣ⲃ̣ⲁ ϩ̅ⲛ̣̅ ⲟⲩ-
ⲃ̅ⲛ̅ⲛⲉ ⲉⲙⲡⲟⲩ̣ϯ ⲡⲉ̣ⲛⲓ-
ⲡⲉ ⲉⲣⲟⲥ ⲉⲛⲉ̣ϩ̣ ⲙ̣̅ⲡⲟⲩ̅ⲥ̅ⲕ̅-
ⲃⲁ ⲛ̅ϩⲏ̅ⲧ̅ⲥ̅ ⲉ̣ⲛ̣ⲉ̣ϩ̣· ⲛ̅ⲅ̅ⲣⲉⲭ̣
ϩⲉⲛϣⲉ ϩⲓⲧⲛ̣ ϩ̣ⲛ̣ⲃ̣ⲁ̣ ⲉ̣ⲧⲁⲁⲩ {ⲉⲩ}
ⲉⲩⲗⲓⲕ ⲛⲧⲁⲗⲁ̣ϥ̣ ⲉⲭⲱⲟⲩ ⲛ̅ⲅ̅-
ⲧⲱϩ ⲙ̅ⲙⲟⲟⲩ ϩ̅ⲙ̅ ⲡⲃⲁ ϣⲁⲛⲧ̅ϥ̅-
ⲃⲱⲗ ⲉⲃⲟⲗ v ⲧⲟⲩⲉⲣⲏⲧⲉ ⲉⲧϣⲱⲛⲉ
ⲧϭⲓⲭ ⲉⲧ̅ⲙ̅ⲙⲁⲩ ⲧⲉ ⲉϣⲁⲥⲧⲁ̅ϩ̅ⲥ̅
ⲉⲙⲡ̅ⲕϣⲁϫⲉ ⲛ̅ⲅ̅ⲣ̅ ϣⲟⲙ̅ⲛ̅ⲧ̅-
ⲧⲉ ⲛ̅ⲛⲟⲩϣⲏ ⲉⲅⲧⲱϩ ⲙ̅ⲙⲟⲕ
ⲉ̣ⲙⲡ̅ⲅ̅ϣⲁϫⲉ ⲉⲙⲡⲕⲓ ⲙⲙⲟⲕ ⲉⲗⲁ-
ⲁⲩ ⲛ̅ⲅⲡⲓⲣ̣ⲟⲩⲧ ⲉⲃ̣ⲟⲗ ⲅ̅ ⲟⲩⲧ̣ⲱ̣ ⲛ̣ⲅ̣-
ⲥⲟⲩⲧⲱⲛ̅ⲅ ⲉⲕⲛ̅ⲕⲟ̅ⲧ̅ⲕ̅ ϩⲓ ⲟ̣ⲩ-
[ⲥ]ⲉ̣ⲟⲟⲩⲛ ⲉⲣⲉⲟⲩⲧⲱⲃⲉ ϩⲁ[ⲣⲟⲕ]

14/1 [ⲉ]ⲧ̣ⲃⲉ ⲡⲉⲥ̣ⲭⲓⲟⲛ ed.pr. **3** ⲛ̅ϩⲙ̅ⲭ̅ⲁ̣ⲥ ed.pr. **5** ⲅⲣⲁ̣ⲙ̣ⲁ ed.pr. **6** [ⲃ]ⲗ ⲃ̣ⲁ ϩ̅ⲙ̅ⲟ̣ⲩ ed.pr. **7** ⲉⲙ-ⲡⲟ̣[ⲩ]ϯ̣ ed.pr. **8** ⲉ[ⲛⲉϩ ⲉⲙ]ⲡ̣ⲟ̣ⲩ̣ⲥ̅ⲕ̅ ed.pr. **9** ⲛ̅ϩⲏⲧ[ⲥ c. 9]ⲛ̅ⲅ̅ⲟ̣ ⲉ̣ⲭ̣ ed.pr. **10** ϩⲓ ⲡⲗ̣[c. 9]ⲗⲁⲩ ed.pr. **11** ⲉⲩⲗⲓⲕ̣ ⲛⲧⲁⲗⲟ̣ⲟ̣ⲥ ed.pr. **12** ϣⲁⲛⲧ̣ⲩ̣- ed.pr. **14** ⲧ̣ϭⲓⲭ ⲉⲧ̅ⲙ̅ⲙⲁⲩ̣ ⲧ̣ⲉ ed.pr. **15** [ⲉ]ⲙⲡ̅ⲕϣⲁϫⲉ ed.pr. ⲛ[ⲅ]ⲣ̅ ed.pr. **16** ⲛ̅ⲛⲟⲩϣ ·: ⲉⲅⲧⲱϩ ed.pr. **17** ⲙⲡ̅ⲅ̅ϣⲁϫⲉ ed.pr. **17–18** ⲉⲗⲁ̣|ⲟ̣ⲩ ed.pr. **18–19** ⲛ̅ⲅ̣ⲡ̣ⲓⲣⲟⲩ̣ⲧⲉ̣ⲃ̣ⲟⲗⲅ̣ⲟⲩ | ⲟⲩⲧⲱⲛ̅ⲅⲉⲗ̣ⲛⲕⲟⲧ̅ⲕ̅ϩⲓⲟ̣ⲩ̣ ed.pr. **20** [.]ⲟⲟⲩⲛⲥ̣ⲣ̣ⲉ̣ⲟⲩⲧ̣ⲱ̣ⲃⲉ̣ϩ[c. 5] ed.pr.

§31 (*Coptic*)

For sciatica, a proven (remedy): (take) an ounce of wax, an ounce of old vinegar, a cup of clear (?) radish oil, (5) two grams of aloe, a frond from a palm-tree before iron has ever touched it, before fronds have ever been taken from it, and you tie up some wood (10) with some fronds, to place them in a vessel, and raise (the wood) over (the wet ingredients) and stir them with the palm-frond until it dissolves. The leg that is in pain, it is that hand that anoints it, (15) without you speaking, and you continue for three nights to stir by yourself, without speaking, without approaching anyone yourself, and you catch the stars (?) three times in this way, and you stretch yourself out, lying down in a (20) bath with a brick under you.

Commentary

§1: p. 2/1–9. The text begins in the middle of a recipe for a medicinal procedure involving some magical names to be spoken over oil and written, along with ritual signs, on a metal sheet, probably to be rubbed on and attached to, respectively, some ailing human limb as an amulet. The beginning and rubric for the procedure will have stood on the lost p. 1, including the specification of the intended context of use. As the following §2 applies a broadly similar procedure to gout, it is at least possible that §1 shared the same application.

2/1 ⲁⲩⲱ. The ⲁ is obscured by a fold-over in the facsimile but has been confirmed on original.

ⲕⲟⲩϊ. The normalization to ⲕⲟⲩⲓ ⲕⲟⲩⲓ by ed.pr. in app. is unnecessary, as the simple adverbial use is attested: see *CD* 93b s.v.

2/3 ⲡⲉⲧⲁⲗⲗⲟⲛ. For ⲡⲡⲉⲧⲁⲗⲟⲛ, by haplography of the Coptic definite article and dittography within the Greek loanword πέταλον, as also ⲡⲉⲇⲁⲗⲗⲟⲛ below (2/7). On the basis of other attestations of this word in Greek ritual texts (see *Suppl.Mag.* II 81.3 n. and the excursus to §2), the transferred sense "leaf" or "thin sheet" of metal is all but assured in place of the etymological "leaf" of a plant, for which φύλλον is more often found (cf. the medical recipe *O.Crum* 487, front, 7, ⲫⲩⲗⲗⲁ). For the loanword in Coptic compare P.CtYBR inv. 1791, second text (ed. Emmel 1994, 351–353 no. 3), 2, ⲡⲉⲧⲁⲗⲱⲛ; *P.Macq.* I 1, p. 7/6–7, ⲡⲉⲧⲁⲗⲟⲛ (ⲙ̄)ⲛⲟⲩⲃ "the golden leaf" described as being "bound upon your loins" in the invocation of Baktiotha and other deities that comprises the first 11 pages of that codex; another transcription can probably be discerned in the fragmentary P.Fribourg AeT inv. 2006.4 (ed. Müller 2009, 66–68), front, 1–2, to be supplemented e.g. [ϫ̣ⲓ] ⲛⲁⲕ ⲛⲟⲩⲡⲉⲧⲁ[ⲗⲟⲛ] (from the photograph; [ ]ⲛⲁⲕⲛⲟ̣ⲕ̣ ⲡⲉⲧⲁ[ ], ed.pr.), with a following enumeration of signs and magical words. The loanword appears to have taken on another, specifically codicological sense: in *P.Fay.Copt.* 44, an inventory of biblical and other books in which interpunction has been introduced (ⲛⲧⲁⲛⲥ⳧ⲥⲓ, 1), some of the volumes are characterized by the presence or absence of ⲡⲉⲧⲁⲗⲟⲛ (ⲙⲡⲉⲧⲁⲗⲟⲛ, ⲛⲁⲧⲡⲉⲧⲁⲗⲟⲛ), whose meaning remains obscure (cf. Förster 2002, 641) but might relate to binding with wooden boards.

ⲁⲛⲁⳍ. The name resembles Greek ἄναξ, appropriate in itself in invocations (cf. e.g. *PGM* III.219, a supreme god as ἄναξ κόσμοιο), but does not necessarily derive directly from it in view of sequences such as αβεραμεν θωουθ λερθεξ αναξ εθρελυοωθ (*PGM* II.125–126). With exemplars including the sequence λιξ τετραξ among the well-known "Ephesian letters" (*Ephesia grammata*, on which see Bernabé 2013 and Edmonds 2013) and the famous Αβρασαξ, new coinages of magical words ending in -ξ/-ⳍ (or related writings of /ks/) were common: in Coptic, e.g. ⲁⲣⲁⳍ ⲃⲁⲣⲁⳍ ⲥⲁⳍ ⲑⲁⳍ, the "four powers" (ⲛ̄ⲇ ⲛⲉⲧⲉⲛⲁⲙⲓⲥ) placed at the disposal of an angel invoked in erotic magic in P.Heid. inv. K 683 (ed. *P.Bad.* V 140), 25.

2/3–4 ⲥⲁⲃⲣⲏⳍ. Not otherwise attested; a new coinage as in the preceding ⲁⲛⲁⳍ is also possible (see the note there).

2/4 ⲁⲡⲏⲙⲉⲛⲱⲛ. There is perhaps a distant relation between this word and Greek ἀπήμων "unharmed", "without pain", which would suit the condition that the procedure seeks to produce. Traces of transliterated Greek might also be detected in the following ⲡⲉⲣⲓ (περί, p. 2/4), ⲁⲛⲁⲕⲉⲛⲟⲛ (ἀνακαινῶν, p. 2/5–6: see the note there), and ⲟⲛⲏⲥⲓⲛ (ὄνησιν, p. 2/6 with the note). For comparanda in later Coptic series of magical words, partly derived from transcription of syntactical Greek, see van der Vliet 1991, 222.

2/4–5 ⲡⲉⲣⲓ· ⲧⲣⲁⲣⲁ. The first word at least might be explained as a transliteration from Greek: see the previous note.

2/5–6 ⲡⲉⲧⲁⲛⲁⲕⲉⲛⲟⲛ. The word is perhaps derived by a combination of translation and transliteration from Greek ὁ ἀνακαινῶν, "the one who renews", appropriate in a medicinal context (cf. also ⲁⲡⲏⲙⲉⲛⲱⲛ, p. 2/4 with the note).

2/6 ⲟⲛⲏⲥⲓⲛ. The word could be taken as a transliteration of Greek ὄνησιν, accusative of ὄνησις "advantage", "profit".

ⲛⲉϣⲁⲕⲥⲁϩⲟⲩ. For ⲛⲉⲧϣⲁⲕⲥⲁϩⲟⲩ by simplification of a consonant cluster.

2/7 ⲡⲉⲇⲁⲗⲗⲟⲛ. For ⲡⲉⲧⲁⲗⲟⲛ, on which the note on p. 2/3 above. The same spelling in πεδ- is reflected in the internal reference to "what is inscribed on this leaf" in the invocation *Suppl.Mag.* I 42.40 (τὰ ἐ̣[γγ]εγραμμένα τῷ πεδάλῳ τούτου).

2/8 ⲭⲁⲣⲁⲕⲧⲏⲣ. An early instance of this loanword from Greek χαρακτήρ, in its specialized sense to denote ritual signs. On the latter and their tradition and development, see Gordon 2014, *P.Oxy.* LXXXII 5304 2/32 and the commentary there, Dzwiza 2019, and Zellmann-Rohrer 2020d.

2/8–9 *signs*. The first two signs, a circle divided into quarters (resembling the hieroglyphic sign Gardner O49: walled settlement or crossroads), each filled with a ring, is found several times in Greek ritual texts (see Zellmann-Rohrer 2016, 11 with further references; there is also a form without the rings among the signs at p. 8/7–13 below); here there may be a relation to the spatial conception of a four-cornered universe (see p. 10/3–4 below with the note). The next two (9) resemble the Greek chi-rho monogram ☧ but need not signal a Christian context (cf. p. 11/6 below with the note), as this sign is attested as an abbreviation in its own right (χορός, χρηστός, χρῶ). There follows a group resembling Greek πη, then what suggests an epigraphic E rotated 90 degrees, then Greek οι. Especially as the preceding line refers to "names (ⲣⲁⲛ) and signs", it would be tempting to see in this sequence a variation of the writing ΠΙΠΙ, which constitutes an attempt to represent the Jewish divine name YHWH as written in archaic Hebrew letters (Andrade 2015, 206, 222). Such a writing, however, is so far unattested in Greek or Coptic magical texts. Three signs formed by adding ringed termini to the Greek χ and a Greek ρ close out the composition.

§2: 2/10–17. A 44-day course of treatment for gout by inscription of ritual text and signs on a silver sheet. Rinsing with seawater apparently will have produced a liquid with healing properties, accompanied by the utterance of the same ritual text. For the Greek tradition of ritual remedies for gout, see further the excursus to §2.

2/10 πρὸς ποδάγραν δόγιμον. The last word is for δόκιμον, where the orthography with γ is consistent with the pronunciation of a native speaker of Egyptian. A comparable rubric with a transliteration of the same Greek term ποδάγρα is among the applications of the prayer of Seth, son of Adam, in P.Mich. inv. 593 (ed. Worrell 1930, 247), ⲉⲧⲃⲉ ⲡⲉⲧⲟ ⲙⲡⲟⲧⲁⲕⲣⲁ ⲛ̄ⲛⲁⲑⲣⲟⲛ (to be spoken over ibis-blood and wine, as an unguent). The adjective δόκιμος describes a medical procedure further on at p. 3/15–16 as "proven", and it is applied to two procedures among the Greek magical papyri: a method for invisibility, "A proven (method to obtain) invisibility", ἀμαύρωσι δοκίμη (*PGM* I.247), and a recipe with a similarly constructed rubric as here, "A proven (method) of Pibechis for demoniacs", πρὸς δαιμονιαζομένους Πιβηχεως δόκιμον (*PGM* IV.3003); for Coptic transliterations see p. 14/1 below with the note there.

2/10–11 *signs*. The first sign in 10 is indistinct but may have been duplicated by the second, in a better state of preservation, which resembles the Greek metrological abbreviation ⲧ︤ (for the talent weight, τάλαντον), shown more clearly at the end of the sequence (p. 2/11). The first, or possibly first two at the beginning of the next line have also deteriorated but may involve the Greek letter χ, seen also in p. 8/9. There follow three signs resembling the Greek abbreviation ȹ for ὥρ(α) "hour", the letter ϛ, and the letter ζ with the addition of ringed termini, respectively. Then come three instances of a sign resembling the Greek symbol ⳁ for the grain-measure ἀρτάβη "artaba" with an additional horizontal at bottom, before an angular sign with ringed terminus at right, two signs resembling Coptic ϩ, and another the Greek ⲗ mentioned above.

2/11–12 αρδαβαι α̣μακουμ. No close parallels have yet been identified. The second element resembles the Greek transcription of the name of the biblical prophet Habakkuk (Αμβακουμ); compare perhaps also the transcription of the Aramaic imperative qūm "arise" as κουμ spoken by Christ to resurrect the daughter of the archisynagogos (Mark 5:41), an outcome not inappropriate in turn for one recovering from gout. Neither relation, if accepted, need suggest any religious orientation of the present collection towards Judaism or Christianity. A specialization of Jewish exorcists of the Roman period in the treatment of gout via incantations (ἐξᾴδει, literally "to draw out by incantation") is nevertheless claimed in the tragic parody of Lucian, in which the gout-goddess mocks their attempts (*Podagra* 173) alongside those who resort to incantations more generally (ἐπαοιδαῖς) and medical therapies drawn from the "Kyrrhane" (τῆς Κυρράνης). The latter may be an early reference to the collection of occult properties of naturally occurring substances circulating in Byzantium as the *Kyranides* (Κυρανίδες [*alias* Κοιρανίδες], on which see the discussion of **Context in the Practice of Medicine and Healing** in the introduction), a tradition related to material elsewhere in the Michigan codex (§§23, 26–28).

2/12. The astrological indication, to time the treatment with the waning of the moon, provides an analogy in turn for the disappearance of the gout; see further the excursus to §3.

ἀργυρᾶν. The noun λάμναν "thin sheet" is to be understood, cf. *PGM* X.26 (λαβὼν λάμναν χρυσᾶν ἢ ἀργυρᾶν) and the note on ⲡⲉⲧⲁⲗⲟⲛ above (p. 2/3).

2/15 τὸ ὄνομα. The referent must be the magical words at p. 2/11–12; the lengthy and syntactical invocation of Isis beginning at p. 2/17 could not accurately be so described.

λεῖαν ἐνεργές. The same advertisement is given in a Greek recipe in *PGM* XII to produce an amuletic ring, with the promise of general success, "a ring for every action and undertaking", δακτυλίδιν πρὸς πᾶσαν πρᾶξιν καὶ ἐπιτυχίαν (203).

§3: **2/17–3/15.** A new section must originally have begun at least by ἐπικαλοῦμαί σε, probably with the loss of a preceding rubric. The following Greek invocation of Isis, which contains also a Coptic section transcribing some traditional Egyptian epithets of Hathor, Isis, and Bastet (p. 3/1–8) paralleled in turn in one contemporary Greek and one later Coptic invocation (see the excursus to §3), bears no relation to the treatment of gout, which was the concern of §2, but rather concerns disorders of the female womb; see further the excursus to §3. Further proof of the division is the introduction of an entirely separate section of instructions accompanying the indication at p. 3/13–15, paralleling those in the latter part of §2 (p. 2/12–17).

2/18–19 τὴν βασιλεύουσ̣α̣ν ἐν τῷ τελείῳ μέλανι. The meaning of this epithet of Isis is open to multiple interpretations. Most recently van der Vliet has proposed an astral context (the "blackness" of the night sky), where Preisendanz had translated the phrase in the parallel in *PGM* VII as "im ganzen Schwarzland (Ägypten)", but the substantive μέλαν "ink", the black color of garments elsewhere attributed to Isis, and the "dark part" as euphemism for the pudendum may also be considered: see further the excursus to §3. For the invocation of Isis as queen see *P.Oxy.* LXXXII 5304 2/1 with the commentary.

2/19–3/1 ἡ δέσποινα̣ θεῶν, οὐρανοῦ γένεσι. The last word may stand for γένεσις, by an omission of terminal sigma not uncommon in contemporary Greek texts (see e.g. ἀμαύρωσι for ἀμαύρωσις in *PGM* I.247, discussed in the note to p. 2/10 above), but a shift to the vocative may also be considered, which would allow the form to be taken as written; the normalization to the accusative tentatively offered by ed.pr. is unjustified. Van der Vliet (see the excursus to §3) proposes a more radical correction to ἡ δέσποινα ⟨τῶν⟩ θεῶν ⟨τοῦ⟩ οὐρανοῦ, ⟨ἡ⟩ γένεσι⟨ς τοῦ οὐρανίου κόσμου⟩, "mistress of the gods of heaven, origin of the heavenly universe", which appears unnecessary; ed.pr. appears to take γενέσι as an alternate form of the dative γενέσει, rendering "from birth", but a noun in apposition to Isis makes for better parallelism, with a neat chiastic order across the two genitives.

p. 3/1–2 ⲁⲑⲉⲣⲛⲉⲕⲗⲏⲥⲓⲁ. The sequence beginning with this compound, which was felt to be Coptic by the copyist (as indicated by the writing of ⲧⲛ̄ⲧⲱⲣⲉϣ with superlineation at p. 3/4 below), is drawn from an invocation of Hathor (ⲁⲑⲉⲣ for *Ḥw.t-Ḥr*), as identified by van der Vliet (see the excursus to §3). The vocalization appears at first anomalous—ϩⲁⲑⲱⲣ is the attested absolute form, cf. also the variant ϩⲉⲑⲱⲗ attested in F (*DELC* 291b)—but is explained as a construct form of the name probably paralleled in a Ptolemaic land-register of the Memphite nome, in which Αθερμα̣χ(ιος) and Αθερνεβθφηι, the latter equated with Isis, are among the divine beneficiaries of temple land: *BGU* VI 1216.2 and 100 (cf. also 88–89) respectively. Compare also the absolute form ⲟⲩⲥⲓⲣⲉ/ ⲟⲩⲥⲓⲣⲓ "Osiris" (e.g. *PGM* IV.11 and 128) with the construct form ⲟⲩⲥ(ⲉ)ⲣ- in the compounds ⲟⲩⲥⲉⲣⲟⲩⲉⲛⲁⲃⲣⲉ (*wsỉr-wn-nfr*) (*PGM* IV.128), ⲟⲩⲥⲣⲟⲩⲉⲛⲁϥⲣ (*wsỉr-wn-nfr*) (P.Brit.Mus. EA 10808, ed. Osing 1976b with Love fc. a, l. 17), and ⲟⲩⲥⲣϭⲛⲧⲉⲙⲛⲧ (*wsỉr-ḫnt.i-ỉmn.tỉw*) (ibid., 40). The vocalization without /h/

is explained by its transmission in Greek script, where /h/ would not have been rendered: compare αθροηρ, perhaps from *Ḥw.t-Ḥr wr.t* (*PGM* XII.470), which also exhibits such a construct form αθ(ε)ρ-; for οηρ, compare ⲡⲟⲩⲣ from *pꜣ wr* (*PGM* IV.126). By comparison with the following compound, ⲛⲉⲕⲗⲏⲥⲓⲁ should derive from an Egyptian nb.t-toponym pattern, "Lady of such-and-such place", but the consonantal cluster is distinctly un-Egyptian. A considerably corrupt form of *nb.t-ḳis* "Lady of Qus" (*LGG* 8, 356), a traditional epithet for Hathor, is conceivable: a Graecized vocalization *ⲛⲉⲃ-ⲕⲟⲩⲥⲥⲁⲓ would explain more than an Egyptian vocalization *ⲛⲉⲃ-ⲕⲱⲥ, with the loss of ⲃ comparatively unproblematic. Nevertheless, the intruding ⲗ remains unexplained; *prima facie* a relation to Greek ἐκκλησία "church" seems less likely in context, but via the older sense of this noun "Hathor-of-the-assemblies" (ⲁⲑⲉⲣ-ⲛ(ⲛ)ⲉⲕ(ⲕ)ⲗⲏⲥⲓⲁ) is at least possible, perhaps related to private religious associations of the Ptolemaic and Roman periods (this suggestion is owed to Barbara Richter). The versions in *PGM* VII, αθερνεκλησιχ, and T.Köln, ⲑⲉⲣⲛⲓⲕⲗⲏⲥⲓⲁ (see the excursus to §3), do nothing to clarify matters. A transliteration of *nb.t-ḳrs.t* "Lady of the Burial" would appear superficially viable, but /r/ has long been lost in the vocalization of this word (cf. *S* ⲕⲱⲱⲥ(ⲉ)), as /r/ is especially weak as the second component in a consonantal cluster—hence the rarity of /k/, /ḳ/, and /g/ before /r/ and /l/ in Egyptian. That such a cluster was not easily vocalized by an Egyptophone is evidenced in orthographies such as κῖτας "keys" (O.Garstang 2 [ed. *P.Worp* 8], 9) for κλεῖδας. For the exercise in futility that is trying to reconstruct the exact phonology of transliterated names corrupted in textual transmission, and the dangers of uninformed guesswork, see the opening remarks in Quack 2019a.

3/1 ⲁⲑⲉⲣⲛⲉⲃⲟⲩⲛⲓ. The second phrase as divided by the present copyist clearly derives from *Ḥw.t-Ḥr nb.t Ỉwn.t* "Hathor, Lady of Dendera" (*LGG* 8, 355), as identified by van der Vliet (see the excursus to §3). The Lower Egyptian vocalization of ⲟⲩⲛⲓ is notable.

3/2–3 ⲗⲁⲃⲓⲥⲁⲭⲑⲓ. The version of this complex of names in the Köln lead tablet (discussed in the excursus to §3) has the comparable ⲗⲁⲃⲏⲥⲁⲭⲑⲏ, which would have had the same pronunciation in spoken Greek of this period. The etymology has not yet been explained, but a tentative analysis may be advanced here. An earlier version may have contained the element *l(ꜣ)by* (*CDD* n 1, 6), which could denote either a lioness or a she-bear (cf. Coptic ⲗⲁⲃⲟⲓ: *DELC* 94a–b)—compare the earlier epithet of Hathor *ḥwn.wt* "the young lioness", with several derived forms (*LGG* 8, 369). In the context of an invocation of Hathor, the creature may be identified as the lioness, given the antecedent of the Egyptian *Myth of the Sun's Eye* in which the goddess is said to have transformed herself into that animal (*DG* 262; as pointed out by Barbara Richter). The following element ⲥⲁⲭⲑⲓ could be explained as a participle or nisbe-adjective qualifying the lioness, which in this mythical context might be expected to express rage or aggressive force (perhaps therefore e.g. *sḫty(.t)* "smiting"), though a convincing identification has not yet been made. The name of the goddess Sekhmet (*Sḫm.t*) must remain a more remote possibility in view of the spelling: the reflex ⲥⲁϫⲙⲓ would be expected (*DELC* 203a).

3/3 ϫⲱⲙⲟϫⲟⲱϫⲓ. The initial element ϫⲱⲙ- could relate to the better-attested form κομ- "creator" in κομφθω (*PGM* III.142 =*PGM* III.A recto 5/32 according to the new reconstruction of Love 2017), best-known in the compound *ḳmꜣ-tꜣ* "Creator of the Earth" (*P.London-Leiden* recto 7/6), but also in κομφνουν, i.e. derived from Egyptian *ḳmꜣ pꜣ nn.w* "Creator of the Primeval Ocean", which Quack has proposed underlies *g-ꜥ-m-p-h-r-w-r* in *P.London-Leiden* recto 28/2, or κομνουν (*PGM* IV.1323), i.e. *ḳmꜣ-nn.w*, as well as the gloss κομρη on *ḳmꜣ-rꜥ* "Creator of Re" (*P.London-Leiden* recto 12/15; cf. also recto 8/9): see Quack 2004, 486–487, with numerous variants. These compounds are very much in the vein of traditional Egyptian deities such as Kematef, i.e. *ḳmꜣ-iꜣw.t≠f* "The one who created his moment", or epithets thereof, such as *ḳmꜣ-p.t* "The one who created the Sky". Griffith's deduction that *ḳmꜣ* "to create"—obsolete in Coptic—may have been reinterpreted as "shaker", cf. S ⲕⲙⲧⲟ "earthquake < earth-shaker" (1900, 93; see also *CED* 59), is consistent with the string of epithets κομφτο κομασιθ κομνουν ὁ σίσας καὶ σίων τὴν οἰκουμένην "Creator/Shaker of the Earth, Creator/Shaker of the Snake (?), Creator/Shaker of (the) Primeval Ocean, the one who shook and shakes the world" (*PGM* IV.1323–1324), yet compare *ḳmꜣ-rꜥ r ti.t-ḫpr r ḳmꜣ* "Creator of Re, who created Creation" (*P.London-Leiden* recto 8/9). In turn, the element ϫⲟⲱϫⲓ is reminiscent of χωουχε, glossed in demotic *g-h-ꜥ-w-k-h-e*, from *kk.wt* "Goddess of Darkness" (*P.London-Leiden* recto 16/10), comparable to χυχ from *kk.w* "God of Darkness": see Quack 2004, 500, with numerous variants. Perhaps ϫⲱⲙⲟϫⲟⲱϫⲓ may derive ultimately from a transliteration of a hypothetical *ḳmꜣ-kk.wt* "Creator of the Goddess of Darkness" (with notable Lower Egyptian vocalization of the final vowel, not otherwise attested).

ⲓⲥⲓ· ⲥⲟⲩⲥⲏ. An emendation to ⲥⲱⲑⲓ on the basis of Ἶσι Σῶθι "Isis-Sothis" (*ꜣs.t Spd.t*) in a version of this invocation in *PGM* VII is proposed by van der Vliet (see the excursus to §3), supported by Nagel (2019, 829), and remains attractive. These orthographies need not be interpreted as Greek versions of the Egyptian theonyms, e.g. vocatives, as ⲓⲥⲓ ⲥⲟⲩⲑⲏ would be a perfectly viable rendering of Egyptian vocalization in alphabetic transliteration. One might still hesitate over ⲥⲟⲩⲥⲏ, however, in favor of a magical word, deformed from a different antecedent (cf. perhaps σουσινεφι(εν) in *PGM* IV.601–602), a compound containing the noun ⲥ(ⲓ)ⲟⲩ "star" (e.g. *sbꜣ/sw*) and perhaps ⲥⲏⲩ "time", "day" or even (ⲓ)ⲥⲏ "Isis", the latter pronounced identically in the contemporary language as (ⲓ)ⲥⲓ (cf. ⲏⲥⲓ, *PGM* IV.94, 141; for comparable compounds with the element ⲥⲓⲟⲩ "star" see *DELC* 200a), or a reinterpretation relating to such a name.

3/3–4 ⲙⲟⲩⲛⲧⲏ. Perhaps to be analyzed as ⲙⲟⲩ-ⲛ(ⲟⲩ)ⲧⲏ, a transcription of an underlying Egyptian *mw.t-nṯr* "mother of the god" (cf. H ⲛⲟⲩⲧⲏ "god"), where ⲙⲟⲩ- evidences a construct form in a lexicalized compound. This common epithet of Isis (suggestion of Barbara Richter; see *LGG* 8, 33) would refer principally to Horus (for whom see p. 6/4 below). An underlying *mw.t-nṯr.w* "mother of the gods" is less likely given the absence of final ⲣ (cf. ⲛ̄ⲧⲏⲣ *nṯr.w* "gods" below, p. 5/3), although the invocation of Isis in the Greek portion above addresses her as "mistress of the gods, origin of heaven". A transcription of the name of the divinity Montu is another possibility (compare the Greek transcription of the Egyptian personal name Παμωνθης, from Pꜣ-Mnṯ) but seems a poorer fit for the context.

3/4 ⲧⲛ̄ⲧⲱⲣⲉⲱ. Probably a transcription of an underlying Egyptian *tꜣ nṯr.t ꜥꜣ.t* "the great goddess" (*ⲧⲉ-ⲛⲧⲱⲣⲉ-ⲱ, the supralinear stroke here representing ⲉ), as already recognized by van der Vliet; compare the lexicalized *pꜣ nṯr-ꜥꜣ* transliterated as ⲡⲛⲉⲧⲟ in *PGM* III.421 (= *PGM* III.B verso 3/15 in the new reconstruction of Love 2017). A Greek version of the epithet served in turn as a personal name in Roman Egypt: Θεὰ Μεγίστη, *O.Theb*. 145.3.

3/4–5 ϊⲱⲃⲁⲥⲧ: ⲃⲁⲥⲧⲁϊ· ⲣⲓⲃⲁⲧ: ⲭⲣⲓⲃⲁⲧ. The parallel version in *PGM* VII has Βουβαστις· ευρελιβατ; that the goddess Bastet (*bꜣs.tit*), traditionally associated with Hathor, is referenced here is suggested also by a parallel in an invocation of "the greatest goddess" (τὴν μεγίστην θεόν) in *PGM* XII.390–395 (as already recognized by van der Vliet): θαθαβαθαθ πετενναβουθι πεπτου Βαστ Ειησους Ουαιρ Αμουν ουθι ασχελιδονηθ βαθαριβαθ (cf. also p. 3/7 below). The initial ϊⲱⲃⲁⲥⲧ may be parsed ϊⲱ ⲃⲁⲥⲧ; transliterating an exclamatory particle ϊⲱ (elsewhere ϊⲟ, for which see the note on p. 10/1–2 below) followed by the name of the goddess; ϊⲱ is more likely from Egyptian *hy* "Hail!", cf. S ϩⲁ(ⲉ)ⲓⲟ but especially F ⲁⲓⲟ/ⲁⲓⲁ (omitted /h/ is also consistent with a stage of textual transmission in Greek transliteration), which can be followed directly by a theonym, than *ꜣw(y)* "Greetings!", attested otherwise only in its prepronominal form in Old Coptic transliteration as ⲉⲟⲩⲱⲧ⸗ϥ/ⲟⲩⲧⲱ⸗ⲩ (*ꜣw(e)ṯ⸗f/ꜣw(e)ṯ⸗w*) followed by a theonym (*DELC* 49a). Parallels include *h(y) inp* "Hail Anubis!" (*P.London-Leiden* recto 2/18; 18/15; 18/17; 18/21), *hꜣy by sr* "Hail Ba-soul of the Ram" (ibid. 10/28; 27/6), and *h(ꜣ)(y)* before a string of magical names (ibid. 14/9; 23/24). The form ⲃⲁⲥⲧ accords most closely with an Egyptian, as opposed to Graecized, vocalization.

3/5 ⲑⲉⲣⲏⲥⲓⲃⲁⲧ. The correct reading was already proposed against ⲟ̣ⲉⲣⲏⲥⲓⲃⲁⲧ of ed.pr. by van der Vliet (see excursus to §3) by comparison with the Köln tablet. The element completes the sequence begun by ⲣⲓⲃⲁⲧ: ⲭⲣⲓⲃⲁⲧ·, a string of magical names rooted in ⲃⲁⲧ, perhaps from ⲃⲁⲥⲧ "Bastet" (see the previous note); analysis as ⲑⲉⲣⲏ ⲥⲓ ⲃⲁⲧ "Therē son (sꜣ) of Ba(s)t(et)" remains possibile.

3/5–6 ⲭⲁⲙⲁⲣⲉⲓ. The sequence resembles the well-known ακραμμαχαμαρει *logos*, for which see *P.Monts.Roca* IV 61.1 with the commentary for further parallels and Brashear 1995, 3578 for various proposed etymologies.

3/6 ⲥⲟⲩⲉⲣⲏ. The version in *PGM* VII has σουηρι, derived from Egyptian *(ꜣ)s.t wr.t* ("Isis the great", cf. *LGG* 2, 478), as recognized by van der Vliet. The Old Coptic predecessor would presumably have been *(ⲏ)ⲥ(ⲉ/ⲓ)-ⲟⲩⲉⲣⲏ, cf. ⲟⲩⲣ (*wr* "the great", "great one") in *PGM* IV.126.

3/7 ⲑⲁⲑ· ⲃⲁⲑⲁⲑ. The syllables ⲃⲁ and ⲑⲁⲑ are repeated in various permutations in the Köln tablet (see the excursus to §3); van der Vliet also compares αθθα βαθθα (cf. ⲑⲁⲣⲑⲁⲑⲁⲃⲁⲁⲑⲑⲁ also in the Michigan text), which is explicitly equated with Isis in *PGM* IV.1078–1079; cf. also p. 3/4–5 above. A reference to yet another ancient Egyptian god may underlie the sequence, Thoth to match the consonants, or Tat (Τατ), the son of Hermes in the Hermetic Corpus—whose name perhaps derives from Egyptian *ḏd* (Ray 2011, 269–270)—in which case ⲃⲁⲑⲁⲑ could reflect *bꜣ ḏd* "Ba-soul of Tat".

3/9 μήγραν. The presence of this writing for μήτραν may be a pure copying error, as the interchange of /g/ and /t/ is not well attested; compare however the forms ⲛ̄ⲕⲛⲟⲩϫ̄ⲧ̄ (p. 11/15) and ⲛⲟϫ̄ⲧ̄ϥ̄ (p. 13/9) for -ⲛⲟⲩϫⲕ and ⲛⲟϫⲕ⸗ (ⲛⲟϫϭ⸗) respectively.

τῆς δεῖ(νος) ἣν ἔτεκαν ἡ δεῖ(να) (ⲇ̣ cod. bis). Read ἔτεκεν for ἔτεκαν. The phrase amounts to a formulaic identification of the patient by the mother's name (metronymic), following traditional Egyptian magical practice, which is also found in a heavily abbreviated form as ⲇ̣ⲇ̣ at p. 4/5 below and in the Coptic portion of the codex (p. 8/3), where the more neutral ⲛⲓⲙ ⲡϣⲉ ⲛⲓⲙ also appears (p. 10/5–6). On the magical use of the metronym see Curbera 1999 and *P.Oxy.* LXXXII 5304 2/4–5 n.; for this specific formulation in an apotropaic context, e.g. Zellmann-Rohrer and Martínez-Chico 2021; the formulaic relative clause with ἔτεκεν renders Demotic *r:msi̯*: Dieleman 2010.

3/10 εἰς τὸ κατὰ φύ(σιν) γενέσθαι. In place of the unlikely Greek-Bohairic Coptic combination ⲕⲁⲧⲁⲫϯ ⲉⲛⲉⲥⲑⲁⲓ read for the latter portion by ed.pr. (Meyer renders "attain the [condition] from god", following the text of ed.pr., but in a note [p. 359] proposed "the natural position", which is adopted without comment by Pernigotti, "in posizione naturale" [1995, 3715]), an entirely Greek continuation of the rest of the Greek instructions can be identified. The phrase εἰς τὸ κατὰ φύσιν is well attested in constructions with verbs denoting restoration in Greek medical authors: Galen makes use of the idiom εἰς τὸ κατὰ φύσιν ἐπανέρχεσθαι for "recover" several times (e.g. *De methodo medendi* 10:507 Kühn), and it continues in later authors, e.g. Aetius of Amida, *Iatrica* 12.4 εἰς τὸ κατὰ φύσιν ὁ κάμνων ἐπανέρχεται "the sick person recovers", cf. also ibid. 5.53

of the patient's complexion (χρῶμα) changing "from the unnatural to the natural" (ἐκ τοῦ παρὰ φύσιν εἰς τὸ κατὰ φύσιν) as a sign of recovery. A later, unpublished Byzantine medical recipe applies the related phrase "bringing (back) to its natural condition" (εἰς τὸ κατὰ φύσιν ἄξαι) to disorders of the womb specifically (πρὸς ἀναδρομὴν μήτρας: Vatican, Bibliotheca Apostolica Vaticana cod. Vat. gr. 299, f. 457r, prescribing the application of pig dung).

3/12 'βασανίστως. For ἀβασανίστως. The loss of initial α, whether by mechanical error of the copyist or genuine phonetic variation, seems inevitable; there is no evidence of an adjective βασάνιστος, though the sense could perhaps be accommodated ("in a proven manner"; cf. p. 2/10 with the note). For the aphaeretic form compare πεсχιοн, derived from Greek 'σχίον as variant of ἰσχίον, at p. 14/1 and τί for ὅτι at 7/14, with the notes there.

3/12–13 ἤδη β̅ ταχὺ β̅. Each member of this formulaic expression of urgency is to be repeated twice; the abbreviation probably renders an Egyptian one with *sp-sn* "twice", see p. 8/4 below with the note.

3/13 ἐρίδη. For ἐριδίου, apparently formed from an indeclinable syncopated ἐρίδι(ν), paralleled in a documentary text from Roman Egypt (*O.Florida* 16.7). Wool pads (κⲁⲙⲉ) soaked in medicinal preparations are prescribed a number of times in later Coptic medical texts for uterine disorders: see *CD* 105a.

3/15 θεράπευσον. The closing continues the sequence of aorist imperatives while adding an applied boast of efficacy, as more explicitly given throughout Greek and Coptic magical-medical recipes and in the present codex at pp. 2/10, 3/15–16, and 14/1. The verb θεραπεύω, for which see also p. 4/5 and 4/11 below, is applied via direct transliteration of the present-tense imperative ⲑⲉⲣⲁⲡⲉⲟⲩⲉ in a Coptic amulet for tonsillitis, P.Ant. inv. 15.11.13 (ed. Delattre 2014), 28.

§4: 3/15–19. A plaster for splenitis, with the title and first portion of the directions for time of application in Greek, before the ingredients are listed in Coptic. A similar bilingual interaction involving the treatment of splenitis is on record in P.Utrecht Copt. Ms. B3.8, ed. van den Broek 2017: a Greek iatromagical recipe with the indication "for spleen pain" (πρ(ὸς) σπληνὸς πόνους) has been copied on a sheet of papyrus along with two Coptic texts, one perhaps an invocation. Splenitis is treated there by the inscription of ritual text and signs on caper-root, attached to the patient as an amulet, one part of the root having been soaked in very sharp vinegar (ὄξει δριμυτάτῳ, cf. ⲍ̅ⲙ̅ⲭ ⲉϥⲭⲏϥ in the present text, p. 3/18–19) before application.

3/16–17 ἀπὸ πρωΐας ἕως ὅ(ρας) ϛ τῆς ἡρέρας. For the writing ὅ(ρας) see the following note. The time and duration of application for plasters for splenitis is also specified in Marcellus Empiricus, *De medicamentis* 23.19, as from morning to the seventh hour of the day (*adpositum mane medicamentum in horam septimam esse patieris*), after which the patient is to sit in the hot chamber of the bath; similarly in [Galen], *De remed. parab.* 14:524 Kühn, a κατάπλασμα, to be applied from morning to the eighth hour (ἀπὸ πρωῒ ἕως ὥρας η´). The use of barley flour and vinegar in spleen plasters is found also in [Galen], *De remed. parab.* 14:377 Kühn; Theodore Priscianus, *Euporiston* 2.28 (ed. Rose 1894, 183); and among the anonymous Latin iatromagical recipes in the sixth-century Leiden, Universiteitsbibliotheek cod. VLQ 9, ed. Piechotta 1887, ix §127.

3/17 ὅ(ρας). For ὥρας. The abbreviation by simple unmarked ο is unusual; the suspension of the following ρ as e.g. ορ might be expected (cf. also ἡμ for ἡμέρα "day" in P.Louvre AF 12530, ed. Richter 2014, 165–183 no. 3, verso 96). Compare however the simple ω for ὥ(ρας) in an astrological graffito from Dura-Europos, *TEAD* VI 652 (p. 132), 5, θ´ ὥ(ρας) νυκτερ(ινῆς) "the ninth hour of the night".

3/17–18 ⲉⲓⲱⲧ. For parallels for the use of barley in splenitis plasters in Graeco-Roman medicine see the note on p. 3/15–19 above; for medicinal use of barley in Coptic texts, see Till 1951a, 60 no. 45.

3/18 ⲟⲝⲩⲅⲅⲓⲛ ⲛ̄ⲣⲓⲣ. The compound is a hybrid, with a loanword from Greek ὀξύγγι(ο)ν, itself from Latin *axungia*, and Coptic ⲣⲓⲣ. Pig fat is rare in Graeco-Roman or Coptic medical recipes, occurring also at p. 12/16 below (Coptic ⲕⲛ̄ⲛⲉ in place of the loanword) and in a prescription against swellings in P.Berl. inv. 8109 (ed. *BKU* I 25; cf. Beltz 1984, 88–91), 9–10. Boar or pig gall (*fel apri uel suis*) is prescribed to be drunk for splenitis in a late ancient medical collection attributed to Pliny, *De medicina* 2.13.7 (ed. Önnerfors 1964), and figures among the ingredients of an ointment for erysipelas (*ignis sacer*) in an interpolation to Theodore Priscianus, *Euporiston* (ad 1.23), ed. Rose 1894, 282.

3/18–19 ϩ̄ⲙⲭ ⲉϥϫⲏϥ. The phrase probably renders Greek ὄξος δριμύ or, given the following ⲧⲟⲛⲟⲩ, δριμύτατον, the latter being prescribed also in an iatromagical recipe for splenitis in a bilingual Greek-Coptic recipe-collection on a single sheet (see the note to p. 3/15–19 above). Vinegar so qualified is prescribed in a range of other medical applications in Coptic: see *P.Med.Chassinat* 81/161 (ed. p. 190; a kollyrium), 127/265 (p. 257; for psoriasis), 171/342 (p. 291; for rheum), 198/365 (p. 298; for skin fungus), 214/386 (p. 305; for removal of thorns), 217/391 (p. 308; for skin fungus); as well as *P.Ryl.Copt.* 106 verso 41–42 and in general Till 1951a, 54–55 no. 31.

3/19 ϩⲙⲟⲩ. For the medicinal use of salt in Coptic texts see Till 1951a, 91–92 no. 132.

§5: 3/19–21. A medical recipe, now entirely in Coptic, to prevent the growth of eyelashes via application of the blood of two different animals at the waning of the moon, the latter probably providing an analogy for the diminution of the hairs. More specifically the goal may be the cure or prevention of trichiasis, an excessive or abnormal, inward growth of the eyelashes. The procedure is paralleled in [Galen], *De remed. parab.* 14:349 Kühn; Marcellus Empiricus, *De medicamentis* 8.181; and Theodore Priscianus, *Euporiston* 1.12 (ed. Rose 1894, 42); an anonymous Byzantine collection of "healing wisdom" (*iatrosophion*) in the manuscript Paris, Bibliothèque nationale de France cod. gr. 2316, f. 360r, ed. Oikonomu-Agorastu 1982, 66 no. 143, aims to prevent hair growth more generally via application of the mingled blood of bat, snail, and frog. Bat's blood is recommended on its own in the *Kyranides* (2.28), and a later Coptic parallel involving vulture's blood is found in *P.Med.Chassinat* 200/367 (p. 299).

3/19 ⲉⲧⲃⲉ. A common opening in the titles of medical prescriptions in Coptic, see e.g. *P.Borg.Copt.* 278; P.Mich. inv. 593b (ed. Worrell 1935b, 187–192); P.Berl. inv. 8109 (ed. *BKU* I 25; cf. Beltz 1984, 88–91), recto 16 (probably to be supplemented also at recto 13 and verso 8).

3/20 ⲃⲟⲩϩⲉ. For the meaning, see Till 1951a, 14 no. 1, correcting *CD* 48a s.v. ("eyelid").

ⲥⲛⲟϥ. For medicinal use of blood in Coptic texts, see Till 1951a, 51 no. 19.

3/20–21 ϭ[ⲓ]ϭⲗⲱ. The blood of the bat (ⲥⲛⲟⲩϥ ⲛ̄ⲕⲁⲛⲕⲗⲱ) is used to write amulets for ⲟⲩϩⲁⲗⲁϩⲟ (a disease of the skin? Cf. *CD* 649a) in P.Cair. inv. 45060 (ed. Kropp *AKZ* I, text K), 29–30, also with a specification of timing on the lunar calendar (there the sixth day). The boiling of a bat in water (ϭⲁⲡ ⲡϭⲓⲛϭⲓⲗⲱ ⲗⲉϩ[ⲙ]ⲉϥ ϩⲓ ⲙⲁⲩ), which is to be applied in turn to the flesh ([ⲧ]ⲱϩⲥ ⲉⲧⲥⲁⲣ̣ϩ̣ⲥ), figures in a collection on occult properties of the parts of birds, P.Berl. inv. 8117 (ed. *BKU* I 26), 20–22: the indication is lost but was probably medicinal.

3/21 ⲕⲟⲩⲣⲓⲥ. A loanword from Greek κόρις (cf. Förster 2002, 434), as in the parallel text in [Galen] cited above; "shrimp", ed.pr., tentatively, referring to the Doric form of Greek καρίς, but rightly doubting whether "the shrimp [has] any visible blood?" The same objection might be raised against the κόρις as insect if it were not assured by the parallels; apparently the blood is more properly that of the victims that it has bitten before being caught and crushed.

ⲉⲣⲉⲡⲟⲟϩ ϭⲱ̣ⲝ̄ϥ̄. For the lunar indication see the note on 3/19–21 above; from the Graeco-Roman tradition there is a recipe similarly aimed at controlling eyelash growth among the anonymous iatromagical recipes in the sixth-century

Leiden, Universiteitsbibliotheek cod. VLQ 9, ed. Piechotta 1887, xii §149, in which a paste made from leeches is applied. For lunar indications in Coptic medical texts see further *P.Med.Chassinat* 99/193–194 (p. 212: on the basis of ⲉⲣⲉⲡⲟⲟϩ ϭⲱ̣ϫ̄ϥ̄ in the present text, ⲉⲣⲉ ☽ ϭⲱϫⲉϥ should be rendered "when the moon [☽ for ⲡⲟⲟϩ] is waning"; the ingredient is the brain (ⲁⲛⲅⲉⲫⲁⲣⲟⲥ) of an animal whose name is given in cryptographic script and remains obscure, perhaps ϩⲟⲗ ⲙⲟⲟⲩ "river dog", that is, the beaver (Greek κυνοπόταμος), the occult properties of whose body parts are discussed in the *Kyranides*, 2.19); see further ibid. 98/192 (p. 211: snake skin), 102/199–204 (p. 219: a compound powder), and in general Chassinat's commentary at p. 57, to which add now P.Heid. inv. K 685 (ed. Meyer 1996), p. 17/11–16.

§6: **p. 4/1–12.** A recipe for the cure of fever via an incantation drawn from analogically appropriate verses of Homer (4/1–4: *Iliad* 3.33–35) and an invocation of the angel Gabriel, alongside the tying of knots. See further the excursus to §4, and for ritual approaches to fever in Greek-language texts, *P.Oxy*. LXXXII 5306–5310 with references to additional literature.

4/2 ἀνέντη. Graphic confusion for ἀνέστη, which is an at least conceivable, if less satisfactory and unattested, variant for ἀπέστη in the Homeric verses cited here.

4/4 κ(αὶ) τρίτε. Ed.pr. offers a normalization to κ̄ τρίτη, followed up with a note to the translation, "'Twenty-third'? Perhaps strayed into the text from the Greek original". No linguistic distinction, however, is to be made between the present, entirely Greek recipe and its putative original, and the sequence is better understood as a well-paralleled instruction to repeat an invocation three times: τρίτε probably stands for τρίτον, as abbreviated in εἰπὲ γ̄ in the same recipe at p. 4/9 below; the specification of a "third" day or hour, on which the second invocation is to be made, is also conceivable, but the definite article would be expected (τῇ τρίτῃ sc. ἡμέρᾳ, ὥρᾳ, cf. e.g. *PGM* II.45, 142). The form is perhaps related to the derivational process behind the Coptic reflexes in -ⲉ for personal names in -ος adapted via Greek: a contemporary example is ⲡⲁⲩⲗⲉ for Παῦλος in the bilingual Christian letter *P.Amh*. II 145.28 (cf. Παύλῳ in 2). The number three, beyond its general popularity in magical texts, matches the period of the so-called "tertian", probably malarial fever, named after its recurrence every third day by the ancient reckoning (every other day in modern terms). Ancient Greek fever terminology, with attention to both medical authors and amuletic texts, is surveyed by de Haro Sanchez 2010.

4/5 Γαβριήλ. The angel Gabriel (on whom see further the excursus to §6) played a role in both Greek and Coptic magical texts—see respectively Michl 1962, 239–243 and the commentary to *P.Oxy*. LXXXII 5306.7, and Kropp, *AKZ*

III §§141–142 and the notes to p. 7/19 below—but is not otherwise associated with fever or its treatment in particular. In the more detailed angelological tradition, originally arising in Judaism of the intertestamental period and later developed also in Christian Greek texts of Late Antiquity and Byzantium, fever is assigned explicitly to the angel Sychaēl (alias Sichaēl, Sēchaēl), whereas Gabriel, in addition to his generally elevated position as archangel, is placed in charge of "joy" in connection with his role in the annunciation of Christ's birth: see e.g. the Byzantine exorcistic amulet edited from a manuscript of the mid-fifteenth century (Paris, Bibliothèque nationale de France cod. gr. 2316, ff. 316r–319r) by Reitzenstein 1904, 296, "I adjure you also by (...) Gabriel, the one (who presides) over joy (and ...) Sichael, the one (who presides) over chills and fevers" (ὁρκίζω ὑμᾶς καὶ εἰς ... τὸν Γαβριὴλ τὸν ἐπὶ τῆς χαρᾶς ... Σιχαὴλ τὸν ἐπὶ τοῦ ῥίγους καὶ πυρετοῦ).

θεράπευσον. For the verb in iatromagical texts see also p. 3/15 above.

τὸ ϕϕ. Understand τόν for τό by an omission of the nasal especially common in word-final and pre-consonantal positions; the rest stands for δεῖ(να τῆς) δεῖ(νος) or (ὃν ἔτεκεν ἡ) δεῖ(να), an abbreviated version, condensed to the placeholders for the names alone, of the traditional Egyptian metronym formula, in its fuller form τὸν (τὴν) δεῖνα ὃν (ἣν) ἔτεκεν ἡ δεῖνα "him (or, her), N, whom she, N, bore": see the note on p. 3/9 above.

4/5–6 ἤδη β̅ ταχὺ ταχύ. A hybrid writing of a formulaic closing expression of urgency, for which see p. 8/4 with the note, where it is written in full (similarly in transliteration in the Coptic portion at p. 10/6); the full abbreviation is found above at p. 3/12–13.

4/6–8. The incantation and invocation are accompanied by the tying of knots of a ritually significant number in threads of the same number, probably with an analogical implication for the exertion of the desired control over the present fever. The tying of seven knots, accompanying ritual speech, is prescribed more generally for the cure of swelling and headache in a procedure mentioned by Pliny, Marcellus Empiricus, and some anonymous late ancient recipes (Pliny, *Naturalis historia* 28.48; Marcellus, *De medicamentis* 32.19, 21; and e.g. *Antidotarium Bruxellense* §64, ed. Rose 1894, 380; with Heim 1893, 475–476 no. 38). Seven might have additional significance here as the sum of the periods of the so-called "tertian" and "quartan", probably malarial fevers, recurring every third or fourth day by the ancient reckoning (every other day and every third day in modern terms), for which see the note on p. 4/4 above.

4/8–9. The instruction to face the east while invoking an angel, beyond its general appeal as the direction of Paradise, an angelic abode, is paralleled in an anonymous, unpublished recipe preserved in a Byzantine codex of the late fourteenth century but showing signs of late ancient origins, in this case one Elampryel for help against ophthalmia: Vatican, Bibliotheca Apostolica Vaticana cod. Vat. gr. 299, f. 501r–v, “For all ophthalmia: write and attach, and if it is possible, let the patient also say (it) facing east; to heal, say, ‘I adjure you, Elampryel, great holy one who presides over the eyes, by the God who is stationed above the Cherubim, to scatter and put off every rheum of the eyes and every cataract of this (man) or this (woman)’, twice, ‘quickly’, twice” (πρὸς πᾶσαν ὀφθαλμίαν· γράφε καὶ περίαπτε, εἰ δὲ δύναται, καὶ ὁ κάμνων λεγέτω πρὸς ἀνατολάς· τοῦ ἰᾶσαι λέγε· ὁρκίζω σε, Ἐλαμπρυήλ, μέγαν ἅγιον τὸν ἐπὶ τῶν ὀφθαλμῶν ἐγκείμενον κατὰ τοῦ θεοῦ τοῦ τεταγμένου ἐπὶ τῶν Χερουβὶμ ὥστε ἀποσκεδάσαι καὶ διαχωρῆσαι πᾶν ῥεῦμα ὀφθαλμῶν καὶ πᾶσαν ἐπίχυσιν τοῦδε ἢ τῆσδε, β′, ταχύ, β′).

4/11–12. The phrase ὁ πάσχων to denote the patient, paralleled in the *PGM* only in IV.3013 (within the exorcism-procedure against demonic possession, attributed to Pibechis), is a fixture of the Galenic corpus and becomes much more common in iatromagical texts in the Byzantine tradition. For θεράπευσον see pp. 3/15 and 4/5 above.

§7: 4/13–15. A recipe to ease the growing pains of teeth in children. Treatment for teething is not otherwise known in Coptic medical texts; for adult dentistry see *P.Med.Chassinat* 130/270 (p. 260), 151/305 (p. 272), 184/344–346 (p. 292), and p. 12/18–20 below.

4/13–14 ⲛⲁϫⲉ. The form without ϩ is preferred also at p. 12/17 ⲛⲁⲁϫⲉ (Hand 2). For the omission of ϩ within words, see *P.Bal.* I p. 142 §123g.

4/14–15 ⲧ ⲥϩⲃⲏⲏⲧⲉ ⲛ̄ⲙⲟⲩⲗⲁϩ. Ed.pr. offers a tentative normalization ⲧ ⲥϩⲃⲏ ⲏ ϯⲡⲙⲟⲩⲗ̄ⲁ̄ϩ̄; “Wachsschaum”, Till 1951a, 100 no. 160 (“Was damit gemeint ist, weiß ich nicht”). There is mention of “foam” (ⲥⲃⲏⲏⲧⲉ) in a medical context, in that case probably the removal by skimming of that produced by cooking in honey over a fire, in *P.Ryl.Copt.* 106 verso 45–46, ϭⲟⲡ ⲃ̄ ⲗⲓᵀ ⲛⲉϥⲓⲱ ⲙⲙⲉ ⲧⲁⲗⲟⲟⲩ ⲉⲡⲕⲱϩⲧ ϩⲱⲡ ⲡⲉϥⲥⲃ̣ⲁⲓⲑ̣ⲉ̣, and P.Louvre AF 12530 (ed. Richter 2014, 165–183 no. 3), verso 73–76, ⲛ̄ⲅ̄ⲧⲓ ⲉϫⲱϥ ⲛⲟⲩⲉⲃⲓⲱ ⲛ̄ⲅ̄ⲧⲁ̣ⲁ̣ⲩ ⲉϫⲛ ⲡⲕⲱϩ̄ⲧ̄ ⲛ̄ⲅ̄ⲃⲓ ⲛ̄ⲧⲉϥϩⲃⲏⲧⲉ ⲧⲏⲣⲥ.

4/15 ⲛϥⲧⲉ. Crum recorded ⲛⲉϥⲧⲉ on the basis of *P.Med.Chassinat* as intestinal “swelling or wind” (*CD* 240), tentatively adding the present instance in the addenda at p. xx. The etymology of ⲛ(ⲉ)ϥⲧⲉ is probably grounded in “loosening” or “slackening” (ⲛⲟⲩⲧϥ) but transitioned in its meaning to “swelling”, given the verbal ⲛⲟⲩϥⲧ “swell”, “be distended”, perhaps through semantic inversion. Vycichl appears to associate ⲛⲟⲩϥⲧ not with ⲛⲟⲩⲧϥ but with ⲛⲓϥⲉ “blow”, “breathe” (*DELC* 151a), proposing a verbal noun **nifi.t* “blowing” (of wind) (presumably also meaning therefore “swelling”) from which **nifi(.t)* would derive. This relation, however, is impossible due to the phonology of both the verbal ⲛⲟⲩϥⲧ "swell", "be distended" and "loosen", "settle" and the nominal ⲛⲉϥⲧⲉ "swelling", which show an etymological final /t/. The verb ⲛⲓϥⲉ instead derives from Egyptian *nfỉ* (3ae inf.), Demotic *nf(y)* (*CED* 116), thus nominal *nf* "breath", "wind": compare Demotic *nfy.w n pꜣ ḥf* "breaths (i.e. hissing) of the snake" (*CDD* n 70). The two verbs ⲛⲟⲩϥⲧ "swell", "be distended" and ⲛⲟⲩⲧϥ/ⲛⲟⲩϥⲧ "loosen", "displace" derive from *ntf* "unbind", "loosen" (3rad.) (*CED* 116) and *nft* "slacken", "loosen" (3rad.) (*CED* 113), respectively. The latter, however, is the root form, and thus the two remain closely related and conflated based on the metathesis in Coptic of ⲧϥ in the orthography of the latter.

§8: 4/16–19. A medical recipe to cure swellings of a more general kind in adult patients, via application of salt produced in the refining of gold. The specification of the patient as a man may indicate that the affliction was located in the genitals more specifically, but ⲣⲱⲙⲉ could have generic force as "human" (cf. p. 8/2 below, ⲣⲱⲙⲉ ⲛⲓⲙ, and *CD* 294b–295a). In the organization of the recipes a thematic link was perhaps felt to the "swellings" of the nascent teeth addressed in the previous section (ⲛϥⲧⲉ, p. 4/15).

4/16 ⲉϥϣⲁϥⲃⲉ. For ⲉϥϣⲁϥⲉ; this writing of the infinitive is not otherwise attested.

4/16–17 ϩⲙⲟⲩ ⲛ̣ⲟⲩⲛⲟⲩⲃ ⲡⲏ ⲉϣⲁⲩⲱϣ̄ⲙ̄ ⲛⲟⲩⲃ ⲛ̄ϩⲏⲧϥ̄. Till, who catalogued this passage among his collection of Coptic medical recipes arranged by ingredient, rendered "Goldsalz, (d. h.) das (Salz), in das man Gold geknetet hat" (1951a, 133 no. 4), more idiomatically than ed.pr., "Salt of a piece of gold: that in which pieces of gold are quenched". The by-products of the refining of precious metals feature in a few ritual and medical recipes of Late Antiquity: "gold-smelting soot" (αἰθάλη χρυσοχοϊκή or χρυσοχόου) is prescribed in the preparation of special inks in *PGM* IV.2005, 2104, and 3202–3203; more relevant to the present recipe, "silver dross" (*spuma argenti*) is an ingredient in a plaster for swellings (*ad omnem tumorem*) in an antidotary from a Latin codex of the seventh or eighth century, London, British Library Harley Ms. 5792, f. 275r, ed. Sigerist 1923, 19.

4/18 ⲛⲉϩ. For the medicinal use of oil in Coptic texts, see Till 1951a, 80–82 no. 105.

4/18–19 ϣⲁⲛⲧϥ̄ⲗⲟ. The same verb is applied to the relief of afflicted body parts or recovery of patients promised in the conclusion of medical recipes at pp. 10/16, 10/19, 11/3, 12/16, 12/20, 13/3, 13/5; compare also the direct address to the patient ⲗⲟ in the incantation at p. 6/2 with the commentary. Elsewhere it is common in the former use, e.g. P.Heid. inv. K 686 (ed. Kropp 1966), p. 15/254, ϣⲁⲩⲗⲟ ⲡⲟⲩⲱϣ ⲡⲛⲟⲩϯ; *P.Ryl.Copt.* 104 §3, ϣⲁϥⲗⲟ (for fever); *SB Kopt.* II

1029.8, ϥⲛⲁⲗⲟ (for bleeding); P.TT 157-470 (ed. Richter 2014, 156–164 no. 1), 2/8–9, [ⲕⲟⲗⲏ]ⲣ̣ⲓⲟⲛ ϣⲁϥⲧⲣⲉ ⲡⲣⲱⲙⲉ [ⲗⲟ ⲉϥ]ϣⲁⲛϩⲣⲉⲩⲙⲁⲧⲓⲥⲉ; and in the prayer in *P.Borg.Copt.* 278, p. 241 (ed. p. 627), ⲙⲁⲣⲉϥⲗⲟ ⲛϭⲓ ⲛⲁ̣ⲁ̣ (ibid. ⲥⲉⲛⲁⲗⲟ probably refers to the feet, given the preceding ⲛⲅϯ ⲏⲣⲡ ⲉⲣⲟⲟⲩ ⲛⲅⲗⲟⲟⲗⲉ ⲉⲣⲟⲟⲩ). In several instances of the construction in *P.Med.Chassinat*, the first editor's understanding of the sense may be revised on the basis of such parallels: 68/134 (p. 175), for an upset stomach, both ϥⲛⲁⲗⲟ and the variant ϣⲁⲩⲗⲟ ibid. 6/17 should refer to the patient (p. 62, preceded by ϫⲣⲱ ⲉⲣⲟⲟⲩ, the antecedent of which in context must be the patients); similarly ibid. 14/34 (p. 102), ⲧⲱϩ̄ⲥ ⲡⲉϥⲥⲱⲙⲁ ⲧⲏⲣϥ̄ ϣⲁϥⲗⲟ (Chassinat's "l'enflure disparaîtra" is unjustified, as is "applique-lui, le mal cessera" for ϯ ⲉⲣⲟⲟⲩ ϣⲁⲩⲗⲟ ibid. 38/72 [p. 145]; more accurate is "oins-les, ils guériront" ibid. 19/42 [p. 105], for ⲧⲱϩ̄ⲥ ⲉⲣⲟⲟⲩ ϣⲁⲩⲗⲟ).

§9: **pp. 5/1–6/5.** A recipe comprised of a divine drama—sometimes termed "*historiola*" or "charm", see the excurses to §§9 and 10—, a mythical precedent where the problem concerning the divine protagonist is analogous to that concerning the human patient, and whereby a solution in the mythical precedent is actualized for the human patient by the practice of the ritual. The mythological scene is set in the opening lines where Amun—the protagonist—is first addressed in his associations with the wind (i.e. breath of life) and wave (i.e. flood). Amun then journeys through a mythological landscape on his way to help deliver the infant Horus to his mother Isis, who is suffering in an ongoing labor. He is met by Thoth, who asks him in what form and where is he journeying, and in answering Thoth's questions Amun provides the ritual instructions and commands to be recited to Isis, and thereby the human patient, to ensure that the child is both delivered and suckled. The textual *structure* and *content* as well as mythological and cosmogonic associations and resonances in this divine drama are discussed in detail in the excursus to §9, while the reconstruction and contextualization of its history of textual transmission—including a reconstruction of the pre-Coptic source text—are discussed in **Transmitting Textual Traditions**.

5/1–3. The mythological scene is set by utilizing the motif of presence and absence of the voice of the wind and of the wave (i.e. flood), which is paralleled in both earlier Egyptian (P.Chester Beatty VII = P.Brit.Mus. EA 10687 6/7–7/1, ed. Gardiner 1935, 55–65; pls. 33–38) and Demotic (O.Stras. D 1338, ed. Spiegelberg 1911, 34–37; pl. 6 no. 1) magical texts as well as a later Coptic magical text (P.Saqqara F.17.10, ed. van der Vliet 2018). The relevant portions run, "Voice (or, sound) of wind, (when) there is no wind in it. Voice (or, sound) of water, (when) the Nile has not been born" (*ḫrw ṯꜣw nn ṯꜣw im=f · ḫrw mw n ms.t ḥꜥpi*, P.Chester Beatty VII 6/7–6/8); "Oh heaven, do not create wind (or, breath)! Oh sea, do not create wave (or, flood)!" (*i tꜣ p.t m-iri̯ iri̯ ṯꜣw | i pꜣ ym m-iri̯ iri̯* *hy⸢m⸣*, O.Stras. D 1338 l. 2); "There is wind, there is no wind; there is wave, there is no wave" (ⲟⲩⲛⲧⲏⲟⲩ ⲙ̣ⲛⲧⲏⲟⲩ ⲟⲩⲛϩⲱⲓⲙ ⲙⲛϩⲱⲓⲙ, P.Saqqara F.17.10 ll. 1–2). For a discussion of these partial parallels, see the excursus to §9. For a re-edition of the Coptic text, see the appendix.

5/1 ϩⲣⲟⲩ. The repetitions of the noun in this and the following line include the variant writing ϩⲣⲟⲟⲩ twice, the second time with an additional ⲟ added before ⲟⲩ as an emendation. Van der Vliet's correction of the first spelling to ϩⲣ<ⲟ>ⲟⲩ is, however, unnecessary. For a discussion of these potentially dialectal features, see **Linguistic and Orthographic Features**.

ⲛ̄ⲧⲏ̣ⲟⲩ. Although the translation preferred is "Voice (or, sound) of wind (or, breath)", this construction, in which the modifier following the undefined article phrase lacks the definite article, is attributive, and therefore the more literal rendering would be "breathy voice" or "windy sound." Contrary to both Worrell and van der Vliet, ⲧⲏ[ⲟⲩ] is restored in the second instance given the orthography ⲧⲏⲟⲩ in the first, and adequate space. The cosmogonical associations of the wind and wave with Amun are discussed in the excursus to §9.

ⲛ̄ϩⲟⲓ̈ⲙⲉ. Observations as ⲛ̄ⲧⲏⲟⲩ. The Coptic word is derived from Demotic *hym* "flood", "wave" < Egyptian *h(ꜣ)n.w* "wave", "flood". The cosmogonic associations of the wind and wave with Amun are discussed in the excursus to §9.

The syntax of these opening three clauses is grammatically pre-Coptic and would be ungrammatical in Standard Coptic. It is notable, then, that the partial parallel in the first two lines of P.Saqqara F.17.10—noted in the commentary to p. 5/1–3 and discussed in the excursus to §9—has, by comparison, been syntactically updated so as to be grammatically Coptic: ⲟⲩⲛⲧⲏⲟⲩ ⲙ̣ⲛⲧⲏⲟⲩ ⲟⲩⲛϩⲱⲓⲙ ⲙⲛϩⲱⲓⲙ.

5/2–3 ⲡϣⲙⲛ̄ⲧⲛ̄ⲧⲏⲣ. In the grammar of Standard Coptic, one would expect the construct form of the numeral followed by an undefined noun in the singular or the absolute form of the numeral followed by an attributive construction with an undefined noun in the singular. Indeed, plural forms of nouns do not appear with cardinal numbers. This construction, as well as the use of the lexicalized plural ⲛ̄ⲧⲏⲣ, is, then, evidence of an older grammatical construction, as found in one Demotic parallel: *pꜣ ḫmt nṯr.w* "the three gods" (*P.Krall* 8/9; 8/16), ed. Hoffmann 1996, where it refers instead to Apis, Mnevis, and Pharaoh—erroneously listed as **nṯr.w-ḫmt* in *LGG* 4, 536, which is not attested. For the consideration that this may be an epithet of Amun referring to his tripartite nature, as discussed in the excursus to §9, Korshi Dosoo is thanked. The alternative interpretation of a relation to an unnamed triad is also discussed in the excursus to §9. After all, where references to "the three gods" persist in the textual tradition of Coptic magical texts, triads of named gods are consistently referenced. Consider, "The flame gnaws at the three gods. (Fire) is kindled under the bones of Apis and Isis and Osiris” (ⲡⲕⲱϩⲧ ⲟⲩⲱⲙ ⲛ̄ⲥⲁ ⲡϣⲙⲧⲉⲧⲏⲣ ⲥⲟⲩⲥⲁϩⲧⲉ ϩⲁ ⲛⲕⲉⲉⲥ ⲛ̄ϩⲁⲡⲉ ⲙⲛ̄ ⲏ̄ⲥ̄ⲉ̣̄ ⲙ̄ⲛ̄ ⲟⲩⲥⲓⲣⲉ, P.Mil.Vogl. Copt. 16, ed. Pernigotti 1979; 1999, 4/3–6); “[The flame gnaws] at the three gods, for I will kindle under the bones [of Apis and] Isis and Osiris […]” (…] ⲉⲃⲟⲗ ⲛⲥⲁ ⲡϣⲙ̇ⲧⲉⲧⲉⲣ ϫⲉ ⲧⲓⲛⲁⲥⲁϩⲧⲉ ϩⲁ ⲛⲅⲉⲉⲥ [ⲛ̄ϩⲁⲡⲉ ⲙ]ⲛ ⲏⲥⲉ ⲙⲛ ⲟⲩⲥⲓⲣⲉ̣ […], P.Stras. K. 205 verso frr. A, I, K l. 19). The reconstruction of the latter is based on the parallel in P.Mil.Vogl. Copt. 16 4/3–6, whose potential was not recognized by ed.pr in Hevesi 2019, 46–47, which was itself a correction to Hevesi 2018, 2018, 70–73, where the reference to Apis in P.Mil.Vogl. Copt. 16 4/3–6 was confused with Hapi (2019, 46; 49). The partial parallel in P.Saqqara F.17.10 noted in the commentary to p. 5/1–3 has “the seven voices of the snake heads” (ⲡⲉϩⲣⲱⲟⲩ ⲛⲥⲁϣϥⲉ ⲛⲛⲁⲡⲏ ⲛ̣ϩⲱ̣ϥ̣, ll. 3–4).

5/3 ⲧⲱⲛ. The emendation proposed by ed.pr. to ⲉⲧⲱⲛ is unnecessary.

5/4 ⲣⲏⲣⲉ. Apparently for ⲣⲏⲧⲉ, by the inevitable emendation of ed.pr. It is unclear what the copyist could have understood by ⲣⲏⲣⲉ, but ϩⲣⲏⲣⲉ “flower” is not inconceivable.

ⲧⲟⲩⲣⲏⲥ. For the association of Amun with the south-wind, see the discussion in the excursus to §9.

5/5 ⲟⲩⲧⲉ. Of the three instances in this line the last is best regarded as a copying error, where what follows in the source text was omitted, or where ⲟⲩⲧⲉ was repeated in error. Although the word was interpreted by ed.pr. as a transcription of Greek οὔτε and translated “nor”, which was taken up by Meyer, it is much more likely to be S, F ⲟⲩⲧⲉ “between,” “among”, not least because this word is Egyptian and this text otherwise lacks Greek loanwords (though there are signs of a broader dependence on Greek in the use of Greek numeral ⲍ̄ in §10, at p. 6/10 and 7/2–3, and the Greek transcription of a Hebrew divine name ⲓⲁⲱ ⲥⲁⲃⲁⲱⲑ at p. 7/5), but also because the sense rendered in the dualism is much more appropriate for the context; see also p. 5/7 below with the commentary. This peculiar code-switch on the part of ed.pr. also resulted in an unnecessary emendation at p. 6/1 where he suggested that ⲟⲩⲧⲉ was a mistaken writing of ⲟⲩⲃⲉ.

ⲉϩⲏⲧ. Notable is the etymology, Demotic <u>h</u>t < Egyptian <u>h</u>dj̓, “(to travel) downstream”.

ⲕⲁϣ (...) ⲕⲁⲙ. For an interpretation of the significance of this pairing, see the discussion in the excursus to §9.

5/6 ⲧⲓⲛⲁ ⲉⲃⲱⲧ. Haplography for ⲉⲉⲃⲱⲧ. Van der Vliet emends the text dramatically to ⲧ̤ⲓⲛ <ⲙⲛ> ⲉⲃⲱⲧ “Thinis and Abydos”, but given (i) the first person has already been introduced and (ii) ⲟⲩⲧⲉ is constructed with ⲟⲩⲧⲉ, i.e. ⲟⲩⲧⲉ A ⲟⲩⲧⲉ B “between A and B”, this emendation is both unnecessary and ungrammatical. Crum (ap. ed.pr.) first suggested reading ϯⲛⲁ ⲉⲉⲃⲱⲧ, but ed.pr. also, as van der Vliet, considers this phrase "out of place". Dosoo (2021) considers this a "miscopying" and would emend the text. However, if the preceding ⲟⲩⲧⲉ is instead taken as a miscopying (see commentary to p. 5/5), nothing is missing, nothing needs to be added, and nothing needs to be relocated.

5/7 ⲛ̄ⲧⲉ ⲧⲉϊⲥⲓⲃⲓⲧ ⲥ̄ⲛ̄ⲧⲉ. The duality of "two mountains" and "two hills" further supports the interpretation of S, F ⲟⲩⲧⲉ "between", "among" in 5/5. Without this interpretation, there would be one parallel phrase lacking a further ⲟⲩⲧⲉ. At the beginning of this line the emendation of ed.pr., followed by van der Vliet, of ⲛ̄ⲧⲉ to ⲟⲩⲧⲉ is unnecessary. The use of ⲛ̄ⲧⲉ here, unless simply expressing greater precision, demonstrates that both the "two mountains" and "two hills", clearly defined, were conceptualized as toponyms. For an interpretation of this pairing, see the discussion in the excursus to §9.

5/7–8 ⲉϊⲧⲁⲗⲏⲩ ⲉϩⲧⲟ ϩⲁⲧ. The indefinite article is omitted before ϩⲧⲟ. The phrase is closely paralleled in *P.London-Leiden* verso 33/1, *ỉw=f ṯỉ.t ꜥl'yṯ r wꜥ ḥtr ḥḏ*, where the indefinite article is written, see further **Transmitting Textual Traditions**. Although ed.pr. translated "silver horse", the duality with the black horse is evident, as is the fact that when S, B ϩⲁⲧ is used as an adjective, it most commonly means "white" (*CD* 713b). Ed.pr. also proposed that an emendation was required to ϩⲧⲟ ⲛ̄ϩⲁⲧ, but given that a construct (prenominal) form of the noun S ϩⲧⲟ is possible in A, such a form might also be identified here, see **Linguistic and Orthographic Features**, or this may be further evidence of the influence of pre-Coptic Demotic grammar, where an adjective can follow a noun without attributive marker, see also the note on p. 5/2–3. For an interpretation of the significance of white and black horses, see the excursus to §9.

5/8 ϩⲧⲟ ⲕⲁⲙ ⲉⲛⲉϥϩⲁⲣⲟϊ. Observations as ϩⲧⲟ ϩⲁⲧ. This circumstantially converted preterite construction demonstrates that either a verb or prepositional phrase can follow the converter ⲉⲛⲉ-. The parallel in *P.London-Leiden* verso 33 (see the note on p. 5/7–8) is damaged, and so the exact phraseology of the construction preceding *r wꜥ ḥtr km* is unclear. However, despite the phrasing here, one would expect a verbal construction, likely beginning *ỉw=f*, given that the traces of *r* before *wꜥ* are secure, and thus *ẖr*, or similar, would not be suitable. Here it is also possible that ϩⲧⲟ ⲕⲁⲙ ⲉⲛⲉϥϩⲁⲣⲟϊ stands for ϩⲧⲟⲕⲁⲙ(ⲉ) ⲉⲛⲉϥϩⲁⲣⲟϊ, but ⲕⲁⲙ is itself perfectly Sahidic, see **Linguistic and Orthographic Features**. Ed.pr. translated "[a] black horse being under me", taken up by Meyer and van der Vliet, which makes precisely no sense given that the same speaker has just declared he is "mounted on a white horse". The emendation of this phrase to ⲉⲣⲉ ⲟⲩϩⲧⲟ ⲛ̄ⲕⲁⲙⲉ ϩⲁⲣⲟⲓ, suggested by ed.pr., is also unnecessary, because there is simply an apposition of the nominal subject preceding the circumstantially converted preterit converter, where the pronominal subject of that converter refers back to the preceding nominal subject. For an interpretation of the significance of a white and black horse, see the excursus to §9.

5/9–10 ⲉⲣⲉⲛ̄ϫⲱⲱⲙⲉ ⲛ̄ⲑⲟⲟⲩⲧ ⲛ̄ⲧⲟⲧ: ⲛⲁⲡⲟⲣϯⲟⲩ ϩ̄ⲛ̄ ⲛⲁϭⲓϫ. There is a close parallel in *P.London-Leiden* verso 33/2, *ỉw nꜣ ḏmꜥ [n ḏḥw.tỉ n-ḏr./ḥr-ꜣ].ṯ=f nꜣe pꜣ wr-tỉw ẖn ḳne=f*. Van der Vliet emends the text to ⲡⲟ<ⲩ>ⲣ ϯⲟⲩ, which is both unnecessary and distracts from what can be safely assumed to be a lexicalized epithet, ⲡ-ⲟⲣ- evidencing a construct (prepronominal) form of ⲡ-ⲟⲩⲣ. For a discussion of this parallel, and those preceding (p. 5/7–8), see further **Transmitting Textual Traditions**. For the significance of the "Books of Thoth" and the "Great of Five" as an epithet of Thoth, see the discussion in the excursus to §9.

5/11 ⲉⲉⲧ. This stative/qualitative form betrays its Demotic predecessor *ỉwr.t*, stative/qualitative *ỉwr.ṯ*.

5/11–12 ⲉⲓ̈ⲱⲧ̄ⲡ̄ ⲛ̄ⲛⲉⲧϣⲓⲧ. Given that "closing up" is a positive and desired outcome in context, in parallel to "delivering" in the preceding phrase, the etymology of ϣⲓⲧ can be sought in B ϣⲓϯ "leap", "gush", vomit", which is derived from Demotic and Egyptian *šdi̯* "take (out)", "remove" (*Wb* 4, 560.8–562.19). The lack of the final vowel could be explained by haplography, given the following construction, ⲉⲓ̈ⲧⲣⲉⲥⲟⲟⲩϩⲉ ⲛⲓⲙ ⲣ̄ϣⲁⲩ. This verb, however, does not appear to be attested in any other dialect of Standard Coptic, but has semantic predecessors in Demotic (itself a Lower Egyptian language variety). Dosoo (2021) has also suggested an unattested qualitative form of ϣⲱⲱⲧ "to lack", but this fits less well in context.

5/12 ⲉⲓ̈ⲧⲣⲉⲥⲟⲟⲩϩⲉ. The emendation of ed.pr. to ⲛ̄ⲥⲟⲟⲩϩⲉ is erroneous, as ⲧⲣⲉ- is itself a construct (prenominal) form. For the mythological and cosmogonic associations of Amun and the egg, see the excursus to §9.

5/12–13 ϣⲁⲧ̄ⲛ̄ⲥⲟⲟⲩϩⲉ. Haplography for ϣⲁⲧ̄ⲛ̄ⲛ̄ⲥⲟⲟⲩϩⲉ.

5/13 ⲗϭⲣⲏⲛ. The earliest attestation of this word in a Coptic script is in the Old Coptic Schmidt Papyrus, ed. Satzinger 1975 but cf. also Love fc. e, as ⲗⲁⲣⲏⲛ (line 8). Although thought unattested in Demotic by Richter (2002, 248 n. 13), Zauzich's *ꜣkrn.t* (1983, 172 n. 50) and Vittmann's *ꜣkrn* (1996, 438) are readings of the same attestation (*CDD ꜣ*, 97) which had already been identified by Satzinger (1975, 49 n. 60) in P.Vind. inv. D 10000, ed. Janssen (1954, 28–29), cf. also Zauzich (1983). The relevant clause reads "The infertile (will) rejoice while the child-bearing will be glad because of the good things" (*tꜣ ꜣkrn.t (r) ỉhy r (i.e. ỉw) tꜣ ms.ṯ.t r ršy tbꜣ nꜣ mt.w(t) nfr.t*, 3/2–3) (Zauzich 1983, 167).

ⲁⲩⲟⲩⲱⲧ̄ϥ. For S ⲁⲩⲟⲩⲟ(ⲟ)ⲧϥ/ⲁⲩⲟⲩⲁ(ⲁ)ⲧϥ. This interpretation is much less problematic than that of ed.pr., following a suggestion of Crum (Crum Notebook 87, f. 86), that ⲉⲟⲩⲱⲧ̄ϥ or ⲉⲩⲱⲧϥ "Hail him" should be understood—which was subsequently taken up by Meyer. The present reading would also explain the supralinear strokes over the final ⲧ and suffix pronoun.

The construction with respect to the following ⲑⲟⲟⲩⲧ is noteworthy as in (Standard) Coptic the postponed subject—Thoth—would be introduced principally by the mediator ⲛ̄- or ⲛ̄ϭⲓ, whereas apposition is found principally when an independent pronoun follows. For the parallel attestation of Thoth in other divine dramas, see the excursus to §9.

5/14 ⲁϥⲉⲓ ⲉⲃⲟⲗ ϩⲏⲧ. For ⲁϥⲉⲓ ⲉⲃⲟⲗ (ⲉ)ϩⲏⲧ.

5/15 ⲡϣⲟⲙ̄ⲛ̄ⲧ̄ ⲛ̄ⲏⲥ̄ⲉ̄. This passage requires clarification insofar as ⲡϣⲟⲙ̄ⲛ̄ⲧ̄ appeared as an epithet of Amun at p. 5/2–3 (ⲡϣ̄ⲙ̄ⲛ̄ⲧ̄ⲛ̄ⲧⲏⲣ). Thus, Dosoo (2021) has suggested to emend the text to "Amun, where are you going, o three <gods>?". This is problematic for the following reasons: (i) ⲛ̄ⲧⲏⲣ is missing; (ii) ⲛ̄ⲧⲏⲣ would be ungrammatical in this position because, unlike in ⲡϣ̄ⲙ̄ⲛ̄ⲧ̄ⲛ̄ⲧⲏⲣ at p. 5/2–3, ϣⲟⲙ̄ⲛ̄ⲧ̄ is the absolute form; (iii) ⲡϣ̄ⲙ̄ⲛ̄ⲧ̄ⲛ̄ⲧⲏⲣ is, as discussed in the commentary to p. 5/2–3, a pre-Coptic grammatical construction (cardinal number in a construct form taking a plural noun); (iv) it seems less likely that here Standard Coptic ⲛ̄-(ⲡ)ⲛⲟⲩⲧⲉ is instead missing; (v) given that Amun was addressed at the beginning of the clause, an apposition following the verbal clause—as opposed to directly following his name—is unlikely. Dosoo (2021) has further suggested that a clause is missing, of which ⲛ̄ⲏⲥ̄ⲉ̄ is the object, e.g. "(I replied,) 'To (?) Isis'". However, although ⲛ̄- as a preposition denoting movement towards is attested, this construction is highly unusual, while something substantial would have to have been lost in the history of textual transmission. Regardless, unlike at p. 5/2 ϣⲟⲙⲛⲧ is in the absolute, not construct form, which agrees perfectly with the fact that ⲏⲥⲉ is introduced with the attributive marker. The composition of ⲡϣⲟⲙ̄ⲛ̄ⲧ̄ ⲛ̄ⲏⲥ̄ⲉ̄ is therefore grammatical and so seems correct, and given that this was the form rendered by the copyist, it should in the first instance be taken and interpreted as integral in and of itself. While philologists may be tempted to reconstruct the ideal of a discourse, the complete absence of bidirectional dialogue in §10 demonstrates that such was not seen as necessary by contemporary copyists or practitioners. For an interpretation of the identity and resonances of "the three of Isis" as the three midwives of the god's mother (e.g. Nekhbet, Hesat, and Sekhathor) in the ritual of the *God's Birth*, see the excursus to §9.

5/16 ⲉⲥϯⲛⲁⲁⲕⲉ· ϥⲧⲟⲟⲩ ⲛ̄ⲥⲟⲩ. Haplography for ⲉⲥϯⲛⲁⲁⲕⲉ (ⲉ)ϥⲧⲟⲟⲩ. The association of the "pains" here described with those of labor is unambiguous given the textual content preceding this phrase. Compare the "labor pains" here to those discovered by Jesus in a doe in the first magical text of P.Berlin inv. 8313, ed. *BKU* I 1 (cf. Beltz 1983, 65–67), ⲁϥϭⲓⲛⲉ ⲛⲟⲩⲉⲓⲟⲩⲗ ⲉⲥϩⲏⲕ . . . . . . [ⲡⲉ]ⲧⲣⲁ ⲉⲥⲧⲓ̣ⲛ̣ⲁⲕⲉⲥ ⲉⲧⲣⲉⲥⲙⲓⲥⲉ "He found a doe who was afflicted, [lying upon a(?)] stone, suffering (in labor) that she might give birth" (1/5–6). For the use of the undefined cardinal number with ⲥⲏ(ⲟ)ⲩ in an attributive construction, compare ϣⲟⲙⲧ ⲛⲥⲏⲩ ϩⲛ ⲧⲉⲣⲟⲙⲡⲉ "three times in the year" in the Sahidic version of Exodus 23:17. As discussed in the excursus to §9, perhaps the reference to "four" is derived from a source text, which was itself applied; that is to say, in the practice of the ritual this number could be replaced by the number of "times" in which the contemporary patient had been in labor. In the excursus to §9, a parallel is discussed from the Edfu Mammisi where Egyptian *św*, the predecessor of ⲥⲟⲩ, describes the time at which the labor of the god's mother has come to an end.

5/16–17 ⲉⲥϯⲛⲁⲁⲕⲉ· ⲧⲟⲟⲩ ⲛ̄ⲥⲟⲩ ⲏⲣ ⲙⲉⲛ ⲟⲩ' ⲧⲉ. For ⲉⲥϯⲛⲁⲁⲕⲉ· (ⲉ)ϥⲧⲟⲟⲩ ⲛ̄ⲥⲟⲩ (ⲟⲩ)ⲏⲣ ⲙⲉⲛ ⲟⲩ'(ⲏⲣ) ⲧⲉ (see also the following note). Crum (*CD* 489a) books ⲛ̄ⲥⲟⲩ ⲟⲩⲏⲣ "such and such a day" (complete with haplography in ⲛ̄ⲥⲟⲩ (ⲟⲩ)ⲏⲣ), which proves appealing in the first instance as providing a placeholder for the user to add the day of the patient's labor: "That she has been in suffering (in labor) is for so-and-so long, and how many is it?". But ϥⲧⲟⲟⲩ interferes, and this understanding would rely on something being missing before or after ϥ-ⲧⲟⲟⲩ, resulting an undesirable emendation to the existing text. The gender of the copula could be seen as unexpected, but Crum collects several examples of the use of ⲧⲉ as the generic copula "often" used with non-feminine subjects (*CD* 391b). Dosoo (2021) parses ϥⲧⲟⲟⲩ ⲛ̄ⲥⲟⲩⲟⲩⲏⲣ, translating "he sends (?) for such-and-such a day", by reading ⲧⲟⲟⲩ as ⲧⲁ(ⲟ)ⲩⲟ, which is phonologically impossible, and does not account for ⲙⲉⲛ.

5/17 ⲏⲣ ⲙⲉⲛ ⲟⲩ' ⲧⲉ. For ⲟⲩⲏⲣ ⲙⲉⲛ ⲟⲩⲏⲣ ⲧⲉ, due to haplography across the line break, the first of which was identified by Crum ap. ed.pr. The problematic phrase caused difficulties for ed.pr., who simply cited Crum's suggestion of "on the how-manyeth (day)" in a note. Especially given the lectional sign following ⲙⲉⲛ ⲟⲩ, this phrase may be constructed from the interrogative ⲟⲩⲏⲣ followed by the preposition ⲙⲉⲛ and a second interrogative ⲟⲩ separated from the copula ⲧⲉ by apostrophe, or, if the lectional sign marked an abbreviation instead, a second ⲟⲩ(ⲏⲣ); compare the construction ⲟⲩⲏⲣ ⲙⲛ ⲟⲩⲏⲣ "so-and-so many" (Layton 2000, 61 §73). This construction is thereby a placeholder for the number of days in which the patient has been in labor. See also the previous note.

5/17–18 ϥⲡⲟⲗ̅ϭ̅ ⲉⲛⲧⲱⲃⲉ ⲉⲙⲓⲥⲉ. Understand (ⲉ)ϥⲡⲟⲗ̅ϭ̅. This clause is taken as a circumstantial following the preceding bipartite nominal sentence, with an initial haplography of ⲉ with preceding ⲧⲉ. Not only would reading this clause in isolation limit the sense that can be drawn from it, but a connection between the two clauses is favorable based on a proposed parallelism with the preceding verbal clause, itself expanded by a temporal adverbial clause. In spite of the emendation of ed.pr. in the notes to the translation, followed by Meyer, to ⲧⲱϣⲃⲉ "seal", the textual content preceding this phrase, and the following reference to "birth" (ⲉⲙⲓⲥⲉ for S ⲙ̄ⲙⲓⲥⲉ), make clear that the text may be understood as written, A (and sometimes S) ⲧⲱⲃⲉ "brick". Dosoo (2021) emends quite substantially to ⲟⲩⲇⲉ ⲛ̄ϥⲡⲱⲗϫ ⲛ̄ⲛ̄ⲧⲱⲃⲉ ⲙ̄ⲙⲓⲥⲉ ⲁⲛ and translates "yet he does not divine (?) his bricks of birth", unlikely given the absence of Greek loanwords in both §§9 and 10, apparent omission of ⲁⲛ, and unnecessary in light of the parallel discussed here, which also explains the pre-Coptic grammar exhibited in this clause. Furthermore, given that the object marker is written consistently ⲛ- or ⲛ̄- in this manuscript, it seems unlikely that ⲉⲛ-ⲧⲱⲃⲉ writes both the object marker and plural definite article. In light of B ⲡⲟⲗϫ, ⲡⲟⲗ̄ϭ̄ could instead be understood as the construct (prenominal) form of S ⲡⲱⲗϫ followed by ⲉⲛⲧⲱⲃⲉ as direct object. As discussed in what follows, the translation of this phrase accords with an older meaning of ⲡⲱⲗϫ, from Demotic *plg*/*plk*, not with its contemporary Coptic meanings, which may help to explain this construction (an object marker or following preposition is not attested in Demotic). Note also that *tby msi̯* "birth bricks" occurs without attributive marker in the following Demotic example, perhaps explaining—at least in the context of this text's Vorlage—the exceptional orthography ⲉ- for the object marker in this construction. Incorporating the preceding ⲧⲉ with this verb is not possible, i.e. ⲧⲉϥⲡⲟⲗϭ, because the nominal form is masculine. The meaning of the otherwise enigmatic idiom "releasing the birth bricks" is clarified by the use of the verb *plg*/*plk* in direct association with bricks (*tby* < *ḏbꜣ.t*) in *P.Harkness*, ed. Smith 2005, dating to 61 CE. At the very beginning of this composition of afterlife texts for the benefit of a deceased woman Tanaweruow, the text reads: "You will board (i.e. the bark). It is Isis who has rescued [you]. It is Neith who has given you a bark. It is the great gods of your town who have released (*plg*) your brick (*tby*)." (1/2). This last phrase is interpreted by ed.pr. as referring directly to the "birth brick" (*tby msi̯*) upon which an individual's lifespan would be inscribed—as paralleled in other afterlife texts in hieratic (*msḫn.t*) and Demotic (*tby msi̯*), see Smith 2005, 89. As a result, the birth brick itself is also used to refer to labor and childbirth figuratively—see Roth 1992, 146; Roth and Roehrig 2002, 136–137—as noted by Smith (2005, 89). Thus, while in *P.Harkness* the reference is to the deceased's (re)birth, in the present text the reference to "releasing the birth bricks" refers to facilitating the birth of offspring directly, where *tby msi̯* (ⲧⲱ(ⲱ)ⲃⲉ ⲛⲙⲓⲥⲉ) translates earlier Egyptian (and hieratic) *msḫn.t* "birth brick", which carries the literal etymological meaning of "place of alighting". For a discussion of birth bricks and the Egyptian conceptualization that a child's lifetime and fate was decided at the moment of birth, and written upon the birth bricks, see the excursus to §9.

5/18 ⲉⲥⲧⲱ. Taken by ed.pr., on the advice of Crum, as the Greek ἔστω, "Let it be", "So be it". However, as considered above at p. 5/5, the insertion of a Greek loanword in a text that otherwise lacks Greek loanwords is problematic.

Korshi Dosoo is thanked for proposing the interpretation ⲉⲥⲧⲱ "if", literally ⲉ⸗ⲥ-ⲧⲱ+ "it being given" (*CD* 493a): see now Dosoo 2021. An attractive explanation previously considered was haplography with following ⲙ̄ⲡⲉⲕ-, and thus an interpretation as ⲉ⸗ⲥ-ⲧⲱⲛ "Where is she?" (focalized). This analysis is problematized by ⲙ̄ having to serve double duty for both the omitted ⲛ and circumstantial converter required in S ⲉ⸗ⲥ-ⲧⲱⲛ ⲉⲙ̄ⲡⲉⲕ-, while the interrogative is otherwise seen as ⲧⲱⲛ (p. 5/3; 5/15).

5/18–6/2. For the ubiquitous trope of finding a deity or their name in the Egyptian tradition, see the excursus to §9. In Coptic magic more specific reference is made in some narrative incantation motifs to the provision of alternative ritual means, including further invocations, as a substitute for the presence of a deity or knowledge of the latter's name: P.Schmidt 1, ed. Kropp, *AKZ* I, text A, lines 14 and following, P.Schmidt 2, ed. ibid., text B, lines 29 and following, P.Berl. inv. 8313, ed. *BKU* I 1 (cf. Beltz 1983, 65–67), verso, lines 2 and following. The motif of internal prescriptions of incantations, probably following on from this late ancient background, continues in Greek texts of the medieval period (Zellmann-Rohrer 2019a, 290–291) with specific parallels including incredulous questions from the deity, who eventually comes along to resolve the affliction, as to why such methods had not already been deployed: e.g. a procedure for relief of general "pain", in which it is recounted how Mary the *theotokos* was disturbed by the patient's cries and asked, "'Isn't there anyone else, with (hands with) fingernails, with five fingers? Let him take hemp, three times let him adjure it and three times let him bind it, let him cut it, let him cast it into the depths of the earth, into the depths of the sea, as the waves of the sea are scattered" (ἕνε ἄλλος μετάνυχος πενταδάκτυλος; νὰ πάρῃ κανάβι, γʹ φορὲς νὰ τὸ ἐξορκίσῃ καὶ γʹ φορὲς νὰ τὸ δέσῃ, νὰ τὸ κόψῃ, νὰ τὸ ῥίξῃ εἰς τὰ ἄβυσσα τῆς γῆς, εἰς τὰ ἄβυσσα τῆς θαλάσσης, ὡς σκορπίζονται τὰ κύματα τῆς θαλάσσης, ed. Almazov 1901, 321 no. 35; re-collated).

5/20 ⲟⲩⲱϣⲏⲛ̄ ⲛ̄ⲛⲉϩ ⲛ̄ⲉⲓⲛⲉ ⲉⲃⲟⲗ ϩ̄ⲙ̄. Ed.pr. offers a rather bizarre interpretation in his notes, suggesting that the "oil of bringing forth" is that utilized in divinations involving oil-gazing, and hence the entire magical text serves "scrying" or "oil-gazing" to produce "visions", resulting in the "queer appearances" that he believed to follow in the next section. The textual content thus far, however, makes unambiguous reference to childbirth, which can easily be connected to an oil that is specifically "for bringing out"—presumably the child. Given that ⲛⲉϩ ⲛ̄ⲉⲓⲛⲉ ⲉⲃⲟⲗ ϩ̄ⲙ̄ is not syntactical on its own, and that ϩⲙ̄ is clearly assimilated to a following non-syllabic ⲡ or ⲙ, the conclusion that something has been omitted by the copyist over the page-turn is inevitable. Rather than several words (Dosoo 2021), perhaps this omission was as simple as ⲡϣⲏⲣⲉ "the child". The prescription of specific liquids to aid delivery is also attested in the Mesopotamian divine drama for childbirth *A Cow of Sîn*—discussed in the excursus to §10. In that composition there is a direct pun between the "oil from a jar" (*šaman pūri*) prescribed to aid the delivery of the divine cow Geme-Sîn, who is suffering in labor, and the words "heaven" (*šamû*) and "calf" (*būru*) (Veldhuis 1991, 21–22).

p. 6/1 ⲛ̄ⲅⲧⲁⲁϥ. Crum originally suggested the reconstruction [ⲛ̄ⲅⲧ]ⲁⲁϥ (Crum Notebook 87, f. 87) without the benefit of autopsy; ed.pr. later confirmed the first three letters on the original, obscured by a fold. The "it" (⸗ϥ) presumably refers to the "oil" (ⲛⲉϩ) of p. 5/20.

6/1–2 ⲡⲗⲉⲃⲉⲛ ⲛ̄ⲧⲉⲥϫⲓⲥⲉ ⲉⲡⲉⲥⲏⲧ. The first noun, for S, B ⲗⲉⲃⲁⲛ, is otherwise attested only in the literal sense of a "cable" used to draw along canal-boats (Vycichl, *DELC* 94b–95a), but the following qualification implies a transferred sense, of an anatomical cable at the back of the woman, i.e. the spine or ridge of the spine. This rendering suits the place upon which "a little oil for bringing out" should be applied, downwards along the back. Vycichl's suggestion that this is an Arabic loanword is untenable given its presence in this text. Dosoo (2021) instead considers Vycichl's identification of ⲗⲉⲃⲁⲛ as an Arabic loanword as evidence that this is not the word to be read here, but in turn does not offer an alternative etymology. Given Arabic لبان noted by Vycichl, perhaps the most parsimonious explanation is that this lexeme instead entered Egyptian from a Semitic root earlier, and this is simply its earlier attestation in written form. Otherwise, it could simply be an Egyptian lexeme that is unattested before Coptic.

6/2 ⲛ̄ⲕ̸ϫⲟⲟⲥ. Corrected from -ϫⲉ-: the copyist may have been confused as to whether the construct (prenominal) or prepronominal form of the verb should be written—or if the prenominal form was first intended, even whether the verb was ϫⲱ, ϫⲟ, or ϫⲓ—but a skip of the eye ahead to the following conjunction ϫⲉ is also possible.

ⲁⲗⲟ. Although ed.pr. took this word to mean "child", the expected orthography is S, B, F ⲁⲗⲟⲩ, B, A, ⲁⲗⲁⲩ and F ⲁⲉⲓⲗⲟⲩ, and although there are some dialectal features which might imply the orthographic convention ⲟ for ⲟⲩ in this text, such as ⲟⲩ for ⲟⲟⲩ in ϩⲣⲟⲩ (p. 5/1) and ⲟ for ⲟⲟ in ⲛ̄ⲧⲟⲧ (p. 5/9)—see **Linguistic and Orthographic Features**—, the most parsimonious reading would be the second person singular feminine imperative form of ⲗⲟ, i.e. ⲁⲗⲟ. The feminine form fits a direct address to the patient, a woman who is in labor, i.e. that her labor may soon cease. Given the semantic range of ⲗⲟ, another viable translation would be "Be healed! Be healed there!" as the concept of healing itself derives from something harmful "ceasing". As noted below, the use of this verb as marking the outcome of a procedure or treatment, such as anointing, in Coptic magical texts favors the former in this context. This interpretation also aids the understanding of these two statements as the first in a string of imperatives directed towards the woman in labor. The use of this verb in magical texts with medical applications is also widely paralleled. In the present text see the commentary to p. 4/18–19; elsewhere, for example, treatment 24 in the codex *P.Macq.* I 1, p. 15/16–19, for a wart which describes the ingredients of a remedy and provides the ritual instructions ⲧⲁϩⲥⲟⲩ· ⲥⲟⲩⲁⲗⲟ "Anoint them. They cease", or the treatment for impaired vision in P.Brit.Mus. inv. EA 10391, ed. Kropp, *AKZ* I, text M, 59, whose beneficiaries "will cease" to be ill or "get relief".

6/4 ⲡⲟⲩϣⲏⲣⲉ. The emendation of ed.pr. to ⲙ̄ⲡⲟⲩϣⲏⲣⲉ is unnecessary, see *CD* 58b.

6/5. Crum's suggestion that p. 6/3–4 (ed.pr. lines 82–83) are addressed to Isis, whereas 6/2 (81) is addressed to Horus, noted by ed.pr., is based on a misreading of ⲁⲗⲟ as "child", i.e. the boy Horus, which is rejected for the reasons given above. ϩⲛ̄ ⲧϭⲟⲙ ⲙ̄ⲡϫⲟⲉⲓⲥ ⲡⲛⲟⲩⲧⲉ need not be connected directly to the preceding clause. This later addition could be considered as applicable to all six of the preceding imperatives—see further the excursus to §9.

§10: **6/6–7/11.** Another recipe comprised of a divine drama, for which term see the note to **§9**: 5/1–6/5, above. The mythological scene is set in the opening lines, where the Cow of Amun—the protagonist—is first addressed while going out to pasture and returning to the fold. Unlike in §9, there is no clear structure of a bidirectional dialogue, but the Cow of Amun is warned against "evils" that would prevent her from "producing milk" before she is joined by three herders. These herders appear in a dirty and disorderly state, reflecting the unideal situation of the Cow of Amun being unable to suckle her young. Two commands are given that provide the resolution, the first perhaps by the three herders, the second by Iao Sabaoth, which involves further journeying across a mythological landscape to encounter and herd "the two brothers". The textual *structure* and *content* as well as mythological and cosmogonic associations and resonances in this divine drama are discussed in detail in the excursus to §9, while the reconstruction and contextualization of the history of textual transmission—including a reconstruction of the pre-Coptic source text—are discussed in **Transmitting Textual Traditions**.

6/6 ⲧⲉϩⲉ ⲛ̄ⲁⲙⲟⲩⲛ. For the identity and associations of the Cow of Amun—Amunet the consort of Amun as well as a host of other goddesses who are equated with *ỉh.t* "the (heavenly) cow" and *ỉh.t-wr.t* "the great (heavenly) cow"—see the excursus to §10. The vocative use of the direct article is particularly common in direct addresses to (manifestations of) deities in Egyptian-language texts.

6/6–7 ⲧⲙⲁⲁⲩ̈ ⲛ̄ⲛ̄ⲧ̄ⲃ̄ⲛⲟⲟⲩⲉ. For an analogy between the "herd" and "humanity" in Egyptian conceptions, which supports the interpretation that this epithet could refer to the Cow of Amun's associations with the "womb" and a primaeval creator goddess who created the sun-god and thereby all his descendants, see the excursus to §10.

6/7, 6/8–9 ⲁⲩϩⲱⲛ ⲉⲧⲟⲟⲧⲉ. “They have commanded you (f.)”, where the third-person plural subject is interpreted as being one and the same as the three herders introduced at p. 6/15, could also be understood in the passive voice: “You (f.) have been commanded”.

6/7–8 ⲉⲧⲟⲟⲧⲉ ϩⲧⲣⲟⲩ ⲉⲣⲁⲉⲓ. Haplography and scribal error across the line-break for ⲉⲧⲟⲟⲧⲉ ⲉϩⲧⲟⲟⲩⲉ ⲉⲣⲁⲉⲓ, as partly noted by ed.pr. The error perhaps stems in part from the copyist’s skipping ahead to ⲉⲧⲟⲟⲧⲉ ϩⲓ ⲣⲟⲩϩⲉ (6/9), and indeed it could also be that the ⲧ in ϩⲧⲣⲟⲩⲉ was corrected from ϩⲓ. The preceding verb ϩⲱⲛ is best taken in its specific sense with ⲉⲧⲟⲟⲧ⸗ “to command”, especially in view of the following instructions; ed.pr. rendered “[t]hey have approached thy (f.) hand”, upon which Meyer improved with “[t]hey have drawn near you”, given that cows do not have hands, but did not consider that ϩⲱⲛ “to command” takes the preposition ⲉⲧⲟⲟⲧ⸗, whereas ϩⲱⲛ “to approach”, does not.

6/9 ⲉⲣⲁⲃⲱⲕ ⲉϩⲟⲩⲛ ⲉⲧⲣⲥ̣ⲱ. The emendation of ed.pr. to ⲉⲧⲣⲉⲩⲥⲱ “to cause them to” or “let them drink”, taken up in the translation of Meyer, is unnecessary (although stemming from an understandable desire for a duality between this second of two phrases). At p. 6/7–8 the female subject has been commanded at dawn to come out to pasture, and at 6/8–9 the female subject is commanded in the evening to return to the stable.

6/11–12 ⲡⲃⲛ̄ⲧ ⲛ̄ⲡϣⲱⲡⲉ. Ed.pr. read ⲛ̄ⲡⲟ̣ⲱ̣ⲡⲉ̣ for ⲙ̄ⲡⲟⲟⲡⲉ “of (the month of) Paope”.

6/12–13 ⲡⲓⲱⲧ ⲉⲙⲡⲁⲧϥ̄ⲣ̄ ⲥⲏⲃⲉ. Literally “the barley, in that it has not yet made blade”, rather than “in that it has not yet made reed”, as ed.pr., reading ⲥⲏϥⲉ.

6/13 ⲛ̄ⲧⲏϭⲙⲉ. Perhaps haplography for ⲙ̄ⲛⲧⲏϭⲙⲉ, or even ⲛ̄ⲛⲧⲏϭ ⲙ̄ⲙⲉ, “(the) genuine” or “precious plants”, as otherwise the purpose of the supralinear stroke marking the syllabic consonant would be unclear. Ed.pr. mentions a suggestion of Stefanski that a singular definite article had been omitted, but this seems less likely than the omission of the plural, by an easy haplography. As the following description makes clear, the plants are anything but “precious”, for in addition to endangering the cows, they cannot even offer useful products for animal herding. This qualification by opposite recalls a style of euphemism used in Greek healing and apotropaic incantations in the Byzantine tradition, in which diseases are denoted by positive epithets in place of their true names, avoiding which may be seen in turn as a further means of defense: e.g. “the sweet one” (τὸ γλυκύ) for epilepsy, in the treatise on magical uses of the Psalms, ed. Zellmann-Rohrer 2018, 121 (text PV §6), with further parallels ibid. n. 4; and in popular conceptions of disease more broadly, “blessing” (εὐλογία) for plague lesions in the seventh-century collection of *Miracles* of St. Artemius performed at Constantinople (§34, ed. Papadopoulos-Kerameus 1909, 52.12–14).

6/13–14 ⲉⲙⲉϥⲣ ⲕⲉⲗⲉⲗⲉ ⲛ̄ϣⲱⲥ. Either a haplography for ⲉⲙⲉϥⲣ ⲕⲉⲗⲉⲗⲉ ⲉⲛϣⲱⲥ (by omission or with ⲉ represented by the supralinear stroke of ⲛ̄), or an attributive construction—"a shepherding crook". However, as above, the former interpretation is favored given the presence of the supralinear stroke.

ⲕⲉⲗⲉⲗⲉ. Stefanski's proposed emendation to ⲕⲁⲗⲓⲃⲉ ap. ed.pr. (adopted also with hesitation by Meyer) is unnecessary, as the word, whether taken as "wooden staff" (i.e. a shepherd's crook) or "sounding-board" used in herding, makes good sense in context. The former would suit best the spelling as transmitted (Vycichl, *DE* 78a s.v.) and the rest of the members of the sequence, being essentially variants of a wooden pole used in different ways in herding. It would be possible but not necessary to regard the word as an alternate spelling for the better-attested ⲕⲁⲗⲉⲗⲉ "sounding-board", best known in a specifically Christian context, "a sonorous wooden board struck to assemble congregation", as well as in monasteries to summon the monks to prayers and meals, perhaps used for the same purpose in herding as bells or whistles nowadays. A close relationship to ⲕⲁⲗⲉ, as proposed by Vycichl (*DE* 78a s.v.), also locates this lemma within the Egyptian (*ḳꜣ(ꜣ).t*/*ḳꜣr.t*) and Demotic (*ḳlꜣ(.t)*/*ḳli.t*/*ḳrr*/*ḳri*) lexicon.

6/14 ⲙⲉϥⲣ̄ ϣⲃⲱⲧ ⲛ̄ⲉⲗⲟⲓ̈ϩ. As at p. 6/13–14 above, either a haplography for ⲙⲉϥⲣ̄ ϣⲃⲱⲧ ⲉⲛⲉⲗⲟⲓ̈ϩ (by omission or with ⲉ represented by the supralinear stroke of ⲛ̄), or an attributive construction—"cow-herding staff". Again as above, the former interpretation is favored given the presence of a supralinear stroke; ed.pr. assumed an omission of ⲛ. The rare ⲉⲗⲟⲓ̈ϩ (repeated in 6/16, 19 below) has recently gained an attestation in a letter from a Theban monastic milieu: O.Uppsala VM 1487 (ed. Engsheden and Winkler 2017, 105–112 no. 2), 22. See also the discussion of ⲉⲗⲟⲓ̈ϩ as an epithet of Anubis in Love fc. e §5.1.2.5.

6/15 ⲙⲁϥⲣ̄ ϫⲟⲟⲕⲉϥ ⲛ̄ⲉⲙⲉ. As in the two parallel phrases in 6/13–14 and 6/14, either a haplography for ⲙⲁϥⲣ̄ ϫⲟⲟⲕⲉϥ ⲉⲛⲉⲙⲉ (by omission or with ⲉ represented by the supralinear stroke of ⲛ̄) or attributive construction—"herding goad"; ed.pr. again assumed an omission of ⲛ.

ⲁⲩⲉⲓ ⲉϫⲱⲓ̈. The "they" that have "come upon" the first-person speaker are not the "seven obstacles", but in fact "my shepherd, my cowherd, my herdsman", as they are described as having their garments torn and mouths drooling on the front of their shoes (p. 6/16–18), before it is asked at p. 6/19 why "you (pl.)" are fleeing.

6/17 ⲉⲣⲁⲩ ϩⲁ ϫⲓϩ ϩⲏⲧϥ̄ ⲙ̄ⲡⲉⲩⲧⲟⲟⲩⲉ. Understand ⲉϩⲏⲧϥ̄ for ϩⲏⲧϥ̄. Although ed.pr. followed Stefanski's suggestion to emend the text to read ⲉⲣⲉ ⲡⲉⲩϩⲟⲓ̈ⲧⲉ пнϩ ерє оγϩⲁϭє ϩнт̅ϥ̅ м̅пєγтооγє, translating "A cord being in the midst of their sandal(s)", which was followed in turn by Meyer, Crum's explanation of the passage (*CD* 796b) does not require any correction to the text, therefore producing the most economical understanding and translation: literally "in that their mouths are under spittle, upon its front, i.e. their shoes" (є-рⲁ⸗γ ϩⲁ ϫιϩ ϩнт⸗ϥ м-п-єγ-тооγє). The prepronominal form of ро is most commonly рⲱ⸗, but M features the form ро⸗ from рⲁ, with the shortened front vowel in this closed syllable perhaps influenced by the suffix pronoun. The rarity of mentions of drooling in incantations (in contrast to prescriptions relating to the occult properties of spittle during fasting) might suggest an otherwise unlikely parallel in a Mandaean text preserved in a copy from modern Iraq: as a sign of desire, it is said of the victim of erotic magic cast on a man on behalf of a woman, "N. shall come after N., his mouth open and his saliva flowing" (Drower 1943, 167 no. 25). Here it may figure more general eagerness or unkempt bodily condition resulting from haste. Spittle only otherwise appears in a recipe in Demotic from *P.London-Leiden*, in a recipe against the bite (*phs*) of a dog (*wḥr*) (recto 19/1–9); as the practitioner claims to be spitting out the blood of a black dog, i.e. of one of the 10 dogs belonging to Anubis, so must the "venom" (*mtr.t*) and "saliva" (*ḏꜣk*) be extracted from the patient. The text is to be recited over a medicinal preparation of garlic with gum, which is applied to the wound. In earlier Egyptian magical texts, spittle is described as something whose lack is negative: in the recipe against a scorpion's sting of P.Leiden I 349, ed. de Buck and Stricker 1940, (x+1/9–x+2/1), a divine drama describes Horus as having been bitten, "at night, when there was no wood, no fire, no spell (*šn.t*) for Horus to recite (*šnꞽ.t*) nor spittle (*psg*) to spit (*psg*)" (x+1/10–11). Although it is the fetching of such a "spell" (*šn.t*) that provides the resolution for Horus in the divine drama, the parallelism in the motif of the absence of certain emissions from the mouth—whether to be spoken or spat—is notable.

6/17–18 пєγтооγє єϥтнϭ н̅ⲗⲁϩмєϥ н̅кєм. Literally "their pair-of-shoes, in that it is bound (or, fastened) with black *lahmef*". Following the suggestion of Stefanski, ed.pr. understood єϥтнк н̅ⲗⲁϩмϥ н̅кⲁм, translating "fastened with … of grass". The parallel phrase at p. 7/1—constructed in a dualistic manner as other phrases, above—пєктооγє тнк н̅ⲗⲁс н̅кⲁм "their shoes, being bound (or, fastened) with (a) reed needle (or, black flax)", suggests a similar meaning for the phrase ⲗⲁϩмєϥ н̅кєм here, or that ⲗⲁϩмєϥ was mistakenly written for ⲗⲁс. The difficulty is that ⲗⲁϩмєϥ is firmly attested elsewhere with an entirely different sense, apparently relating to wages: it was booked by Crum as "meaning unknown, ? relates to pecuniary matters (hire, wage)" (*CD* 150a); for that group of attestations, see most recently the discussion of the caption to a scene among the medieval wall paintings in a church at Tebtunis (Walters 1989, 202) in Zellmann-Rohrer 2019b. The pecuniary sense of ⲗⲁϩмєϥ is conceivably formed from the verb ⲗⲱϩⲙ "boil" (cf. Hebrew *leḥem* "food", "bread", Arabic *laḥm* "meat", with *leḥem* and *laḥmā* standing by extension for "provisions", "salary" in Aramaic: Jastrow 1903, 704a s.v.; for the derivation of ⲗⲱϩⲙ from *lẖm* see Vycichl, *DE* 102a; the derivation by suffixed *⸗f*, on which see Osing 1976a, 1: 326, is paralleled by that in suffixed *⸗s* for ⲗⲁϩⲙⲉⲥ "cooked food" [Vycichl, *DE* ibid.]; for a further parallel involving the latter derivational pattern, see Love 2016, 41 n. 131). Crum already suspected that two etymologically distinct words might underlie the attestations collected for the original lemma on ⲗⲁϩⲙ(ⲉ)ϥ but dealt with the present instance only as a brief entry in the addenda to his *Dictionary* (*CD* xviii), of which it would remain the only attestation. The difficulty could be resolved in two ways: either the pecuniary sense on its own might suffice to account for the phrasing, if the composer of an earlier version of this incantation intended a pun on the Egyptian *ꜥnẖ* "life" and *sẖ n pr-ꜥnẖ* "sandal-strap" (this suggestion is owed to Andreas Winkler); or the present copyist conflated into ⲗⲁϩⲙⲉϥ an original ⲗⲁⲥ (ⲛ)ⲙⲁϩⲉ "tongue (or, length) of flax".

6/18–19 ⲁϩⲣⲟⲕ ⲉⲕⲡⲏⲧ. The phrase, literally "What concerns you, in that you flee", has the more idiomatic sense "Why are you fleeing" in the construction of ⲁϩⲣⲟ⸗ followed by a circumstantial. Compare the construction at p. 6/20–7/1, where perhaps scribal error across the page has obscured the sense, and therefore a following circumstantial clause is lacking. However, it could also be that ⲁϩⲣⲟ⸗ there was intended simply to be followed by a prepositional phrase. Parallels to this interrogative construction in the discourse between deities are found throughout the Egyptian magical tradition, compare Old Coptic ⲁⲣⲟ̅ (*PGM* IV.96) and Demotic *ỉḫ r-r⸗* (P.Brit.Mus. EA 10378 verso 5/x+5), and see further Love 2016, 33 n. 78.

6/20 ⲛⲉⲕϩⲟïⲧⲉ. The use of the singular possessive article in this phrase with reference to garments contrasts with the plural possessive article in the preceding phrase with reference to shoes (ⲡⲉⲩⲧⲟⲟⲩⲉ); see also the following note.

p. 7/1 ϩⲏⲧ̅ϥ̅. For ⲉϩⲏⲧ̅ϥ̅. As in the preceding note, the shift of pronominal referents from singular to plural continues, which may have stemmed from a copying error, or deliberately as the result of a shift in the dialogue from addressing the shepherd, cowherd, and herdsman as a triplet to a unity of synonyms for livestock-husbandman, to an unspecified one of them in particular, or to someone else entirely. Given this, and the discussion above on p. 6/18, the emendation of ed.pr. to ⲉⲣⲉ ⲟⲩϩⲁϭⲉ ϩⲏⲧϥ ⲙ̅ⲡⲉⲕⲧⲟⲟⲩⲧⲉ ⲉϥⲧⲏⲕ ⲛ̅ⲗⲁⲥ ⲛ̅ⲕⲁⲙ is to be rejected.

7/1–2 ⲧⲏⲕ ⲛ̅ⲗⲁⲥ ⲛ̅ⲕⲁⲙ. For the interpretation of this construction, see the note on p. 6/18.

7/2–3 ⲍ̄· ⲛ̄ⲉⲥⲟⲩ ϩⲏⲣ· ⲍ̄ ⲛ̄ⲉⲥⲟⲩ ⲕⲁⲙⲉ. Given that there is no construct form of the noun S ⲉⲥⲟⲟⲩ—although the present (reduced) orthography ⲉⲥⲟⲩ suggests that this may indeed be one—, the present forms perhaps belong to established compounds, in which the opposition of "black" in the latter and "white" in the former instance, as understood by ed.pr., seems not unlikely, see also **Linguistic and Orthographic Features**. The further suggestion to understand a copying error of ϩⲏⲣ for ϩⲁⲧⲉ, however—made to ed.pr. by T.G. Allen—is improbable. Although Crum booked ϩⲏⲣ as a stative form "meaning doubtful, opp(osite of) black", this understanding stemmed from the comparable instance of this word in two later cases (*CD* 696b). In P.Copte 44 (ed. Munier 1930), f. 83r, the former element of ϭⲁⲃϭⲏⲃ ⲉⲧϩⲏⲣ is given as the equivalent of Greek ⲉⲣⲉⲃⲉⲛⲑⲱ, i.e. ἐρέβινθος "chickpea", and glossed in Arabic as *ḥimmiṣ maqlī* "fried chickpea". In P.Copte 44 f. 63r, ϭⲁⲃϭⲁⲃⲉ ⲉⲧⲕⲏⲙ is glossed with Arabic *ḥimmiṣ ʾaswad* "black chickpea", equivalent to Greek ἔρβινθος μαυρόν (*sic*). As observed by Boles (2015, 62), although these two stative forms were perceived by Crum as rendering opposites, this is certainly not the sense conveyed by the Arabic gloss, suggesting that ⲉⲧϩⲉⲣ is in fact an unattested stative form ϩⲏⲣ+ from S, B ϩⲣⲱ "oven", "furnace" (2015, 62 n. 166). But consider also the Semitic loanword *ḫrr*, which finds its way into Egyptian as "white lead" (*ḫꜣ-rw-rw*) (Hoch 1994, no. 349). The attestation of ϩⲧⲟ ϩⲁⲧ and ϩⲧⲟ ⲕⲁⲙ earlier in the present codex (p. 5/8) makes a copying error of ϩⲏⲣ for ϩⲁⲧ unlikely—even though the apposition of the two terms in a dualistic phrase seems apt.

7/3 ⲍ̄ ⲛ̄ϩⲉⲱ́. The suggestion of Stefanski ap. ed.pr. that ⲛ̄ϩⲉⲱ́ could also render a form of ⲉⲓⲱ seems unlikely given the orthography; Crum's analysis of the form as ⲛ-ⲉϩⲉ-ⲱ, literally "great cow(s)", is preferable. This is therefore an otherwise unattested lexicalized compound.

7/5 ϫⲉ ⲡⲉϫⲉ ⲓⲁⲱ· ⲥⲁⲃⲁⲱⲑ. Iaō represents the transliteration of the Hebrew divine name of the Jewish divinity YHWH, introduced to Coptic via Greek: see in general Aune 1996; Andrade 2015; Wilkinson 2015, 169–177; for its appearance in Coptic magic (cf. 8/1 below), Kropp, *AKZ* III §217; for a derived and subordinate divinity counted among Aions and angels, ibid. §§36, 46, 136 and further Michl 1962, 216 no. 102; for the use of the name as an epithet of Christ, under Gnostic influence, ibid. §49. For medical applications, see e.g. the fragmentary incantation in *P.Sarga* 20.4–5, [ⲛ]ⲣϫⲟⲟⲥ ϫⲉ ϊⲁⲱ ϊⲁⲱ [ ]ⲡ̣ⲱⲛⲉ ⲉⲧϥⲛϩⲏⲧϥ [ ]; for Greek texts, the commentary to *P.Oxy*. LXXXII 5304 2/7 and 5308.6–7. Sabaōth derives from an epithet of this deity conventionally rendered "of hosts" (*ṣəḇāʾôṯ*), transliterated Σαβαωθ already in the Greek versions of Hebrew scripture (e.g. Isaiah 6:3); see also the commentary to *P.Oxy*. LXXXII 5305 2/12, 3/7; Kotansky, Kovács, and Prohászka 2015, 139; and for Coptic, Kropp, *AKZ* III §217.

The attribution of commands to this deity is also paralleled in a later Coptic incantation against reptiles in *P.Ryl.Copt.* 104 §4, where it is claimed, "The mouth of the Lord Sabaōth is the one that has said this: let no reptile bite me—I, (so-and-so)—, but let all reptiles of the earth be like stone and iron before me, for it is the mouth of the Lord Sabaoth that has said these (words), and the words of the Lord are true" (ⲧⲁⲡⲣⲟ ⲡ̣ⲟ̅ⲥ̣̅ ⲥ̅ⲁ̅ⲃ̅ⲁ̅ⲱⲑ ⲧⲉⲛⲧⲁⲥϫⲟ ⲡⲁⲓ: ϫⲉ ⲙⲡⲉⲣⲧⲣⲉ ⲗⲁⲁⲩ ⲛϫⲁⲧⲃⲉ ⲗⲟⲕⲥⲧ ⲁⲛⲟⲕ ⲁⲗⲗⲁ ⲙⲁⲣⲉ ⲛϫⲁⲧⲃⲉ ⲧⲏ̣ⲣⲟⲩ ⲙⲡⲕⲁϩ ϣⲱⲡⲉ ⲛⲱⲛⲉ ⲙⲡⲁⲉⲙⲧⲟ ⲉⲃⲟⲗ ⲛⲧⲉⲛⲉⲧϩⲓϫⲛ ⲡⲕⲁϩ ⲧⲏⲣⲟⲩ ϣⲱⲡⲉ ⲛⲑⲉ ⲛⲟⲩⲱⲛⲉ ⲙⲛ ⲟⲩⲡⲉⲛⲓⲡⲉ ⲙⲡⲁⲉⲙⲧⲟ ⲉⲃⲟⲗ ϫⲉ ⲧⲁⲡⲣⲟ ⲡ̅ⲟ̅ⲥ̅ ⲥ̅ⲁ̅ⲃ̅ⲁ̅ⲱ̅ⲑ̅ ⲧⲉⲛⲧⲁⲥϫⲉ ⲛⲁⲓ ⲁⲩⲱ ⲛϣⲁϫⲉ ⲙⲡϫ̣ⲟⲉⲓⲥ ϩⲛⲙⲉ ⲛⲉ, 12–18; incorporating the new readings of Anne Grons from her forthcoming re-edition). The divine commandment in that case may relate to the curse pronounced upon the snake in Genesis (3:14–15).

7/5–6 ⲣ̅ ⲡⲉⲙϩⲓⲧ ⲛ̅ⲁⲃⲱⲧ ⲣ̅ ⲡⲣⲏⲥ ⲧⲓⲛ. With omission of the genitive before ⲧⲓⲛ, i.e. for ⲛ̅ⲧⲓⲛ. Contrary to Dosoo (2021), the prenominal form of the verb ⲉⲓ̈ⲣⲉ used as an imperative cannot here have the meaning "be", i.e. "be north", because this would instead require an imperative followed by a circumstantially converted adverbial clause. There is a partial parallel for the geographic instructions in the Old Coptic portion of *PGM* IV, "He (i.e. Thoth) said to her, 'Arise, my daughter Isis, [and] go south of Thebes (and) to the north of Abydos'" (ⲡⲉⲧϭⲁϥ ⲛⲁ́ⲥ ϭⲉ ⲧⲱ́ⲩⲛⲓ ⲧⲁ̣ ϭⲉ̣́ⲣⲉ ⲏ́ⲥⲓ̣ [ⲧⲉ]ϭ[ⲉ]ⲓ̈ ⲉⲣⲏ́ⲥ ⲛ̅ⲛⲉ́ ⲉ̀ⲡⲉⲙⲓⲧ· ⲛ̅ⲛⲁⲃⲱⲧ [-ⲃⲟⲩⲧ addition supra lin.], 106–107) until Isis finds a character called Belf—discussed further in the excursus to §9. The claim of ed.pr. that the form ⲁⲃⲱⲧ is "antique", simply because it is not ⲉⲃⲱⲧ as is found elsewhere, is to be rejected: the spelling ⲉⲃⲱⲧ is in the minority (Vycichl, *DE* 39b–40a), while a subsequent adjustment of a source text in a southern dialect may also be possible, see the discussion of ⲉ for ⲁ in **Linguistic and Orthographic Features**.

7/6–7 ϣⲁⲛⲧⲉⲕ-. The second person masculine singular pronoun marks a change in the character addressed in the divine drama, as does ⲛ̅ⲕ- at p. 7/9, suggesting that the section p. 7/5–11 is a later addition, discussed in the excursus to §10.

7/7–8 ⲡⲁⲓ̈ⲥⲟⲛ ⲥⲛⲁⲩ ⲉⲩⲱϣ ⲉⲩⲡⲏⲧ ϭⲁϩⲏⲧ ⲉⲡⲏⲧ ⲛ̅ⲥⲱⲟⲩ ⲉⲩⲡⲏⲧ ⲥⲁⲣⲏⲥ. Understand ⲥⲁϩⲏⲧ for ϭⲁϩⲏⲧ in light of the following ⲥⲁⲣⲏⲥ. Ed.pr. attempted to restore sense by emending ⲉⲡⲏⲧ to ⲉⲕⲡⲏⲧ. This infinitive construction, however, must be a continuation of the initial instruction attributed to Iaō Sabaōth (7/5): the addressee is commanded to "make (for) the north of Abydos" and "make (for) the south of Thinis" to chase or pursue the "two brothers" fleeing in that direction. Hence the construction is a purpose clause introduced by ⲉ- which connects with the imperatives of ϭⲛ and ⲣ. For an interpretation of the identity and associations of the "two brothers", see the excursus to §10.

7/9 ⲃⲱⲕ. In addition to its more common intransitive sense, this verb can also have the causative meaning "to send forth" (*CD* 30a), which makes good sense in the context, not least because it accounts well for the following ⲉⲃⲟⲗ.

7/10–11 ϫⲉⲕⲁⲁⲥ ⲉⲣⲉ (...) ⲛⲁ-. An unusual substitution of the Second Future for the Third in a purpose clause, perhaps for emphasis on the following ⲡⲉϥ-ϣⲏⲣⲉ as result of the successful birth.

§**11**: 7/11–7/15. Despite the lack of a new title or instructions, the syntactic Greek at p. 7/13–15 makes clear the presence of a new recipe, unrelated to the preceding, whose aim in turn is the control of bleeding. The imperative κάτεχε "restrain" naturally indicates the presence of a single divinity to whom it is addressed, who should be sought in the sequence of the six-times-repeated Ανουσφ through ανουσφιβιαχ (see the following note); for the contents and traditional background see further the excursus to §11. The juxtaposition may have been suggested by the obvious danger of bleeding during pregnancy, the concern of the previous section.

7/11–13. The element ανουσφ is unparalleled in Greek or Coptic texts. After its six repetitions on its own, it is conjoined with -ιβιαχ, which could suggest an Egyptian etymology via re-division as -φιβιαχ: *pꜣ-hb(ỉ)* "the Ibis (i.e., Thoth)" and either *ꜣḫ.t*, another term for "Ibis", or *ꜣḫ* "effective one (i.e., transfigured Akh-spirit of a deceased)", but the initial ανουσ- would remain unexplained.

7/14 ἐν ποιῷ μέλει. This placeholder formula, where originally the specific location of the bleeding was to be specified in the oral performance of this invocation, is paralleled in the procedure for erotic magic in *PGM* IV.327, giving the archetype for a performative statement to accompany the piercing of each limb of an effigy, περονῶ τὸ ποιὸν μέλος τῆς δεῖνα. The term μέλος might suggest external bleeding as the result of injury; internal bleeding resulting in the vomiting (?) of blood is addressed in the Coptic medical recipe in *P.Mon.Epiph.* 574, [ⲉ]ⲧⲃⲉ ⲟⲩⲁ ⲉϥϣⲱⲛⲉ ⲉⲡ̣ⲉϥⲥⲁ ⲛ̄ϩⲟⲩⲛ ⲉϥⲛ̣ⲁ̣ⲛⲉϫ ⲥⲛⲟϥ ⲉϩⲣⲁ̈ⲓ (1–3).

τοῦ ⲇⲇ. A highly abbreviated form of a formula with placeholders for identification of a person, here the patient whose bleeding is to be staunched, by name and mother's name (metronym), as found also in the Coptic portion further on; see pp. 3/9 and 4/5 with the commentary.

τί. For ὅτι; on the form cf. e.g. P.Lond. inv. 2173 (ed. Zellmann-Rohrer 2017b, 156–166 no. 4), 20, τὶ ἂν ἦ̣ "whatever there is".

7/15 Δαμναμενεύς. For the identity of this divinity, and the motif of commands attributed to higher powers, see the excursus to §11.

§12: 7/16–8/4. An invocation of the Sun and three angelic powers, with the goal of winning favor and other benefits for the user especially before one particular target; there are signs in turn of translation from a Greek exemplar, which begin with the loanword used for the title. For the traditional background, see further the excursus to §12.

7/16 ⲭⲁⲣⲓⲧⲓ. An abbreviation of ⲭⲁⲣⲓⲧⲓⲥⲓⲟⲛ, a loanword from Greek χαριτίσιον, a phonetic spelling in turn for χαριτήσιον. The latter is common as a rubric in Greek ritual texts, e.g. *PGM* XXXVI.274, and internal reference to the desired effect is sometimes also made via this term in invocations, e.g. *P.Oxy*. LXV 4468 verso 1/16 δωρήσατέ μοι χαριτήσια "grant me (the results of) *charitesia*"; see further the excursus to §12.

7/17. For the salutation of the Sun with ⲭⲁⲓⲣⲉ (Greek χαῖρε) and its combination with the traditional Egyptian reference to "those who are with you" (ⲛⲉⲧⲛ̄ⲙ̄ⲙⲁⲕ) see the excursus to §12.

7/18 ⲡⲉⲧⲉⲡⲱϥ ⲡⲉ ⲡⲉⲭⲁⲓⲣⲉ. Ed.pr. rendered "Hail to that which is thine", suggesting the deletion of the second ⲡⲉ- and the beginning of a new salutation with ⲭⲁⲓⲣⲉ, but the relative clause is readily comprehensible as written, with nominalized ⲡⲉⲭⲁⲓⲣⲉ to denote the salutation itself, as subject of ⲡⲱϥ instead of an undefined antecedent. Such a construction is paralleled in the invocation of Anubis in *P.London-Leiden* recto 21/7 as "he to whom this earth belongs" (*pꜣ nti pꜣy=f pꜣy pꜣy kḥ*, i.e., *ⲡⲉⲧⲉⲡⲱϥ ⲡⲉ ⲡⲉⲓ̈ⲕⲁϩ). The nominalized form ⲡⲉⲭⲁⲓⲣⲉ is attested also in P.Vind. inv. K 192 (ed. Stegemann 1934, 12–14 text I; with Till 1935, 196–200 and Polotsky 1937, 120–127), 14–15.

7/19 ⲙⲓⲭⲁⲏⲗ. For the archangel Michael in Coptic magical texts see Kropp, *AKZ* III §§138–140; for Greek texts see further Michl 1962, 243–251, and the commentary to *P.Oxy*. LXXXII 5306.7. The earliest attestation of Michael in an Egyptian-language magical text in the Old Coptic script is *PGM* IV.16 (ed. Love 2016, 17; for discussion, see ibid. 20 n. 27; 29). The absolute earliest attestation of Michael in an Egyptian-language magical text is in the partial parallel to the Old Coptic example in Demotic in *P.London-Leiden* recto 21/1–9, in which Michael features among a string of transcribed divine names: a mix of the Jewish Iaho, Sabaho, Atonai, Iauiu (*y-ʿ-w-y-w*[Go], perhaps an alternate transcription of *yʿ-i͗wi̯.w*, i.e. Yahweh: see Quack 2004, 484), and the fellow-angels Sabael and Mistemu (perhaps from Hebrew Mastema, possibly attested in Σαταμα in *PGM* IV.390 and certainly in ⲙⲁⲥⲧⲉⲙⲁ in P.Brit.Mus. EA 10376, ed. Crum 1934a, 15–16: see Quack 2004, 490), and the Egyptian Anubis. These beings are to be invoked and "hailed": *ꜣwe.t̰=f* (…) *m-y-k-h-ʿ-e-l*[Go] (ibid. 6). In the Michigan text, ⲭⲁⲓⲣⲉ stands roughly in place of *ꜣwe.t̰=f*, an archaic form in itself, which can be found in the transcription ⲉⲟⲩⲱⲧϥ in the Old Coptic example in *PGM* IV. Michael also appears in conjunction with Osiris in that manuscript: in one case there is an address to "Harkentechtha, who appears beside Lord Osiris" and "Michael, Archangel of Angels" (2355–2357). In *PGM* VII.1009–1016, Michael is invoked in a procedure for dream-divination alongside Sabaoth, Raphael, and Gabriel, to "enter" and "bring a response" to the practitioner. Over the course of the Coptic tradition, no doubt in connection with his veneration among the saints (including the same Fayum region that produced the Michigan codex, see e.g. Walters 1989, 205; and in general, Michl 1962, 251), Michael attracted such lengthy invocations as that to which the miniature codex P.Heid. inv. K 686 was devoted (ed. Kropp 1966), dated to the second half of the tenth century, and prescribed for a range of ritual aims.

ⲅⲁⲃⲣⲓⲏⲗ. For Gabriel see the notes to p. 4/5 above. The archangels Michael and Gabriel are invoked together in P.Heid. inv. K 518 (ed. *P.Bad.* V 131; cf. Meyer and Smith 1994, 161–164 no. 77), in which they are asked to "fill the heart" of the female target "with every fiery desire, and every longing and every passion and every lust" to make her come to the beneficiary (ll. 6–9).

7/20 ⲥⲉⲙⲉⲥⲓⲗⲁⲙⲯ. As Σεμεσιλα(μ)ψ the name is widespread in Greek ritual texts; for some proposed etymologies, see Brashear 1995, 3598 and A. Mastrocinque in *SGG* I p. 104; for Coptic, Kropp, *AKZ* III §207.

ⲙⲁϯ. As invocations of angelic powers to grant various aspects of favor are attested with simple ϯ (see the excursus to §12), this form is taken as a doubled imperative composed of ⲙⲁ-ϯ, for which see *CD* 392b, rather than a variant (as B) for ⲙⲁⲧⲉ.

p. 8/1 ⲓ̅ⲁ̅ⲱ̅. For the divine name see the note on p. 7/5 above; for the motif of requesting power and other positive qualities as attributes of divinities, see the excursus to §12.

ⲁⲃⲣⲁⲥⲁⲝ. An originally Gnostic divinity, whose name bore additional, intrinsic power through its designation of the number of days in the year (365) via the psephistic value of its letters as numerals: see Michl 1962, 201–202 no. 4 and the commentary to *P.Oxy.* LXXXII 5305 3/8 for this background and his role in Greek-language ritual texts; for Coptic in particular, Kropp, *AKZ* III §203, and most recently the amulet against tonsillitis, P.Ant. inv. 15.11.13 (ed. Delattre 2014), 27.

8/2 ⲥⲁⲃⲁⲱⲑ. For the divine name see the note on p. 7/5 above.

ⲛ̅ϩⲣ̅ⲛ̅. Standard S would have ⲛⲁϩⲣⲛ-. Ed.pr. suggested an emendation to ⲛ̅ⲛⲁϩⲣ̅ⲛ̅, but in that case there would be a superfluous ⲛ.

8/3 ⲕⲟⲓ̈. An abbreviation of the loanword from Greek κοι(νά). The earliest attestation of this Greek loanword in an Egyptian-language magical text is probably to be found in *PGM* IV.25 and 87 in the abbreviated writing κο (Love 2016,

17; 23 n. 47; 25; 26 n. 60); for attestations in Coptic documentary texts in general: Förster 2002, 424–425. Its original sense in Greek would suggest an instruction such as "continue (a sequence of requests or magical words) *ad libitum*", but in some cases it is associated counterintuitively with the place where the user is to insert the particulars of the scenario of use: see P.CtYBR inv. 1206 recto 3/1 with the note in the edition of Zellmann-Rohrer 2020a, 33–44.

ⲁ̣ⲁ̣. For the abbreviation see p. 7/14 above.

8/3–4 ⲡⲉⲩϩⲟ ⲛ̄ⲥⲁ ⲡⲁϩⲟ. There are no precise parallels for this phrase in *charitesia*; more broadly it is asked that an angel bring comparable benefits to the user's "face" in P.Lond.Copt. Or. 6796 (2–3) recto (ed. Kropp, *AKZ* I, text G), 95–96, ⲥⲁⲣⲁⲫⲟⲩⲏⲗ ⲙⲁⲣⲉϥϯ [ⲧⲁⲓ̈ⲟ ⲙⲛ̄] ⲟⲩⲉⲟⲟⲩ ⲙⲛ̄ ⲟⲩϩⲙⲟⲧ ⲉⲡⲁϩⲟ. Crum (*CD* 647a) cites the present phrase among comparable adverbial phrases ϩⲟ ⲙⲛ ϩⲟ, ϩⲟ ⲟⲩⲃⲉ ϩⲟ, and ϩⲟ ϩⲓ ϩⲟ, all of which seem to have entered Coptic via translation primarily from the Old and occasionally the New Testament: it is probable that this instance is one more reflex of a Hebraism, rendering *pānîm el-pānîm* "face-to-face" (here i.e. "them being face-to-face with me"). The relationship between "grace" (ⲭⲁⲣⲓⲥ) and the "face" (ϩⲟ), whether giving to (beneficent) or taking from (malign), respectively, is attested broadly in the Coptic magical tradition. In a formulary recipe seeking favor, or love, in P.Macq. inv. 588 (ed. Dosoo 2018), the command is "You will give grace to the face of [...]" (ⲉⲕⲁϯⲭⲁⲣⲓⲥ ⲉⲡϩⲟ ⲛ̣[ ], 12). Correspondingly, recipes for "favor" (ⲭⲁⲣⲓⲥ) commonly require that users "anoint" (ⲧⲱϩⲥ) their "face" (ϩⲟ): see, for example, the recipe titled ⲟⲩⲭⲁⲣⲓⲥ "Favor" in P.Leid. inv. F 1964/4.14 (ed. Green 1987), verso 2–3, as well as in an application of a prayer in a formulary "on account of your people and the people of your village" (ⲉⲧⲃⲉ ⲛⲉⲕⲣⲱⲙⲉ ⲙⲛ̄ ⲛⲉⲕⲣⲙⲛϯⲙⲉ) in P.Mich. inv. 593 (ed. Worrell 1930, 249), presumably to gain their favor more specifically. By comparison, in the formulary recipe for a curse in P.Heid. inv. K 500+501 (ed. *P.Bad.* V 123), 52–84, the command is to "take the grace from his face for all the days of their (*sic*) life, so that everyone who sees him will hate him and pass him by" (ϫⲉⲧⲛⲁⲃⲉⲓ ⲧⲉⲭⲁⲣⲓⲥ ϩⲉⲛ ⲡⲉϥϩⲟ ⲛⲛⲉϩⲟⲟⲩ ⲧⲏⲣⲟⲩ ⲙⲡⲉⲩⲱⲛⲁϩ ⲟⲩⲱⲧ ⲛⲓⲙ ⲛϣⲁⲃⲛⲁⲩ ⲉⲣⲟϥ ⲉϥⲉⲙⲉⲥⲧⲟϥ ⲛϥⲥⲁⲧⲧⲁⲃ ⲛⲥⲟϥ, 62–64). In an applied curse against several individuals, P.Louvre E 14.250 (ed. Drioton 1946), the idiom is that "None of them will be able to see the face of another among them" (ⲛⲛⲉⲟⲩⲁ ϩⲓ̈ⲟⲟⲩ ⲉϣⲛⲁⲩ ⲉⲡϩⲟ ⲛ̇ⲛⲟⲩ̣[ⲁ ϩ]ⲓ̣̈ ⲛⲉⲩⲉⲣⲏⲩ, recto 11–12, 23 and verso 8). This curse is combined with its inverse in the formulary of P.Heid. inv. K 679 (ed. *P.Bad.* V 142), where the command is "You (pl.) will take the grace [from] his face and you (s.) will give to him the grace of his anus with destruction and hatred and scattering and reversal" (ⲧⲉⲧ̇ⲛ̇: ⲃⲓ ⲧⲉⲭⲁⲣⲓⲥ [ⲉ]ⲡⲉⲃϩⲁ: ⲧⲉⲕϯ ⲛⲁⲃ ⲉⲧⲉⲭⲁⲣⲓⲥ ⲉⲡⲉⲃⲙⲁⲛϩⲉ ⲙⲁⲁⲥ:· ϩⲓ ϣⲟϥ ϩⲓ ⲙⲁⲥϯ, 10–11). Similar to the preceding example, the aim is that "None of all those who dwell with him will be able to look at the face <of> NN" (ⲛⲉⲗⲟⲟⲩ ⲛⲣ̣ⲱ̄ⲙⲓ̣ ⲉⲛⲓⲃⲓ̣ ⲛ̣[ⲉⲧⲟ]ⲩ̣ⲁϩ: ⲛϩⲏⲧϥ ⲛⲉϣ ϭⲱϣⲧ ⲉⲣⲟϥ : ⲉⲡϩⲁ ⲛⲓⲙ, 12–13). Finally, a command might not only “take grace away” but also prevent someone “receiving grace”, perhaps even to counter a beneficent recipe, for example in the formulary recipe for a curse in P.Heid. inv. K 681 (ed. *P.Bad.* V 139), the command is that “Her face will not receive grace, nor her work” (ⲛⲉⲡⲉⲥϩⲁ ϫⲓ ⲭⲁⲣⲓⲥ : ⲟⲩⲧⲉ ⲡⲉⲥϩⲱⲃ, 45–46).

8/4 ⲏⲇⲏ ⲃ̄· ⲏ ⲧⲁⲭⲩ ⲃ. The ⲏ might be suspected as an uncancelled false start of an erroneous repetition of ⲏⲇⲏ (compare the hybrid of full and abbreviated forms of this formulaic closing at p. 4/5–6, ἤδη β̄ ταχὺ ταχύ, and the Coptic transliteration ⲏⲇⲏ ⲏⲇⲏ ⲧⲁⲭⲩ ⲧⲁⲭⲩ at p. 10/6), but it can be maintained as a transcription of the Greek conjunction ἤ (see p. 13/7 below). The rest is an abbreviated writing (as also p. 3/12–13 above) of the ἤδη ἤδη, ταχὺ ταχύ common in the Greek magical papyri and related ritual texts (see Jordan 2006, 166), in a style probably influenced by Egyptian, represented in *P.London-Leiden* recto 10/9; 11/21; 20/4; 21/43, “‘in haste’, twice, ‘quickly’, twice” (*ys sp-sn tkr sp-sn*). The full form *ys ys tkr tkr* is in fact not found in any extant Egyptian texts.

§13: 8/5–13. An amulet, internally labeled as such with the rubric φυλακτήρ(ιον), for stomach- and headaches. The mechanism is the inscription of a composite of text and ritual signs on a tin sheet, including sequences of the seven Greek vowels progressively diminished as an analogy for the deletion of the affliction: see further the excursus to §13.

8/6 εἰς κασσίτερ(ον). Understand “a thin sheet of tin”, with a similar ellipse as in εἰ ἀργυρᾶν above (p. 2/12 with the note). Tin was favored for the inscription of amuletic texts according to surviving formularies (see the note on *Suppl.Mag.* II 94.37; by contrast, an inscription for use in erotic magic in the Coptic formulary P.CtYBR inv. 1791, second text [ed. Emmel 1994, 351–353 no. 3], is to be written ⲉⲩⲡⲉⲧⲁⲗⲱⲛ ⲛ̄ⲕⲁⲥⲓⲧⲏⲣⲛ̄ [2]), though in the archaeological record it is rare in that role (Kotansky, *GMA* p. xvi: no attestations; cf. now *SEG* LXIII 862 on pewter), in comparison to large numbers of lamella-amulets in gold and silver. The famous “Getty hexameters”, amounting to amuletic incantations in Greek from Sicilian Selinous of the fifth century BCE, refer internally to inscription on tin (*SEG* LXIV 680.2–3) despite being preserved on a lead tablet.

8/7–13. The central design framed within a rectangular, double-piped and hatched border consists primarily of ritual signs (for which in general see p. 2/8–9 with the notes) but includes at bottom left a group that may be resolved as κοι, i.e. the abbreviation for κοι(νά) encountered above as a loan-word in the Coptic portion at p. 8.3 (see the note there), and which at an earlier stage may have belonged to instructions following the design in a formulary, to insert the “particulars” of the current healing scenario such as the patient’s name and precise pathology (for instructions alongside and within exemplars for gem-motifs and their finished products see recently Faraone 2020). The majority of the rest of the design is Greek letters with or without the addition of ringed termini: in the first line, σ (in its lunate form c) υ ϛ λ χ, in the second, υ υ ζ σ (again lunate), in the third, σ ι, in the fourth ι η ϛ. Three of the ring-signs, the last two in the third line and the first in the fourth line, are more abstract shapes. The first sign in the first line and third and fourth in the second, finally, resemble the cross-roads or walled-settlement hieroglyph, for which see p. 2/8–9 above with the note.

Flanking this design and its border are two sequences of the seven Greek vowels, each repeated in a wing-like formation with the deletion of the last letter of the previous line: for the background of this motif see the excursus to §13.

§14: pp. 9/1–17 + 10/7–11. A medical recipe for the treatment of kidney-stones, via a combination of a medicinal potion and ritual action, the wallowing of the patient in a horse-wallow (see further the excursus to §14), before immersion in a hot bath. The procedure takes up the entirety of p. 9; the continuation on p. 10 apparently had to fit around a separate text previously copied in six lines of originally blank space there (§15), a general-purpose invocation for divine assistance (see further below).

9/1 ⲡϣⲱ ⲛⲟⲩⲙⲏ. The correction ϣ̄ⲛ̄ⲟⲩⲁⲙⲟⲙⲉ suggested by Crum ap. ed.pr. is unnecessary, as the text can be understood as written. The similar ⲡϣⲱ ⲛⲙⲏ, literally "urine-sand", is found among additional applications for a treatment for splenitis in *P.Med.Chassinat* 65/125–128 (p. 173), a compound potion whose ingredients include honey and wine, as in the Michigan text. The phrase probably renders terminology from Graeco-Roman medical literature of Late Antiquity: in a section of the *De medicamentis* on kidney disorders, Marcellus Empiricus prescribes remedies that can "also draw out the so-called 'gravelly sand'" (*quae etiam quasi harenam sablosam interdum detrahit*, 26.2) or "sand-like bits of stones" (*detrahere ... fragmina quaedam lapidum quasi harenam*, 26.10) or cause the stones to dissolve into sand (*medicamentum ... cuius beneficio in harenam soluuntur lapides*, 26.11). On the condition see further Till 1951a, 26 no. N1.

9/2 ⲫⲓⲗⲁⲛⲓⲥ. The ingredient has not yet been definitively identified, but the meaning seems better sought in Greek than Coptic, which yields nothing plausible. A deformation of the plant-names φυλλανθές or φυλλάνθιον (both obscure, and the former only a conjectural reading in Theophrastus, see LSJ s.v.) is conceivable, but an otherwise unattested compound of φύλλον and ἄννησον, "anise-leaf", may be preferable as anise is recommended to treat urinary disorders in Graeco-Roman medicine: dysuria in Hippocrates, *De mulierum affectibus* §90, and kidney-stones in Marcellus Empiricus, *De medicamentis* 26.2 (cf. the previous note), 26.10, and 26.135.

9/3 ⲉⲃⲣⲓⲁⲁⲙ. As ⲁⲁⲙ figures in *P.Med.Chassinat* 225/403–404 (p. 316) in a remedy for indigestion, and the following series of ingredients is concerned with seeds, the analysis of this compound as ⲉⲃⲣⲓ-ⲁⲁⲙ "*aam*-seed" is preferable to the explanation of ed.pr. via ϣⲉ ⲛ̄ⲁⲃⲣⲁϩⲁⲙ. For the former Chassinat compares ancient Egyptian *ˁˁm*, a plant attested in medical papyri, unidentified at the time of writing (see also Till 1951a, 106 no. 1; *DE* 9a); more recently it has been associated with carom (*ajwain*, *Tachyspermum ammi*, the Greek ἄμ(μ)ι): *CDD* ˁ 43–44. ⲉⲃⲣⲓ-, which recurs twice in the following lines, seems therefore to be an otherwise unattested construct form of S ⲉⲃⲣⲁ, compare especially F ⲃⲣⲉⲉⲓ.

9/4 ⲉⲃⲣⲓⲥⲉⲗⲓⲛⲏ. A compound of ⲉⲃⲣⲓ- "seed" (see the previous note) and a loanword from Greek σέλινον; see further Till, 1951a, 94 no. 144.

9/5 ⲉⲃⲣⲓⲉⲙⲓⲥⲉ. A compound of ⲉⲃⲣⲓ- "seed" (see the note on 9/3) and ⲉⲙⲓⲥⲉ "dill". For dill as a medical ingredient in Coptic texts, see Till 1951a, 53 no. 25.

ⲛ̄ⲅ̄ϯ. The pendant conjunctive without preceding verbal form may simply assume an elided imperative such as ϫⲓ, but it could also be seen to translate one of the participles common in the syntax of Greek medical recipes (e.g. βαλών), especially as the construction is found also at pp. 13/15–16 and 14/9 below; such a function of the conjunctive in translating Greek is also found in the Demotic magical papyri.

9/5–6 ⲛ̄ⲅ̄ϯ ⲉⲃⲓⲱ ⲛ̄ⲥⲱⲟⲩ. This mixing instruction is closely paralleled in the Coptic medical recipes P.Louvre AF 12530 (ed. Richter 2014, 165–183 no. 3), verso 72–74, ⲛ̄ⲅ̄ⲧⲓ ⲉϫⲱϥ ⲛⲟⲩⲉⲃⲓⲱ; P.Berl. inv. 22190 (ed. *BKU* III 393), 6, [ ] ϩⲓ ⲉⲃⲓⲓⲱ ⲛ̄ⲅ̄ⲭⲣⲱ; P.Berl. inv. 8109 (ed. *BKU* I 25; cf. Beltz 1984, 88–91), recto 12, ϯ ⲛⲁϥ ϩⲓ̈ ⲉⲃⲓⲱ ϣⲁϥⲗ̣ⲟ̣ (ϣⲁ̣ϥ̣[ ], Beltz); and possibly the medical notes on wall-plaster from Wadi Sarga, *P.Sarga* 21.8. In Greek medical recipes honey frequently occupies the final place in lists of ingredients, where it serves as a thickening and binding agent, improves the palatability of medicinal potions, and may contribute antiseptic properties, whether recognized at the time or not. For the medicinal use of honey in Coptic texts, see further Till 1951a, 65–66 no. 60; cf. also p. 12/17–18 below.

9/6–7 ⲛ̄ⲅ̄ⲧⲣⲓⲃⲉ ⲙ̄ⲙⲟⲟⲩ ⲙ̄ⲛ̄ ⲛⲉⲩⲉⲣⲏⲩ. The verb is a loan from Greek τρίβω, not uncommon in Coptic medical recipes: e.g. *P.Med.Chassinat* 174/334 (p. 288), ϯⲣⲃⲉ ⲙ̄ⲙⲟⲟⲩ ⲙ̄ⲛ ⲛⲉⲩⲉⲣⲏⲩ (a styptic powder); *P.Borg.Copt.* 278, p. 244 (ed. p. 630), ⲛⲅ̄ⲧⲣⲓⲃⲉ ⲙⲙⲟⲟⲩ ⲛⲅ̄ⲭⲣⲱ (recipe for a skin-ointment); and P.Mich. inv. 593a (ed. Worrell 1935b, 192–194), 18, ⲛ̄ⲅ̄ⲧⲣⲓⲃⲉ ⲙ̄ⲙⲟ̣ⲟ̣ⲩ ϩ̣ⲓ̣[ ] (for splenitis); *SB Kopt.* I 6.30, ⲧⲣⲓⲃⲉ ⲙⲙ̣[ⲟⲟⲩ] (uncertain context).

9/8 ⲍ̄ⲛ̄ⲕⲉ. For medicinal uses of beer in Coptic texts, see Till 1951a, 50 no. 14.

9/9 ⲏⲣ̄ⲡ ⲛ̄ϭⲱⲛ. The adjective ϭⲱⲛ, derived from ϭⲛⲟⲛ, is also used substantively for "mild wine" at p. 10/11 below (ⲉⲕⲥⲉ ϭⲱⲛ); see also *CD* 821b s.v. ϭⲟⲛ. Further specifications of wine are given at p. 10/18 below; for wine as a medicinal ingredient in Coptic texts in general, see Till 1951a, 101–102 no. 166.

9/10 ⲕⲁⲗⲱⲥ. A loanword from Greek via direct transliteration of the adverb καλῶς, as in the medical recipe in *P.Ryl.Copt.* 106 verso 58 and the iatromagical recipe in P.Berl. inv. 8319 (ed. *BKU* I 9), 21 (spelled ⲕⲁⲗⲟⲥ) (similarly P.Berl. inv. 4894, ed. *BKU* I 27, 3; *P.Med.Bouriant* p. 214), and as found also in later Coptic documentary texts: see e.g. the letter *O.Frange* 53.18, and in general Förster 2002, 371. The nexus τρίβε καλῶς reflected here, following on from ⲛ̄ⲅ-ⲧⲣⲓⲃⲉ in the previous line, is in fact found in mixing instructions in Greek medical recipes, e.g. Alexander of Tralles, *Therapeutica* 1.10, 1:473 Puschmann; even more common are the related τρῖψον καλῶς, e.g. Paul of Aegina, *Epitome* 4.21.3, and τρίψας καλῶς, e.g. [Galen], *De remed. parab.* 14:498 Kühn. In Coptic ritual recipes proper, καλῶς is also found as a loanword, especially in specifying the quality of the recipe: in the formulary healing recipe of P.Heid. inv. K 686 (ed. Kropp 1966), for "a man who has been bound (i.e. through a curse) so that he will not be able to join (i.e. sexually) with his wife" and for "a cattle pasture which has been enchanted against you", the recipes are described as having the effect that "It always releases (i.e. the curse) well" (ϣⲁ(ⲃ)ⲃⲱⲗ ⲉ-ⲃⲁⲗ ⲕⲁⲗⲟⲥ) (260 and 267); in the formulary recipe for a curse in P.Heid. inv. K 682 (ed. *P.Bad.* V 137), it closes the ritual instructions for the inscribing of the signs and the offering of frankincense: "It has come to a good conclusion" (literally, "reached its end well", ⲁϥϫⲟⲕ ⲉⲃⲟⲗ ⲕⲁⲗⲟⲥ, 46–47); in a general-purpose formulary recipe in P.Köln inv. 10235 (ed. Weber 1972), the practitioner identifies himself with the statement "I am NN", before seeking assistance "whether love or hatred, whether favor or condemnation, whether binding or loosing, whether killing or saving, whether assembling or scattering, whether establishing or [disestablishing] or watching, well" (ⲕⲁⲗⲱⲥ̣) (33–37); and it is even used to specify the quality of the retribution enacted against someone in the applied curse of *P.HermitageCopt.* 70, where one command states "You (s.) will strike Prēstasia (f.) and Tnounte (f.) and Ebōneh (m.), in haste, well! (ⲕⲁⲗⲱⲥ)" (11–12).

9/11 ⲟⲩⲱⲛ. For ⲟⲩⲟⲩⲱⲛ, not necessarily haplography as this simplification is seen elsewhere in the codex and may represent a genuine phonetic feature; see further the introduction. By comparison, nothing is omitted in ϣⲟⲙ̄ⲛ̄ⲧ̄ ⲛ̄ⲟⲩⲱⲛ earlier in the same line because the cardinal number replaces the article in the attributive construction where a noun follows.

9/12 ⲙ̄ⲏⲛⲉ. Haplography for S ⲙ̄ⲙⲏⲛⲉ, compare ⲙ̄ⲙⲏⲛⲉ (10/11).

9/13 ⲁⲙⲟⲅ. Ed.pr. suggests correcting to ⲁⲡⲟⲧ, which seems phonetically and palaeographically difficult, and the form is repeated. Crum registered the word under a normalized spelling ⲁⲙⲟⲕ "liquid measure", citing only this text (*CD*, addenda p. xv); similarly Till 1951a, 133 no. 5. Tolerable sense may be gained from a noun (albeit unattested) derived from ⲱⲙⲕ "to swallow" (with prepronominal form ⲁⲙⲕ⸗: *CD* 523a s.v.), hence "swallow", "mouthful". This interpretation has a millennia-long precedent in the Egyptian magical tradition, where "swallowing" potions are perhaps best known in the ubiquitous Graeco-Roman Horus *cippi*. This practice is even described in the third person in Egyptian sources, such as in a legend of magical practitioners narrated by Siousire in the cycle of stories conventionally titled *Setne II*; in one episode, Hor, the son of Tanehes ("The Nubian (woman)"), a magical practitioner from Kush, is described as undertaking numerous different ritual acts, one of which is "swallowing magic" (*ỉw⸗f ʿm n ḥyḳ*) (6/5). "Swallowing" in the Egyptian magical tradition is discussed in Ritner 1993, 102–110, and the Hor episode at 108 n. 529.

ⲕⲉⲗⲓⲥⲧⲣⲁ. A loanword from Greek κυλίστρα, a "wallow" for horses (LSJ 1008 s.v., with variant καλίστρα), as proposed by Till 1951a, 133 no. 5; ed.pr. thought of κλεῖστρον "bolt" in his commentary (34 n. 1), which makes for unsatisfactory sense. On the ritual significance, see further the excursus to §14.

9/15 ⲡⲁϩⲟⲩ. Ed.pr. normalized to ⲡⲁϩⲧⲟⲩ, but sense could still be made of the transmitted writing as a prepronominal form derived from ⲡⲱϩ, a more forceful pulling of the legs (apart?) behind the patient's back, cf. *CD* 280a–281a s.v., although no prepronominal form of this verb is booked in Crum or Kasser (cf. *CC* 46).

9/15–16 ⲡⲉⲕⲣⲁⲧ̄ϥ. Ed.pr. considered a hypothetical ⲣⲟⲧⲃⲉϥ "bed", which was rejected by Till 1951a, 133 no. 5, who preferred to leave the word untranslated. The connection to the verb ⲣⲱⲧⲃ (*CD* 305b) remains attractive (compare the rendering of /f/ with ϥⲃ in ϣⲁϥⲃⲉ at p. 4/16), but the sense should be the more general one of the act of reclining, appropriate also to the outdoor setting of the horse-wallow in which the ritual is to be performed.

9/17 ⲧϩ̄ⲙ̄ⲙⲉ. For this substantive sense of ϩⲙⲙⲉ see *CD* 677b; for medical instructions involving the bath, a feature derived from Graeco-Roman medicine, see the excursus to §14. The latter recur at p. 10/8 below (see the note there) and probably 14/19–20; cf. also 11/13. In Coptic see further the directions in *P.Borg.Copt.* 278, p. 242 (ed. p. 628), of an ointment, "Take them with you to the bath; if the person sweats in the bath, apply (it) to his body, let him rub it in, and then wash him in hot water" (ϫⲓⲧⲟⲩ ⲚⲘⲘⲞⲔ ⲈⲦⲤⲒⲞⲞⲨⲚ. ⲈⲢϢⲀⲚⲠⲢⲰⲘⲈ ϯ ⲂⲰⲦⲈ ϩⲚ ⲦⲤⲒⲀⲞⲨⲚ ϯ ⲈⲠⲈϤⲤⲰⲘⲀ ⲘⲀⲢⲈϤϩⲒⲦϤ ⲘⲚⲚⲤⲰⲤ ⲚⲄϪⲀⲔⲘⲈϤ ϩⲒ ⲐⲢⲘⲰⲚ); similarly ibid. p. 243 (ed. p. 629), "Use in the bath" (ⲭⲣⲱ ϩⲚ ⲦⲤⲒⲞⲞⲨⲚ) and p. 244 (ed. p. 630), "Take them to the bath, anoint their body with (the ingredients)" (ϫιτογ ετςιοογν τωϩς επεγςωμα νϩητογ) and "Anoint in the bath with plenty of oil" (ταϩςϥ ϩν τςιοογν μν ογαϣη ννεϩ); and *P.Med.Bouriant* p. 215, of a drug for a female patient in a procedure to promote lactation, "Let her drink (the ingredients) for three days in the bath" (μαρςςογ νγ νϩοογ ϩν τςιοογνε).

εϩραϊ. The word could mean either "up(ward)" or "down(ward)". Crum books βωκ εϩραϊ "to go up to" as occurring "less often" than βωκ εϩραϊ "to go down to" (*CD* 30a); the patient may be imagined to step down into a tub or pool.

§15: p. 10/1–6. An invocation of a supreme deity with control over the entire universe, by a sequence of three thrice-repeated magical words and the originally Jewish name Ia(ō) Sabaōth Adōnāy, for general assistance. It is distinct from §14 and was probably copied before the former, which then had to be fitted around it: see further the excursus to §15.

p. 10/1 ọc̣φη· οςφη· οςφη. There are no exact parallels for this magical word or the following ϊοςφη, but based on their orthographies and several more general comparanda, etymologies can now be proposed. Both οςφη and ϊοςφη suggest an underlying ο-ςφη and ϊο-ςφη, respectively, which can be supported by three considerations: (i) ςφη is a viable transliteration into Greek script of Old Coptic ʒβε/ʒβη, Demotic *šft*, hieratic *šfy(.w)*, derived ultimately from the traditional Egyptian epithet *šfy.tỉ* "respected one" ("respected" in the sense of a reverence for that deity's awesome might and thus coming to mean "mighty one": *LGG* 7, 73; see also Quack 2004, 501); (ii) ο can be understood as Coptic ω, borrowed into Egyptian from the Greek vocative ὦ already in the 2nd century CE, as attested in the Old Coptic erotic recipes of P.Brit.Mus. EA 10808 (ed. Osing 1976b with Love fc. a), x+2/1; x+2/2, and the shortening of the vowel is easily explained by its presence in a compound or more simply by its history of transliteration; (iii) ϊο is attested independently in a comparable vocative role (see the following note). Thus, the underlying meaning derives from "Hail!" or "Oh! Mighty one!"

ϊοςφη· ϊοςφη· ϊοςφη. See the previous note for the etymology of the underlying ςφη in ϊο-ςφη. The initial element ϊο is likely to stem from Egyptian *hy* "Hail!" (as ϊω, see the note to p. 3/4–5, above, and the references therein; *contra*, *DE* 60b), which can be followed directly by a theonym. A derivation of ϊο from Egyptian *ỉ* "Oh!", which precedes verbal exclamations in Egyptian, is not possible.

10/2 βιβιογ· βιβιογ· βιβιογ·. The element βιβιογ is well-known as a component of magical words and longer sequences (*logoi*) in Greek texts: see in general the commentary of D. Martinez in *P.Mich.* XVI pp. 101–102, and more recently Quack 2004, 479, for the derivation from Egyptian *bꜣ-bꜣ.w* "Ba-soul of

Ba-souls", with parallels to the present text in hieratic, Demotic, and Greek. The combination with (ι)ⲟⲥⲫⲏ here recalls the "σιεπη-logos" discussed by Martinez, including the sequence βιβιου βιβιου σφη σφη (e.g. *PGM* XIII.807), for the etymology of which cf. the preceding notes.

10/2–3 ⲓ̈ⲁ̅ⲥ̅ⲁ̅ⲃ̅ⲁ̅ⲱ̅ⲑ̅· ⲁⲇⲱⲛⲁⲓ. Of this pair of divine names, the result of an original transliteration from Hebrew via Greek, the first is a shortened form of ⲓ̈ⲁⲱ ⲥⲁⲃⲁⲱⲑ, on which see p. 7/5 with the commentary, the second a reflex of Adōnāy ("My lord"), originally an epithet substituted for the tetragrammaton YHWH when the latter was felt inappropriate to utter aloud. It is found already in the Greek version of 1 Samuel (1 Reg.) 1:11 (Αδωναι κύριε ελωαι σαβαωθ); for its appearance in Greek ritual texts, see *P.Oxy*. LXXXII 5305 2/12–13 with the commentary, and in Demotic ritual texts, Love 2016, 19 n. 23–24.

10/3–4 ⲡⲉⲧⲁⲙⲁϩⲧⲉ ⲉϩⲣⲁⲓ̈ ⲉϫⲛ̅ ⲡⲉϥⲧⲟⲟⲩ ⲛ̅ⲕⲟⲟϩ ⲙ̅ⲡⲕⲟⲥⲙⲟⲥ. The last is a loanword from Greek κόσμος (see in general Förster 2002, 436), which is used also in a request for universal favor in P.Lond.Copt. Or. 6796 (2–3) verso (ed. Kropp, *AKZ* I, text H), 51–53, ⲙ̅ⲡⲉⲙⲧⲟ ⲉⲃ̣ⲟ̣ⲗ̣ ⲙ̅ⲡⲕⲟⲥⲙⲟⲥ ⲧⲏⲣϥ ⲙⲛ̅ ⲡⲅⲉⲛⲟⲥ ⲧ̣[ⲏⲣ]ϥ ⲛ̅ⲁⲇ̣ⲁ̣ⲙ ⲙⲛ̅ ⲛ̅ϣⲏⲣⲉ ⲧⲏⲣⲟⲩ ⲛⲍⲱ[ⲏ], and in reference to the creation of the universe in the general-purpose invocation in P.Lond.Copt. Or. 6795 (ed. Kropp, *AKZ* I, text F), 32–35; it appears in proximity to Iao Sabaoth in a still obscure context within a curse on an ostracon from Antinoupolis, P.Ant. s.n. (ed. Bélanger Sarrazin 2017b), 11–12, ⲓ̈ⲁⲱ ⲥⲁⲃⲁⲱⲑ ⲡⲉⲧⲙ.[..] ⲛ̅ⲫⲓ̈ϩⲉ ⲛ̅ⲡⲕⲟⲥⲙⲟⲥ. The four corners of the universe may function as a merism for the entirety of creation: in Greek ritual texts compare the mention of four divine names which are "in the four corners of heaven" (*PGM* VIII.8, τὰ ἐν ταῖ δ′ γωνίαις τοῦ οὐρανοῦ), and in a Christian context, angels as "those who cause light to rise from the four corners of the universe" (*PGM* P 15a.6–11, οἱ ἀνατέλλοντες τὸ φῶς ἐκ τῶν τεσσάρων γωνιῶν τοῦ κόσμου), that is, illuminate the entire world. The Greek transliteration of the name of the protoplast Adam, being an acronym for the four cardinal directions in the same language (ἀνατολή, δύσις, ἄρκτος, μεσημβρία), was held as apotropaically powerful by a similar logic (Zellmann-Rohrer 2018, 128 n. 26): it is to be inscribed in turn on the four corners of a dovecote for its protection from predators in a probably late ancient recipe preserved in a Byzantine agricultural encyclopedia, *Geoponica* 13.8.4 = 14.5 (cf. Heim 1893, 524 no. 173).

10/6 ⲏⲇⲏ ⲏⲇⲏ ⲧⲁⲭⲩ ⲧⲁⲭⲩ. Greek ἤδη ἤδη, ταχὺ ταχύ; for the formulaic closing expression of urgency, see p. 8/4 with the note.

§14: pp. 9/1–17 + 10/7–11, continued.

10/7–8 ⲧⲕⲟⲗⲟⲙⲏⲑⲣⲁ ⲙ̅ⲙⲟⲩϩ̅ⲙ̅ⲙⲉ. The phrase is partly transliterated, partly translated from the Greek θερμὴ κολυμβήθρα, immersion in which is recommended in Aetius of Amida, *Iatrica* 4.46 as part of a treatment for a skin disorder. For the role of the bath see also p. 9/17 above with the note. The Greek adjective θερμή has been rendered with a Coptic compound, in which ⲙⲟⲩ- is in the construct form.

10/11 ⲉⲕⲥⲉ ϭⲱⲛ. Ed.pr. rendered "drinking ...", and the entire phrase is left in ellipses by Till (1951a, 133 no. 5), but it can readily be understood in the context of Graeco-Roman medical and dietetic advice regarding baths and types of wine, discussed above. For ϭⲱⲛ, see the commentary on p. 9/9.

§16: 10/12–16. A recipe to treat disorders of the female womb. A generally comparable procedure is given in P.Berl. inv. 8109 (ed. *BKU* I 25; cf. Beltz 1984, 88–91), recto 13–15, a treatment for menstrual bleeding via fumigation with a substance whose name is lost: [ⲉⲧⲃⲉ] ⲟⲩⲥϩⲓⲙⲉ ⲉⲣⲉⲡⲉⲥⲛⲟϥ ϩⲁⲣⲟⲥ [. . . .]ⲟⲡⲟⲥ ⲉⲡⲕⲱϩⲧ· ⲕⲁⲡⲛⲓⲍⲉ ⲙ[. . . .]ⲱⲥ̄ⲛⲁⲗⲟ; the end is read [ ]ⲱⲥ ⲛⲁⲗⲟ by Beltz, but it may be restored ⲙ[ⲙⲟⲥ ⲕⲁⲗ]ⲱ (Greek καλῶς: see the note on p. 9/10 above) ⲥ̄ⲛⲁⲗⲟ. Vaginal fumigations to treat uterine disorders are recommended as early as the hieratic *P.Ebers* (793–795 [pl. 94/3–8], ed. Lalanne and Métra 2017; cf. Goyon 1984); more particularly, fumigation with animal dung is prescribed in *P.London-Leiden* verso 30/9–11; for Coptic, see Till 1951a, 10 no. 13; 27 no. 5 (citing the Michigan and Berlin texts). Fumigations are also offered as a remedy for displacement of the uterus, "uterine suffocation", and other presumed disorders in the Greek medical tradition: see Faraone 2011, esp. 4–9, and the excursus to §12.

10/12 ⲟⲩⲥϩⲓⲙⲉ ⲉϣⲁⲣⲉⲧⲉⲥⲟⲟⲧⲉ ⲙⲕⲁϩ. A similar indication is given for two suppositories in *P.Med.Chassinat* 24/49 (p. 122), [ⲟⲩⲥϩⲓ]ⲙ[ⲉ ⲉⲧϣ]ⲱⲛⲉ ⲉⲧⲉⲥⲟⲧⲉ ⲉⲥϯ ⲕⲁⲥ, and 167/326 (p. 284) ⲧⲁⲁⲥ ⲟⲛ ⲉⲧⲟⲧⲉ ⲛ̄ⲟⲩⲥⲓⲙⲉ ⲉⲥϯ ⲕⲕⲁⲥ ⲥⲛⲁⲗⲟ.

10/13 ϫⲓ ⲛⲁⲕ. The expression is common at the beginning of Coptic medical recipes, see e.g. P.Berl. inv. 8109 (ed. *BKU* I 25; cf. Beltz 1984, 88–91), recto 11 (but Beltz reads ϫⲓ ⲛⲁⲛⲛⲟⲩ); P.Cair. inv. 42573 (ed. Chassinat 1955), f. 2r/12; *P.Med.Chassinat* 70/137 (p. 177); *SB Kopt.* I 2.1–2.

ⲟⲩⲛⲉϩ ⲛ̄ϭⲓⲱⲟⲩ ϩ̣[ⲛ̣]`ⲙ̣´ⲡ̣ⲟ̣ⲩ̣ⲁϩⲉ. Ed.pr. rendered "some oil, (or) fat, or the (fat) of an ox (?)", based on a tentative normalization to ⲛ̄ⲕⲓⲱⲟⲩ ⲏ ⲙ̄ⲡⲁⲩⲁϩⲉ; Till 1951a, 133 no. 6 (cf. also ibid. 82 no. 105.k) translates only "...-öl". Crum (unpublished manuscript notes, Crum Notebook 87, Griffith Institute Archive, Oxford) reads for the last group ⲛ̄ⲅ . ⲟ̣ⲩ̣ⲁϩⲉ; the ⲅ is possible but not to the exclusion of ⲡ, and no plausible verb form can be identified on Crum's reading. For the application of ⲕⲓⲱⲟⲩ, literally "soft" or "fatty", of which the present ϭⲓⲱⲟⲩ is taken to be an orthographic variant, to oil see *CD* 129b s.v. Oil "from the Oasis" (*nḥḥ n wḥꜣ*) is prescribed for ritual use in *P.London-Leiden*, where its genuineness and purity is also required: recto 3/10 (*nḥḥ n whe ỉw≠f wʿb* in lecanomancy) and 6/2 (*nḥḥ n mʿ.t ỉw≠f wʿb n whꜣ* in lamp-divination, similarly *nḥḥ n whe* at 25/12). In this light, ϭιωογ as written, literally "honored" or "glorified" from ϫι εοογ, might be taken as a reinterpretation of historical *ỉw≠f wʿb* "pure" via the additional sense of ογοπ+ as "holy".

10/14 ϐω ⲛ̄ϩⲉⲗⲱ. The reduction of a consonant cluster to a single dental approximant (apical glide) ⲗ, or its replacement with vocalic ⲉ, in ϩⲉⲗⲱ for S ϩⲗⲗⲱ is otherwise unattested. The Graeco-Roman tradition of popular medicine prescribes women's hair for various indications, see Pliny, *Naturalis historia* 28.70–71, among which the fumes (*nidor*) of burned women's hair (but not of old women specifically) promises relief for "uterine strangulation" (*vulvae morbo strangulatae*). This information is reprised in the Byzantine *Geoponica* (5.48.3, with Faraone 2011, 9), where it is attributed to the natural philosopher and sophist Julius Africanus, with an added indication for preventing miscarriage. Possibly an analogical appropriateness was felt with the post-menopausal condition of the elderly womb, as no longer subject to menstrual bleeding and hence calmer. More broadly in Coptic medical recipes women's hair is prescribed in a hemostatic powder in *P.Med.Chassinat* 174/334 (p. 288), ϥω ⲛ̄ⲥⲓⲙⲉ ⲉϥⲣⲱϫ, there mixed with charcoal (ϫ̄ⲃⲃⲉⲥ, cf. the instructions for fumigation over coals here); see also Till 1951a, 63 no. 52.

10/15 ⲛ̄ⲛ̄ϣⲉ ⲛ̄ⲛⲟⲩϩⲉ. In the first element there is an apparent dittography of the attributive marker. For medicinal use of sycamore in Coptic texts see in general, see Till 1951a, 97 no. 153. The sycamore is also used in connection with hemorrhoids in *SB Kopt.* I 5.31–33, which may relate in turn to the metaphorical association of this affliction with ripe figs in the tradition of Greek medicinal incantations (Zellmann-Rohrer 2019a, 282–283 n. 40).

10/16 ⲕⲁⲡⲛⲟⲥ. A loanword from Greek καπνός (cf. Förster 2002, 378); the directions are not precisely paralleled among Greek recipes, but uterine fumigation similarly described, with smoke from burnt willow leaves, in this case as an abortifacient, is prescribed in the Hippocratic *De mulierum affectibus* §78 (περικαθίσας τὴν γυναῖκα ἐῆν ἄχρις ἂν ὁ καπνὸς ἐς τὴν μήτρην ἐνδύνῃ), and more generally the medicinal use of smoke from a set of aromatic substances is recommended e.g. to treat a cough in [Galen], *De remed. parab.* 14:441 Kühn, τὸν καπνὸν ἐν στόματι δέχηται ὁ πάσχων; on fumigation (ὑποκαπνισμός) in general see Aetius of Amida, *Iatrica* 3.144.

ⲥ̄ⲛⲁⲗⲟ. For the verb and its application at the conclusion of medical recipes, see p. 4/18–19 with the commentary.

§17: 10/16–19. A continuation of §16 with a modified procedure in case of a chronic affliction.

10/17–18 ⲉⲣⲱⲧⲉ \`ⲛⲉ´ϣⲁⲩ. The Michigan text remains the only known witness to the prescription of sow's milk in the Coptic medical tradition; for milk in general, see Till 1951a, 76 no. 95.

§18: p. 11/1–8. A remedy for mental illness, attributed to the result of demonic possession, via an amulet consisting of magical signs—among them one possible sign of Christian influence on the cultic background of the codex, which may however be explained otherwise as a pre-Christian symbol—and text enclosed by an ornamental border in the shape of a traditional Egyptian amuletic stele, to be inscribed on a calculous uterine growth. The traditional background of the demonological diagnosis, the apotropaic motif of the stele, and the implications of the use of the uterine stone are discussed in the excursus to §18.

11/2 ⲑⲗⲓⲃⲉ. A loanword from Greek θλίβω (see in general Förster 2002, 339); the verb describes the harmful effects of demons in Greek texts in a Christian context, e.g. *Apophthegmata patrum*, alphabetic collection, Arsenius 3 (PG 65: 88), and systematic collection, 5.47; Sophronius of Jerusalem, *Narratio miraculorum sanctorum Cyri et Joannis* 54.8.

ⲉⲩⲟ ⲛ̄ⲇⲁⲓⲙⲟⲛⲓⲟⲛ. The phrase is probably a calque on Greek δαιμονιακός "demoniac" or δαιμονιζόμενος "possessed by a demon", via the loanword δαιμόνιον with which both are cognate. The same may be said for ⲟ ⲛ̄ⲇⲁⲓⲙⲱⲛ, used in an obscure context in the letter *O.Medin.HabuCopt.* 157.4–5 (cf. Förster 2002, 159): a certain man has come south and sworn an oath that he is so possessed (ⲛ̄ϥⲣ̄ ⲁⲛⲁϣ ϫⲉ ϥⲟ ⲛ̄ⲇⲁⲓⲙⲱⲛ). In the Coptic-Arabic glossary, ed. Munier 1930, 160.23, ⲡⲉⲧⲟ̇ ⲛ̇ⲇⲁⲓⲙⲟⲛⲓⲟⲛ is glossed in Arabic as "those in whom there are satans" (*alad̲īn bihim al-šāṭīn*). The construction is applied in iatromagical recipes in P.Berl. inv. 8116+8117 (ed. *BKU* I 26), 8116b, 18–19, "Apply (the ingredients) to him who is possessed by a demon, and on whom sorcery has been performed" (ⲧⲁⲁⲩ ⲉϩⲣⲁⲓ ϩⲁ ⲡⲉⲧⲱ ⲛⲧⲉⲙⲱⲛⲓⲱ[ⲛ] ⲙⲉⲡⲁⲧⲁⲩⲉⲗ̣ ϩⲓⲕ ⲉⲣⲁⲃ: reading of Crum, manuscript annotations after collation in his copy now in the Sackler Library, Oxford; ⲙⲉⲡⲁⲧⲁⲩⲉⲛ̣ ϩⲓⲕ .ⲫⲁⲃ, ed.pr.), similarly 26–27, ⲟⲩⲣⲱⲙⲓ ⲉϥⲱ ⲛⲧⲉⲙⲱⲛⲓⲱⲛ. The cursing of individuals with demonic possession is expressed with exactly the same construction, simply using the infinitive rather than qualitative of ⲉⲓⲣⲉ, for example in P.Lond.Copt. Or. 5986 (ed. *P.Lond.Copt.* I 1224), 9, ⲑⲓⲟ ⲙ̄ⲙⲁϥ ⲉϥⲉⲓⲣⲉ ⲙ̄ⲙⲁϥ ⲛ̄ⲇⲁⲓⲙⲱⲛⲓⲟⲛ "Cast him down, with him making himself demonic (i.e. being possessed by a demon)", probably a calque on the Greek middle-voice participle δαιμονιζόμενος. The link between sickness and demons more generally is found e.g. in P.Heid. inv. K 686 (ed. Kropp 1966), p. 14/250, among applications of an invocation of the archangel Michael, ⲟⲩⲣⲱⲙⲓ ⲣⲉ ⲟⲩⲧⲙⲱⲛⲓⲟⲛ ϩⲓⲧ ⲙⲁⲃ "A man tormented by a demon"; in P.Brit.Mus. EA 10391 (ed. Kropp, *AKZ* I, text M), 69–73, in a recipe ⲉⲧⲃⲉ ⲡ̄ⲛ̄ⲁ̄ ⲛⲓⲙ ⲛϣⲱⲛⲉ "for every spirit of sickness" that aims "to cast out demons from so-and-so through the writing (of) so-and-so" (ⲉⲛⲉϫ ⲇⲓⲙⲱⲛⲓⲟⲛ ⲉⲃⲟⲗ ⲉϩⲛ ⲁⲁ ϩⲓⲧⲛ ⲛⲉⲥϩⲁⲓ ⲁ̅ⲁ̅); and in a recipe for an amulet in *P.Macq.* I 1, p. 16/5–6, ⲫⲩⲗⲁⲕⲧⲏⲣ· ⲉⲧⲃⲉ ϣⲱⲛⲉ ⲛⲓⲙ ⲙⲛⲉⲧϣⲉⲛⲧⲉⲙⲟⲛⲓ̈ⲟⲛ. On a loose slip added to the latter codex, a recipe is also found for cases involving "a demon" (ⲟⲩⲧⲉⲙⲟⲛⲓ̈ⲟⲛ).

11/3 ⲥⲧⲏⲗⲏ. A loanword from Greek στήλη, a wide-ranging term for monumental markers in durable materials. In Greek ritual texts the term came specifically to denote a textual amulet, probably related to the Egyptian tradition of amuletic stelae in stone, as e.g. *PGM* V.422, VII.216, and *Suppl.Mag.* I 23.10–11 (see also the commentary there); elsewhere, e.g. as a loanword in the Coptic curse T.Köln inv. 35 (ed. *P.KölnÄgypt.* I 11), 10, it is used in a transferred sense for a list of magical names absent any figural arrangement (ⲛⲉⲓⲣⲁⲛ ⲛ̅ⲧⲉⲓⲛⲟϭ ⲛ̅ⲥⲧⲏⲗⲏ). The accompanying drawing here appears to represent an Egyptian monumental stele, in which the ankh-cross matches the hieroglyphic sign for *ʿnḫ*, ornamentally enlarged, found in the top register (lunette) of some comparanda from the archaeological record. In turn the loanword could also designate a burial marker: *O.Crum* 492 (cf. Förster 2002, 750).

11/4 *signs*. The signs currently visible, more abstract geometric versions of the ring-signs seen above at pp. 2/8–9, 10–11, and 8/7–13, appear to overwrite a now-illegible sequence preceding the magical word in the next line, all of which would have complemented the central motif of the apotropaic stele to the right (11/6). Possibly the overwriting was the work of the second of the two later hands that filled out the manuscript (see the introduction).

11/5 ⲭⲟⲩⲃⲁⲣⲟⲩⲭ. This divine name is not otherwise attested. It might be formed from ⲭⲟⲩⲭ, well-attested in Greek texts (χουχ: Brashear 1995, 3582, and the even more widespread χυχ and χωωχ, ibid. and A. Mastrocinque in *SGG* I p. 112), ultimately deriving from Egyptian *kk.w* "(the primeval) god of darkness" (Quack 2004, 500; cf. ⲭⲱⲙⲟⲭⲟⲱⲭⲓ, p. 3/3 with the commentary), and ⲃⲁⲣⲟⲩⲭ, similarly well-attested (βαρουχ: Brashear 1995, 3602; Kropp, *AKZ* II p. 85), perhaps on the analogy of ⲃⲁⲣⲃⲁⲣⲟⲩⲭ as found in P.Berl. inv. 8322 (ed. *BKU* I 7; cf. Beltz 1983, 72–74), 24.

11/6 *stele*. A rectangular stele with rounded top in a traditional Egyptian style (see the note on p. 11/1–8 above and the excursus to §18), whose central field is filled with letter-like magical signs (cf. p. 11/4 above), from which the sequences ⲟⲩⲟⲕⲁⲓ (for the last two signs, ⲁⲓ in ligature, perhaps also Greek ϡ; the first and fourth instead perhaps even Old Coptic characters, ȝ and <, but the last is more likely the metrological abbreviation for δραχμή, cf. *P.Oxy.* LXXX 5249.5–7), ⲥ|ⲧⲙⲏⲁⲉⲧⲱ|ⲗⲟⲩⲗⲓ̈ⲍ; following the final ⲍ possibly the Old Coptic ୨, then ⲓ̈ⲱ|ϣⲏⲩ, ⲭ where each stroke terminates in rings, ⲧⲓ̈ and ⲟ (before ⲟ perhaps Old Coptic ʝ), ⲥ with similar rings, ⲓⲩⲙⲁⲩ, and ⲁⲡⲗⲏ might be discerned. Syntactic Coptic is added at right angles in the side registers (also edited as p.

11/7 below in addition to the representation in the drawing). The pedimental stele features a cross-like sign, which in context probably belongs to the pre-Christian tradition of amuletic stelae as the ankh-sign and need not be taken as a mark of Christian influence, see the note on p. 11/3; in a medical context a similar sign is used to abbreviate χρῶ "use" in pharmacological prescriptions (*P.Oxy.* LXXX 5230 fr. 2.3 n.).

11/7 ⲡⲉⲧϫⲱⲛⲉ. Better sense could be had from a ⲧ- causative of ϣⲱⲛⲉ (an invocation of "the one who causes sickness"), but no such form is attested; if to be understood as the simple verb, ⲡⲉⲧϣⲱⲛⲉ (as ed.pr.), ⲡⲉϫⲱⲛⲉ would be expected, where the dental stop /t/ (ⲧ) turns the fricative /š/ (ϣ) into a palatal stop /d̠/ (ϫ)—compare the conventional Coptic orthographies, e.g. S, L ϫⲡⲟ "to beget", "bear", where the digraph ϫ renders underlying ⲧ-ϣⲡⲟ (*tỉ.t-ḫpr*) as evidenced in distinct A ⲧϩⲡⲟ, and the abbreviated orthography in filiation formulae of ϫⲏ for ⲧ-ϣⲏ- "the daughter of", common to magical texts.

ⲙⲁ ⲧⲟⲩϫⲉ. The latter construct (prenominal) form stands for the absolute form ⲧⲟⲩϫⲟ.

11/8 ⲥⲁϩ̄ϥ̄ ⲉⲟⲩⲱⲛⲉ ⲛ̄ⲟⲟⲧⲉ. The interpretation of ed.pr., "[w]rite it on a vulva stone", may be maintained against the unnecessary modification of Pernigotti, "[s]crivi ciò sopra un amuleto a forma di vulva" (1995, 3717). Such stones and their removal in a contemporary medical context are discussed by Aetius of Amida, *Iatrica* 16.113.

§19: 11/9–15. A procedure to rid a house of reptiles by fumigation. Very similar recipes, though specifically applied only to scorpions, are given in a Byzantine agricultural encyclopedia, the *Geoponica*: fumigation with realgar, galbanum, and butter or goat-fat (13.9.3); and for snakes in the medieval Latin antidotaries ed. Rose 1894, 393 (*Antidotarium Bruxellense* §178) and Sigerist 1923, 95 (St. Gallen, Stiftsbibliothek cod. Sang. 44, p. 254). A collection of methods for driving a broader set of reptiles from the house is also offered in the *Geoponica*, including fumigation with galbanum (χαλβάνη) and another goat product, the hooves (13.8).

11/10 ϫⲁⲗⲃⲁⲛⲏ. A loanword from Greek χαλβάνη, which is probably also to be restored in the prescription for a plaster in O.Brit.Mus. EA 27422 (ed. *O.Brit.Mus.Copt.* I pl. XLIX), front, 12–13 (with Förster 2002, 863; [ ]ⲗⲃⲁⲛⲉⲓ "frankincense", ed.pr.); on the substance in Coptic medical texts, see Till 1951a, 58 no. 38.

11/11 ⲥⲁⲧ[ⲏ]ˋⲩˊⲣⲁⲕⲏⲥ. A loanword from Greek σανδαράκη, apparently transliterated directly from a genitive form in the Greek original from which the recipe was translated, as also at p. 13/15 below, a derivational pattern characteristic of another early Coptic medical text of the fourth or fifth century, P.TT 157-470 (ed. Richter 2014, 156–164 no. 1), with e.g. ⲯⲓⲙⲓⲑⲓⲟⲩ at 1/5 and 1/11; see further the discussion of **Context in the Practice of Medicine and Healing** in the introduction. On realgar in Coptic medical texts, see Till 1951a, 88 no. 88.

11/11–12 ⲕⲛ̄ⲛⲉ ⲙ̄ⲃⲁⲁⲙⲡⲉ. For medicinal use of fat in general see p. 12/16 with the note. The goat's is not specified elsewhere; cf. the prescription of goat's gall in a recipe recorded on wall-plaster at Wadi Sarga, *P.Sarga* 21.9, ⲟⲩⲥⲓⲱϣⲉ ⲛⲃⲁⲙⲡⲉ (indication lost).

11/13 ⲟⲩϩⲙ̣ⲙ̣ⲉ̣. For the term see p. 9/17 above; here it apparently refers to the steam-room in a bath.

ⲕⲗⲁⲇⲟⲥ. A loanword from Greek κλάδος; as also at p. 12/1 below. In a medical recipe of uncertain context (ⲉⲧⲃⲉ ⲟⲩⲛⲏⲃ̣[ ]) on a chip of limestone, *O.Crum* 487, back, 4, leaves whose further specification is also lost are prescribed with the same loanword, ϩⲉⲛⲕⲗⲁⲇⲟⲥ ⲛ[ ] (cf. Förster 2002, 417; possibly the substrate for a ritual text including ⲡⲣⲁⲛ ⲛ̄ⲓ̄ⲥ̄, ibid., 6). For the transliteration compare also the adjuration by "the branches of tree of life", ⲛⲉⲕⲗⲁⲧⲟⲥ ⲙⲡϣⲏⲛ ⲉⲡⲱⲛⲁϩ in P.Heid. inv. K 686 (ed. Kropp 1966), p. 7/108.

11/13–14 ⲕⲁⲕⲟⲇⲁⲫⲛⲏ. A loanword from Greek κοκκοδάφνη, used also in *P.Borg.Copt.* 278 p. 243 (ed. p. 630), in which ⲕⲱⲕⲕⲱⲧⲁⲫⲛⲏ is prescribed as part of a skin-ointment. Both the latter and the present form are referred to κοκκόδαφνον in Till 1951a, 73 no. 84 ("bay-berry": for the Greek term see *LBG* 848b s.v.), but the cognate feminine κοκκοδάφνη (*LBG* ibid. s.v.) is attested in a Byzantine veterinary recipe, *Corpus Hippiatricorum Graecorum, excerpta Lugdunensia* 12, ed. Hoppe and Oder 1927, where it is prescribed alongside birthwort, myrrh, ivory-powder, and cinnamon for cough in horses. If correctly construed here with the preceding ⲕⲗⲁⲇⲟⲥ, the sense, perhaps by metonymy, must be the berry-bearing tree instead of the berry itself. Laurel boiled in water is prescribed as a repellent of flies and fleas in the Byzantine *Geoponica* 13.12.1–4 and 13.15.1–7; for laurel as a demonifuge, see ibid. 11.2.5–7.

11/15 ⲛ̄ⲕⲛⲟⲩⲭ̄ⲧ̄. For ⲛ̄ⲕⲛⲟⲩⲭ̄ⲕ̄: the variant in -ⲧ is thus far known only from this codex (also p. 13/9 ⲛⲟⲭ̄ⲧ̄ϥ̄); cf. *CD* 249a with corr. p. xx. For the alternation of ⲧ with ⲕ in general, see *P.Bal.* I p. 96 §71A.

§20: p. 12/1–4. Recipe for an ointment for skin-sores; the presence of Greek loanwords and units of measure (the stater, p. 12/2) indicate derivation from the Graeco-Roman tradition, while the use of an ibis-feather as applicator is a nod to the local context (12/4).

12/1 ⲟⲩⲕⲗⲁⲇⲟⲥ. For the loanword, see p. 11/13 above with the note.

12/2 ⲁⲛⲏϣ ⲙ̄ⲡⲣⲏ. The first element is comparable to the F and L form of S ⲁⲛⲁϣ, "oath" or "garland" (*DE* 14a), the latter sense being preferable in this botanical context, deriving from Demotic *ꜥnḫ* "bouquet", "garland", "wreath" (*DG* 64). The plant is also prescribed in *P.Med.Chassinat* 121/256 (p. 242), where Chassinat compares ϣⲏⲛ ⲙ̄ⲡⲣⲏ "artemisia" (lit. "Sun's plant"); Till renders here "Sonnen-*Anesch*-Zweig" (1951a, 106 no. 175.b.3). The name may belong to the tradition of occult names for plants in relation to deities, as e.g. γόνος Ἡλίου "Offspring (or, Seed) of the Sun" for white hellebore in *PGM* XII.432—or simply to the tradition of folk names, consider German *Odinskopf* "Odin's head", i.e. Elecampane (Inula helenium).

ϥⲧⲟ ⲥⲁⲧⲉⲉⲣⲉ. For S ϥⲧⲟ ⲛ̄ⲥⲁⲧⲉⲉⲣⲉ or ϥⲧⲟⲩ-ⲥⲁⲧⲉⲉⲣⲉ.

12/2–3 ϩⲟⲥ̄ⲙ̄ ⲛ̄ⲁⲣⲥⲉⲛⲓⲕⲟⲛ. A hybrid formation of Coptic noun qualified by Greek loanword (ἀρσενικόν). Till renders "Rauschgelb Natron" (1951a, 33 no. Q 27), but the mixture of natron and arsenic seems more probable on the basis of the item νίτρον ἀρσενικὸν κεκαυμένον "burned arsenic-natron" in a list of medicinal substances analyzed by particulate quality in Aetius of Amida, *Iatrica* 2.218, where a color specification would not be expected. For natron and arsenic on their own in Coptic medical texts, see Till 1951a, 79–80 no. 102 and 87 no. 122, respectively, and for the loanword, Förster 2002, 100.

12/3 ⲡⲉⲣⲓⲭⲣⲓⲁ. The verb *περιχριάω whose present infinitive (as also p. 12/10 below) this loanword transliterates is an otherwise unattested by-form of περιχρίω "anoint all over"; cf. the contraction χριω-, apparently from χριάω, in the perfect participles χριωμένον and χριωμένη in the late Byzantine veterinary treatise of Demetrius Pepagomenus, *Iatricon* (recension C §25; and ibid. §26, with recension L §31; ed. Capone Ciollaro 2003), and the form ⲧⲣⲓⲃⲁ (implying an underlying Greek *τριβάω) for ⲧⲣⲓⲃⲉ in a medical recipe in O.Brit.Mus. EA 27422 (ed. *O.Brit.Mus.Copt.* I pl. XLIX), front, 25. Use of a comparable loanword ⲡⲉⲣⲓⲭⲣ/ is made in a medicinal context in P.Mich. inv. 593b (ed. Worrell 1935b, 187–192), 25, (read via digital facsimile; expanded ⲡⲉⲣⲓⲭⲣⲱ by ed.pr.); in the medical recipe-collection *SB Kopt.* I 6.15, [ ]ⲭⲣⲓⲁ ⲛ̣ⲕⲉⲕ̣ⲟⲩ̣ⲓ̣ ϩⲙ̣ⲝ̣ is perhaps to be restored as [ⲡⲉⲣⲓ]ⲭⲣⲓⲁ on the basis of the present text. Some form of the loanword might be suspected to underlie what has been read as [ⲧ]ⲉⲣⲓⲭⲉ ("salt", ed.pr.) in a prescription for an eye-salve in O.Brit.Mus. EA 27422 (ed. *O.Brit.Mus.Copt.* I pl. XLIX), front, 8: from the drawing read perhaps ⲡ̣ⲉⲣⲓⲭⲣ̣. The related noun ⲡⲉⲣⲓⲭⲣⲓⲥⲙⲁ (περίχρισμα) introduces a prescription for pain in the breasts and male genitals in *P.Med.Bouriant* p. 214.

12/4 ⲟⲩⲙⲏϩⲉ ⲛ̄ϩⲓⲃⲱⲓ̈. The same applicator for an ointment is prescribed at p. 12/11 below and in *P.Med.Chassinat* 120/254 (p. 240). In the Graeco-Egyptian magical papyri, the feather of an ibis is also used to apply an ointment, but in those instances to the eye of an individual who desires a direct vision of (theophany and visitation by) a god: see the discussion of these example in the treatment of *PGM* IV.26–51 in Love 2016, §4.1.1.3.

§21: 12/4–11. A medical recipe addressing a variant of the same condition as the preceding, via another ointment.

12/4–5 ⲡⲁⲉⲓϣⲉ. For the condition, see Till 1951a, 33 no. Q26 and *P.Macq*. I 1, p. 15.14 with the commentary.

12/5–6 ⲗⲓⲃⲁⲛⲟⲥ ⲛ̄ⲝⲉⲛⲓⲕⲟⲛ. Loanwords from Greek λίβανος ξενικός, the latter apparently transliterated directly from the accusative case in which it was found in the exemplar translated (see further the discussion of **Context in the Practice of Medicine and Healing** in the introduction); for the substance as medicinal ingredient, see Till 1951a, 101 no. 165. The qualification as "imported" (lit. "foreign") is new; in Greek medical recipes it is found for copper (μίσυ), e.g. Galen, *De comp. med. sec. loc*. 12:733 Kühn.

12/6–7 ⲥⲁϣϥ̄ ⲛ̄ϭⲁⲡⲁⲧ ϩⲓ ⲟⲩⲥⲟⲟⲩ ⲛ̄ⲕⲁⲙⲉ. Ed.pr. took ϭⲁⲡⲁⲧ as a variant for ϭⲁⲡⲉⲧ "palm branch", which fits poorly with the following specification; Crum recognized the sense "collar-bone" (*CD* 827b; see also Westendorf 1965–1977, 463 s.v.), which suits the derivation of this ingredient from sheep, assuming ⲟⲩⲥⲟⲟⲩ for ⲟⲩⲉⲥⲟⲟⲩ in the following. Till thought of a rather radical emendation to ⲧⲁⲡ "horn" (1951a, 66 no. 61.f) based on the following ⲟⲩⲧⲁⲡ ⲛ̄ⲛⲉⲥⲟⲟⲩ. The specification of the color of the animal from which bones are sourced is paralleled in P.Cair. 42573 (ed. Chassinat 1955), f. 2r/16–18, where a ritual preparation for the "displacement" of a target from his house (ⲟⲩⲡⲱⲛⲉ) includes "seven bones from a black dog (f.) and seven from a black horse" (ⲍ̄ ⲛⲕⲓ̈ⲥ ϩⲛ ⲟⲩⲟⲩϩⲁⲣ ⲕⲁⲙⲉ ⲙⲛ ⲍ̄ ϩⲛ ⲟⲩϩⲧⲟ ⲕⲉⲙⲉ).

12/6 ϩⲓ ⲟⲩⲥⲟⲟⲩ. Apparently for ⲟⲩⲉⲥⲟⲟⲩ; ϩⲓ\ⲁ̣/ⲟ̣ⲩⲥⲟⲟⲩ ed.pr. What was read by ed.pr. as a supralinear addition of ⲁ (in app. "Doubtful ⲁ or ⲟ above line") is more likely a flourish or blotting of the right leg of ⲗ in ⲗⲓⲃⲁⲛⲟⲥ in the line above.

12/7 ⲧⲁⲡ ⲛ̄ⲛⲉⲥⲟⲟⲩ. Apparently for ⲧⲁⲡ ⲛ̄ⲉⲥⲟⲟⲩ, where dittography appears more likely than the genitive and plural definite article. "Ram's horn" is also the name of a plant described in *P.London-Leiden* as "an herb which is like a wild fennel bush; its leaves and stem are pricked like the 'love-man' plant" (verso 4/10–13), also compared to styrax (ibid. 15–19).

12/8 ⲙⲏⲙⲟⲟⲩ ⲛⲕⲟⲩⲓ̈ ⲁⲫⲑⲁⲣⲧⲟⲥ. The last is a loanword from Greek ἄφθαρτος, specified perhaps to increase the notional purity of the product. Children's urine is prescribed by Marcellus Empiricus to dry out rheum in the head (*De medicamentis* 4.14, *urina humana, id est puerili*). Perhaps ⲙⲏⲙⲟⲟⲩ here evidences a construct form of ⲙⲏ-, or else again a metathesis of the expected attributive in ⲙ̄ⲙⲟⲟⲩ, given that an attributive would also be expected before ⲁⲫⲑⲁⲣⲧⲟⲥ.

ⲗⲟⲕ. This term for "vessel" or "measure (of liquid)" can be characterized in various ways in ritual texts: both by its material, e.g. *wꜥ lḳ n yl* "a glass *lok*-vessel" (*P.London-Leiden* recto 5/26; 27/26), and as a liquid measure, e.g. *wꜥ lḳ n mw* "a *lok*-measure of water", *wꜥ lḳ n nḥ* "a *lok*-measure of oil" (*P.London-Leiden* recto 10/11; 28/4–5), *wꜥ lḳ n ỉrp* "a *lok*-measure of wine", as well as *lḳ sn.nw* "two *lok*-measures" (*P.London-Leiden* recto 24/11; 12/2). Compare also ⲗⲟⲕ ⲛⲛⲉϩ "*log*-measure of oil" in the Sahidic version of Leviticus (14:10; 14:12; 14:15; 14:21; 14:24), where it renders the Greek κοτύλη in a form in fact etymologically cognate with the original Hebrew *lōg*.

12/9–10 ⲟⲩⲗ̣ⲟⲟⲕⲉ ⲛ̄ⲃ̄ⲣ̄ⲣⲉ ⲉⲥϫⲏⲣ. Rendered "a new, burned (?) ... (?)" by ed.pr.; "ein neues ... Gefäß (oder: zu frischem ... Sesam?)", Till, who elsewhere proposes reading ⲟⲕⲉ (1951a, 108 no. 175.c.9). Here ⲗⲟⲟⲕⲉ is taken instead as a variant writing for ⲗⲟⲕ (on which see p. 12/8 with the note; cf. also ⲗⲓⲕ at p. 14/11 below): compare the plural ⲗⲟⲟⲕ (*CD* xviiib; Westendorf 1965–1977, 76). For the derivation of ⲗⲟⲟⲕⲉ from ⲗⲟⲕ, compare ⲕⲟⲩⲕⲉ "skin" from ⲕⲱⲕ "nakedness < to peel". The qualification as black, or blackened from intense firing of the ceramic, would contribute little from a pharmacological perspective but may have some ritual force as responding to the black sheep whose bones figure among the ingredients (see p. 12/6 above).

12/10 ⲡⲉⲣⲓⲭⲣⲓⲁ. See p. 12/3 above with the note.

12/11 ⲟⲩⲙⲏϩⲉ ⲛ̄ϩⲓⲃ̣ⲱï. See p. 12/4 above with the note.

§22: 12/12–13. A brief medical recipe for an obscure disorder, which both ed.pr. and Till declined to interpret, but which probably concerns the testicles, for which bull's gall is prescribed as an ointment. Broad comparanda for the treatment are Marcellus Empiricus, *De medicamentis* 33.18, in which calf-fat (*adeps uituli*) and natron are applied as a poultice to swellings and other disorders of the testicles, and Theodore Priscianus, *Euporiston* 1.27 (ed. Rose 1894, 82), in which bull's gall (*fel taurinum*) is recommended for disorders of the male genitals (*ueretri dolores*, similarly cow's gall, *fel bubulum*, in [Pliny], *De medicina* 2.20.4); in Paul of Aegina, *Epitome* 3.54.3, goat's gall (τραγεία χολή) is an ingredient in an unguent for sores on the scrotum.

12/12 ⲁⲗ̣. The word, literally "pebble", is taken here as a euphemism for "testicle": see *CD* 4a s.v. c; Till 1955, 331–332 no. 51; Westendorf 1965–1977, 2; *DE* 6b s.v. 3. By a similar transferred sense, a skin eruption might be denoted here instead (*CD* 4b s.v. d, *DE* 6b s.v. 4), but the former sense is preferred in view of the parallels from Graeco-Roman medicine cited in the previous note.

Both senses are so far confined to Bohairic: for the testicles, Leviticus 21:20 (ed. Lagarde 1867: ⲟⲩⲣⲱⲙⲓ ⲉⲣⲉ ... ⲟⲩⲁⲗ ⲓⲉ ⲛⲟⲩⲱⲧ ⲡⲉ ⲛ̀ⲛⲉϥⲁⲑⲣⲉⲩ) and 22:24 (ⲫⲏ ⲉⲧⲗⲁⲥ ⲛ̀ⲛⲉϥⲁⲗ ⲓⲉ ⲫⲏ ⲉⲧⲁⲩϩⲟϫϩⲉϫ ⲛ̀ⲛⲟⲩϥ ⲛⲉⲙ ⲫⲏ ⲉⲧⲁⲩϣⲉⲧ ⲛⲟⲩϥ ⲉⲃⲟⲗ ⲛⲉⲙ ⲫⲏ ⲉⲧⲁⲩⲑⲉⲕⲉⲙ ⲛⲟⲩϥ ⲉⲃⲟⲗ); for skin eruptions, Leviticus 13:38 (ϩⲁⲛⲁⲗ ⲉⲩⲉⲣⲟⲩⲱⲓⲛⲓ ⲉⲩϯ ⲟⲩⲃⲁϣ).

ⲉϥⲟ ⲛ̣. . . . ⲁ. ⲏ̣. If the rendering of the preceding ⲁⲗ as "testicle" is accepted, the circumstantial should indicate some disorder, perhaps lesions, distensions, or failure to descend, but no convincing fit for the traces can be found. The second unread letter is most likely ⲃ or ⲣ; followed by ⲗ or ⲁ; then ⲉ, ⲑ, or ⲥ; ⲧ or ⲅ; the last may be ⲛ as read by Worrell, but ⲅ and ⲡ cannot be excluded.

12/13 ⲡ̣ⲉϥⲙⲟⲧⲉ. Partially obscured by a hard-set crease in the parchment, but there is no trace of superlineation, and so ⲡ is to be preferred to ⲛ.

ⲥⲓϣⲉ. For the use of gall in Coptic medical texts, see Till 1951a, 58–59 no. 41.

§23: 12/13–16. A treatment for rheumy eyes via the application of the ashes of a lizard suspended in vinegar and frankincense. The medicinal use of the green lizard is probably derived from Greek lore on the occult properties of natural substances; p. 13 witnesses a cluster of recipes making use of substances from a single animal, in that case a bull, comparable to the same tradition (§§26–28). A treatise in this genre with a wide circulation in Late Antiquity and Byzantium, the *Kyranides* (for which see the study of **Context in the Practice of Medicine and Healing** in the introduction), discusses the medicinal properties of three different types of lizard (2.14, περὶ ζαύρας), the "sun-lizard" (ἡλιακή), "bronze lizard" (χαλκῆ), and "green lizard" (χλωρά; elsewhere in Greek, χλωροσαύρα). Specifically of the "sun-lizard" it is said that the eyes, removed from a live specimen that should later be released, will cure ophthalmia. It is also recommended that this reptile be blinded with metal pins and allowed to grow back its eyes in confinement, while the pins are fashioned into rings bearing a jasper gem inscribed with an image of a lizard and the word χουθεσουλε (the variants χουθουσελε, κοθεσουλε, κοθουσουλε are also found in the manuscripts), which will both heal and ward off ophthalmia. No such claims are made for the "green lizard" in particular, but in general the green and sun lizards are said to have equal powers (ἡ ἡλιακὴ σαύρα τὰ ἴσα δύναται τῇ χλωρᾷ). In Pliny the Elder, however, similar procedures are in fact recommended for the "green lizard" (*lacerta viridis*, at *Naturalis historia* 29.129–130), which are continued and elaborated by Marcellus Empiricus (*De medicamentis* 8.49–50; cf. also 29.45, where an incantation is added, for which cf. Heim 1892, 533 no. 198). Pliny specifies that such a lizard should be burnt and used as ointment for overactive tearing or other discharge and glaucoma of the eyes. Pliny also recommends the ashes from burned lizards more generally for the former complaint (*Naturalis historia* 29.118; similarly, mixed with wine and honey, in Marcellus Empiricus, *De medicamentis* 8.90). On this tradition, with discussion of attestations of gems inscribed with related formula, see Drexler 1899, 610–616; A. Mastrocinque in *SGG* I p. 62. For medicinal uses of the lizard in the Coptic tradition, see also Till 1951a, 54 no. 29. In Demotic, a medical recipe in a magical formulary recommends the use of a lizard with a "blue-green" skin (*k-ʿ-r-ʿ-y-n-e*[Ko], i.e. καλαΐνη from καλάϊνος) and which has no feet, apparently to be combined with a herb named "ram's horn", pounded once dried, made into a dry powder and applied to "any wound", because "it always heals" (*P.London-Leiden* verso 4/6–15).

12/13 ⲟⲩϩⲁⲃ[ⲗ]ⲉⲉⲗⲉ̣ⲓ. For the form, see Westendorf 1965–1977, 406 s.v. ϩⲁϥⲗⲉ(ⲉ)ⲗⲉ, with variants including ϩⲁⲃⲗⲉⲉⲗⲉ and ϩⲁϥⲗⲉⲗⲓ; for the etymology, *DE* 319b.

12/14 ⲉⲥⲟⲩⲉⲧⲧⲟⲩⲱⲧ. Dittography for ⲉⲥⲟⲩⲉⲧⲟⲩⲱⲧ. The rendering of ed.pr. "while it is fresh" is strained, as the verb is proper to the color of vegetation (*DE* 239a; cf. ⲉϥⲟⲩⲱⲧ at p. 12/16–17 and ⲉⲩⲟⲩⲱ̣ⲧ̣ at p. 13/18 below, which must mean "fresh"): the etymological sense "be green" is also supported by the parallels for medicinal uses of green lizards cited above.

12/15 ⲗⲓⲃⲁⲛⲟⲥ. For the loanword, see the note on p. 12/5–6 above.

12/15–16 \ϩ/ⲣⲉⲩⲙⲁⲧⲓ̈ⲥⲉ. The same derivation from the aorist stem of Greek ῥευματίζω appears in a recipe for a *kollyrium* in P.TT 157-470 (ed. Richter 2014, 156–164 no. 1), 2/9 (§3). The curse in P.CtYBR inv. 1800 (ed. Emmel 1994, 353–355 no. 4), 10, seeks to beset the target with rheum, denoted with ⲟⲩϩⲣⲉⲩⲙⲁ, the Greek ῥεῦμα from which this verb is derived.

§24: 12/16–18. A medical recipe for the treatment of sores on the posterior. Via euphemism the anus (assumed by Meyer), and in turn hemorrhoids or fissures, may be meant more specifically.

12/16 ⲕⲛ̄ⲛⲉ ⲛⲉϣⲱ. For the use of fat in Coptic medical recipes, see Till 1951a, 56–57 no. 35 and p. 11/11–12 above; for that of the pig in particular, p. 3/18.

12/17 ⲉⲩⲁϣⲱⲡⲉ. Most likely the relatively common writing of the circumstantial conversion of the First or Second Future, i.e. ⲉⲩⲛⲁϣⲱⲡⲉ. The omission of ⲛ in the writing of forms of these conjugations is not uncommon in Lycopolitan (in particular): see *P.Bal.* I pp. 151–152 §128–129; 208–209. Here a circumstantial conversion of the Second Future seems most likely as the adverbial element stressed is the "backside" or "anus", literally "place of sitting" (see the following note).

пмаnеϩмоос. Probably a calque on the Greek ἕδρα or ἀφεδρών "seat" (cf. *CD* 680a), which is also used euphemistically for the posterior (not always the anus, as Meyer) in medical contexts, e.g. Aetius of Amida, *Iatrica* 16.127; [Galen], *De remed. parab.* 14:548 Kühn.

12/17–18 **ебιω м̄ме**. For the use of honey in medical preparations, see p. 9/5–6 above with the note. The phrase probably translates μέλι ἀληθινόν, as found in [Galen], *De remed. parab.* 14:547 Kühn.

§25: 12/18–20. A medical recipe for the treatment of toothache via irrigation with donkey's milk. There is a close parallel in a Greek recipe for the same purpose, [Galen], *De remed. parab.* 14:355 Kühn, "Rinse with donkey's milk" (ὀνείῳ γάλακτι διακλύζου), which is also found in a Latin version in Theodore Priscianus, *Euporiston* 1.16 (ed. Rose 1894, 49), "Warm, fresh donkey's milk curtails and alleviates (toothache) immediately" (*lac asinae recens tepidum constringit et mitigat* [sc. *dolores dentium*] *continuo*). For dental prescriptions in general, see p. 4/13–15 above with the note.

12/18 **naaϫе**. The form without ϩ is preferred also at p. 4/13–14 naϫе (Hand 1). For the omission of ϩ within words, see *P.Bal.* I p. 142 §123g.

12/18–19 **еуϭопе**. For оуϭопе ("a small vessel['s worth]") as at p. 10/17 above, probably by simple conflation with the preceding еуті.

12/20 **cnaao**. For the verb at the close of medical recipes in general see p. 4/18–19 above with the commentary there. Here the subject may be the teeth (naaϫе) in a collective singular, but an impersonal construction is also possible.

§§26–28: p. 13/1–8. The succession of recipes prescribing medicinal uses for different parts of the same animal again recalls the occult lore of the *Kyranides* (2.6; see also p. 12/13–16 [§22] above), though there the specific indications for the bull differ: burned bull's vertebrae whiten the teeth; bull's gall promotes fertility; bull's liver as part of a potion is recommended for the same, or as a fumigant or ointment to treat bee- and wasp-stings.

13/3 **овϩе**. For the first and last time in the codex, the word овϩе is used in place of na(a)ϫе, S naϫϩе. While the former is attested from the beginning of Egyptian textual culture, the latter is a later introduction (by the Middle Kingdom; see *DE* 154b and *CED* 119 respectively), but both are attested in all the dialects of Coptic and can refer to the teeth of human and non-human animals. Whether any particular tooth or teeth are referred to by овϩе, or whether this evidences a distinct source text, cannot yet be discerned.

13/4–5 **antнλ̄м̄**. Possibly the contents of the head, or some paste or powder made from the skull, are meant, but given the specification of the brain with a different term at p. 13/7–8 below, the translation "head" is preferred here. For references to animal heads as medical ingredients, see Till 1951a, 65 no. 59.

13/7 ⲁⲧⲕⲁⲥ. For the medicinal use of marrow, see Till 1951a, 74–75 no. 90. The convergence with the B form ⲁⲧⲕⲁⲥ is noteworthy, the latter deriving from a distinct etymology, i.e. ⲱⲧ-ⲕⲁⲥ "bone fat", as opposed to the synonymous S ⲁⲗⲧⲕⲁⲥ, which is not cognate but derives from ⲱⲗ-ⲧⲕⲁⲥ "pain remover" by "a transformation due to the belief that animal marrow is an efficient remedy against pain": see *CED* 5, citing Till (as above).

ⲏ. The Greek conjunction ἤ, used also in a medical recipe for disorders of the liver (ϩⲏⲡⲁⲣ) in *P.Mon.Epiph.* 575.7, 12.

13/7–8 ⲁ̀ⲛ́ⲅⲕⲉⲫⲁⲗⲟⲥ. A loanword from Greek ἐγκέφαλος (cf. Förster 2002, 224). For medicinal uses of animal brains, see Till 1951a, 65 no. 59; and in particular *P.Med.Chassinat* 99/193–194 (p. 212; as cited in the note on p. 3/21 above), where the brain of the beaver is denoted with the same loanword (ⲁⲛⲅⲉⲫⲁⲣⲟⲥ). Two other medical prescriptions use similar spellings of this word to indicate the human brain: P.Brit.Mus. inv. EA 10391 (ed. Kropp, *AKZ* I, text M), 58 (ⲁⲛⲕⲉⲫⲁⲗⲟⲥ), and *P.Ryl.Copt.* 107 (b) (ⲁⲛⲕⲉⲫⲟⲗⲟⲥ).

§29: 13/8–10. A recipe belonging more broadly to the management of a household (as §19 above), specifically to rid it of a pest whose identity remains obscure (see the following note). A recipe in a Byzantine agricultural encyclopedia, the *Geoponica*, recommends the same ingredient, white lead, as an ointment for the bite of gadflies, in case a preceding recipe for a repellent made from bay-berries has failed (17.7).

13/8 ⲕⲉⲓ. According to ed.pr., "probably some sort of reptile" (for a procedure targeting reptiles in general see above at p. 11/9–15 [§19]), while Till reserved conjecture. A parallel for the use of white lead in a Greek recipe might suggest that the target is an insect (there, the gadfly: see the previous note), but no candidates suiting the Coptic term present themselves. If indeed an animal, compare perhaps ϭⲓⲉ, with the B, F form ⲕⲓⲏ: *CD* 803a; the he-goat, a creature of proverbially unpleasant odor in the Graeco-Roman world (e.g. Catullus 69.5–6; Martial 6.93.3, 11.22.7), whose name might also stand by metonymy for a miasmic stench. The more abstract ϭⲁ(ⲉ)ⲓⲉ "ugly one", "ugliness" (*CD* 466a; cf. Dem. *gꜥ* "nasty", "evil", *CDD* g 1) is another possibility, to refer to a noxious creature whose name is omitted by a sort of taboo deformation (cf. e.g. English bruin, etymologically "brown one", in place of "bear").

13/8–9 ⲥⲓⲙⲓⲑⲓⲟⲛ. A loanword from Greek ψιμύθιον (cf. Förster 2002, 895), as also at p. 13/15 below; for the substance in Coptic medicine, see Till 1951a, 51 no. 18; Richter 2014, 164. It is requested in a Coptic letter along with opium and saffron (ⲟⲩϣⲧⲁ ⲛⲟⲡⲓⲟⲛ ⲁⲩⲱ ⲟⲩϣⲏⲙ ⲛ̄ⲕⲣⲟⲕⲟⲥ ⲁⲩⲱ ⲟⲩϣⲧⲁ ⲙ̄ⲯⲓⲙⲓⲧⲑ̣ⲉ, 3–5) for a man said to “have a malady on his face” (ϣⲱ̣ⲛ̣ⲉ ⲉⲡⲉϥϩⲟ, 6): *SB Kopt*. IV 1694. The first editor of the latter presses too hard the “monastic context required by the title ⲡⲁⲥⲟⲛ” (Crislip 2007) applied to the patient, who could be the writer’s literal brother or simply professional colleague in a secular practice; see further the discussion of **Context in the Practice of Medicine and Healing** in the introduction.

13/9 ⲛⲟϫⲧ̄ϥ̄. For ⲛⲟϫⲕϥ (ⲛⲟϫϭϥ); compare ⲛ̄ⲕⲛⲟⲩϫ̄ⲧ̄ at p. 11/15 with the note there.

§30: 13/10–18. A recipe for a medicinal preparation named after its expected color, “black poultice”. The purpose is not specified, but on the basis of parallels from Graeco-Roman medicine it was probably intended as a dressing for wounds, to promote their closure and proper healing. Here oil, vinegar, white lead, and the obscure ϩⲉⲗⲕⲓⲉⲙⲁ are to be combined via heating in a pot. The first three ingredients are found together in a poultice also called “black” (μέλαινα ἄλλη) in a section on “plasters for closing up (wounds)” (περὶ κολλητικῶν ἐμπλάστρων) in Galen, *De comp. med. per gen.* 13:566 Kühn, which includes dried pitch, resin, bitumen, manna, copper sulfate, and verdigris-scrapings.

13/10–11 ⲧⲉⲥⲕⲉ[ⲟ]ⲩⲏ. A loanword from Greek σκευή, “preparation”. This term is sometimes found, as a synonym for the more common σκευασία, in the introductions to medical recipes in the Graeco-Roman tradition, e.g. the title “Preparation of the purgative via fruits” (καθαρσίου τοῦ διὰ μήλων ἡ σκευή) in Alexander of Tralles, *Therapeutica* 7.3, 2:255 Puschmann; Aetius of Amida, *Iatrica* 7.106, “The preparation of the *kollyrium*” (ἡ τοῦ κολλυρίου σκευή); and the headings in Paul of Aegina, *Epitome* 7.15.4–6. For the spelling cf. ⲥⲕⲉⲟⲩⲉ as plural of Gk. σκεῦος, Förster 2002, 735 s.v.

13/11 ⲟ̣ⲩ̣ⲥ̣ⲡ̣ⲗⲉⲗⲓⲛ ⲛ̄ⲕⲁⲙⲏ. The first element is a variant of ⲥⲡⲗⲏⲗⲓⲛ, a kind of poultice (see *CD* 351b s.v.), which matches the Demotic form *s-p-l-e-l-y-n*^{Fl} (for which see *CED* 159; *DE* 194b), attested only in *P.London-Leiden* verso 9/9, derived from Greek σπληνίον “pad”, “compress”, diminutive of σπλήν “spleen”; the Demotic orthography evidences Egyptianizing assimilation of the first ν to preceding λ, as found in the Coptic orthographies. The reading ⲥⲡⲉⲗⲉⲗⲓⲛ by Crum’s suggestion was already acknowledged by ed.pr. but relegated to the apparatus; “Wegen der ... schwarzen ... Umschlag (?)” Till. The titling of medicinal preparations with color-descriptors is known in Graeco-Roman medicine: see the note on p. 13/10–18 above and further e.g. Galen, *De comp. med. per gen.* 13:809 Kühn, a plaster (ἔμπλαστρος) called “Andromachos’s Black Entreaty” (ἡ ἱκεσία μέλαινα Ἀνδρομάχου); a later Coptic medical collection in P.Louvre AF 12530 (ed. Richter 2014, 165–183 no. 3), verso 1–9 (§18) gives “a black plaster". For named drugs in Coptic recipes see also O.Brit.Mus. EA 27422 (ed. *O.Brit.Mus.Copt.* I pl. XLIX), front, 18, "Plaster that is called *karby*[ ]" (ⲉⲙⲡⲗⲁⲧⲟⲛ ⲉϣⲁⲩⲙⲟⲩ[ⲧⲉ ⲉⲣⲟϥ] ϫⲉ ⲕⲁⲣⲃⲩ[ ]; cf. perhaps κάρβων, Latin *carbo* "coal"); *SB Kopt.* II 1043.1, "The savior" (ⲯⲱⲧⲏⲣ).

13/12 ⲝⲉⲥⲧ̣ⲏ̣ⲥ̣. As also at p. 13/13 below, a loanword from Greek ξέστης, itself derived from Latin *sextarius*. Oil is measured in the same unit in some later Coptic documentary texts, e.g. *CPR* II 195.3, IV 160.12; *O.Frange* 604.8; see in general Förster 2002, 555–556.

ⲛⲉϩ ⲙⲉ. Potentially a haplography for ⲛⲉϩ ⲙ̄ⲙⲉ, compare ⲉⲃⲓⲱ ⲙ̄ⲙⲉ at p. 12/17–18. The oil is genuine because it is prepared in the traditional way from olives, not a cheaper substitute (e.g. radish, as at p. 14/4 below). This characterization of a product or material as "genuine" has a long history in Egypt: compare Egyptian *ḫsbd mꜥꜥ* "genuine lapis lazuli", attested already in the New Kingdom, which distinguishes lapis lazuli from an imitation made of faience, which could be passed off as *ḫsbd* "lapis lazuli", *ḫsbd* thereby coming to mean "faience". This construction is applied to olive oil in Demotic in the Graeco-Roman period: *nḥ n mꜥꜥ{.t}* "genuine (i.e. olive) oil" in *P.London-Leiden* recto 14/18; 20/18; 20/21; 20/22; verso 6/3. For the medicinal use of oil in Coptic texts, see Till 1951a, 81 no. 105.b.

13/13 ϩ̣ⲙ̄ϫ̄ⲁⲥ. Apparently ϩⲙ̄ϫ̄-ⲁⲥ "old vinegar", as at p. 14/3, the adjective being sometimes utilized as a "genderless suffix": see Layton 2000, 89–90 §112.

ⲗⲓⲧⲣⲁ. A loanword from Greek λίτρα (cf. Förster 2002, 474–475); depending on what is being quantified, the unit could be either one of weight ("pound"), as more commonly in Greek (and Coptic documentary texts, e.g. of gold, *P.KRU* 55.24, 106.202), or volume ("liter", as apparently for honey in a medical recipe in *P.Ryl.Copt.* 106.45–46, ⲗⲓ^ⲧ ⲛⲉϥⲓⲱ). As the ingredient has not yet been identified (see the following note) and occurs in sequence between two volume measurements (the pint) and one weight measurement (the stater), the choice between the two senses must be left open.

13/14 ϩⲉⲗⲕⲓⲉⲙⲁ. In the facsimile the ⲙ is partially obscured by a fold, but it has been confirmed on the original. The word has so far gone unexplained. A compound with an initial element derived from ϩⲱⲗϭ "be sweet" or ϩⲉⲗϭⲉ "sweetness" (*CD* 673b) might be considered, but the rest is obscure.

13/15 ⲡⲥⲓⲙⲓⲑⲓⲟⲩ. The noun is a loanword derived from Greek ψιμύθιον (for which see p. 13/8–9 above) but transliterated directly from the Greek genitive (ψιμυθίου), as with ⲥⲁⲧ[ⲏ]`ⲩ´ⲣⲁⲕⲏⲥ at p. 11/11 above; see further the note there.

13/15–16 ⲛ̄ⲅⲧⲁⲁⲩ. For the pendant conjunctive, perhaps a sign of translation of the Greek participle, see the note on p. 9/5 above.

13/16 ⲉⲩⲗ̣ⲓ̣ⲕ̣ ⲛ̄ⲗⲟⲟⲕⲉ. Till rendered "in einen [großen (?)] Topf" based on the text of ed.pr.; for the sense preferred here, compare ⲟⲩ̣ⲗ̣ⲟⲟⲕⲉ at p. 12/9 above with the commentary there. ⲗⲓⲕ is presumably a variant of ⲗⲟⲕ, both deriving from Demotic *lḳ*.

13/16–17 ⲛ̄ⲥⲁϩⲧⲉ. Apparently for ⲛ̄ⲅⲥⲁϩⲧⲉ by simplification of the initial consonant cluster; cf. ⲛⲧⲁⲗⲁ̣ϥ̣ at p. 14/11 below.

13/18 ⲉⲩⲟⲩⲱ̣ⲧ̣. Ed.pr. read the final letter without underdot; only a high horizontal remains above the break, and there is no trace of a junction with the vertical, but in context the reading seems inevitable.

§31: p. 14/1–20. The final page is devoted entirely to a complex procedure for the treatment of hip pain (sciatica), including a poultice, immersion in a bath, and ritual observances on the conditions under which plant materials are to be gathered, their exposure to astrological influences, the matching of the hand used to apply the poultice with the side on which the pain occurs, and the avoidance of speech during the treatment. Marcellus Empiricus devotes a chapter to comparable pathologies (*De medicamentis* 25, whose title begins *lumborum et coxarum doloribus et torpori siue sciaticis remedia*, "Remedies for pain and numbness in the lower back and hips, or for those with sciatica"), which offers no precise parallel for the present procedure (for whose background see also the excursus to §31), but broad similarities include the use of wax (25.6, 31, 47), vinegar (25.10, 27–28), herbs gathered at ritually auspicious times with restrictions on whom the patient may touch during the treatment (25.11), herbs gathered (i.e., cut) without iron blades (25.14), administration of medicine over three days (25.14, 17, 25, 30, 32, 38–39), and hot baths (25.9, 12, 14, 22, 32, 42, 46). Sciatica is the target of a popular genre of textual amulets on gems, depicting a man stooping to reap a field of wheat and inscribed with the Greek ’σχίων "for the hips" (cf. the following note): see Bonner 1950, 71–77 (with mention of the present recipe), and recently *SEG* LVIII 1766.

14/1 [ⲉ]ⲧⲃⲉ ⲡⲉⲥⲭⲓⲟⲛ. A loanword from Greek ἰσχίον, via the aphaeretic form ’σχίον encountered in its own right in textual amulets (see the previous note). The same rubric is used in an iatromagical recipe in P.Berl. inv. 8109 (ed. *BKU* I 25; cf. Beltz 1984, 88–91), recto 16–25, [ⲉⲧ]ⲃⲉ ⲡⲉⲥⲭⲓⲟⲛ, with a procedure including inscription of ritual text (ⲛ[ⲅ]ⲥϩⲁⲓ ⲛ̇ⲛⲁ̣ⲓ̈ [c. 6]ⲁ̣ⲝ "and write these (words)", with at least one magical word ending in *-ax*; but Beltz reads ⲛ[. .]ⲥ ϩⲛⲛⲩ[ ]). For the affliction, see further Till 1951a, 29 no. P 7.

ⲧⲟⲕⲓⲙⲟⲛ. A loanword from Greek δόκιμον (cf. Förster 2002, 207–208), for which see p. 2/10 above with the note. A comparable transliteration and claim for a recipe come in one to inflict ticks on cattle, P.Cair. 42573 (ed. Chassinat 1955), f. 2v/21–26, "It is a proven one" ([ⲟ]ⲩⲧⲱⲕⲓⲙⲱⲛ ⲡⲉ); more general advertisements of the efficacy of medical recipes in Coptic include e.g. *P.Ryl.Copt*. 106 verso 30, "A really fine medicine" (ⲟⲩⲡⲁϩⲣⲉ ⲛⲥⲁⲓⲉ ⲕⲁⲗⲱⲥ).

14/2 ⲟⲛⲅⲓⲁ. As also in the following line, a loanword from Greek οὐγκία (cf. Förster 2002, 593–594), itself from Latin uncia, applied as a weight measure in later Coptic documentary texts, e.g. *P.KRU* 21.70 and *SB* I 5589.75 (of gold); for use in Coptic medical texts, see e.g. O.Brit.Mus. EA 27422 (ed. *O.Brit.Mus.Copt*. I pl. XLIX), front, 20–21, and back, 21–23, and Richter 2014, 183, index 5.

14/3 ϩⲙ̄ϫ̄ⲁⲥ. Apparently ϩⲙ̄ϫ̄-ⲁⲥ "old vinegar": for the form see p. 13/13 with the note.

14/4 ⲟⲩⲟⲧϩ̄. For ⲟⲩⲟⲩⲟⲧϩ̄ by simplification; see further the discussion of **Linguistic Features** in the introduction.

ⲛⲉϩ ⲛ̄ⲥⲓⲙ. For the use of radish-oil in Coptic medical texts, see Till 1951a, 81 no. 105.f.

14/4–5 ⲉϥⲙⲟⲕⲉ. Kasser was the first to recognize the form as qualitative of ⲙⲓⲕⲉ, expressing a quality of the oil: "huile limpide, reposée, ayant fait ses dépôts?" (*CC* 27a) with reference to the medical recipe-collection P.Vind. inv. K 5595 (ed. Till 1951b; now *SB Kopt*. I 6), 7, in which he read ⲛ̣ⲉ̣ϩ ⲉϥⲙⲟⲕⲉ (. . ϩ ⲉϥⲙⲟⲕⲉ, ed.pr.), where the presence of ⲛⲉϩ had already been suspected by Till (1951b, 74) with reference to the present text, "eine besondere Eigenschaft des Öls ... etwa 'abgesetzt, abgestanden'" (cf. also Westendorf 1965–1977, 88 s.v.; not taken into account in *DE* 110a). The point is perhaps that the lightest, finest oil, resting on the top of the product allowed to settle in a vat, is to be preferred. The parallel in the Vienna papyrus renders negligible the interpretation of ed.pr. and an earlier one of Till based thereon.

14/5 ⲅⲣⲁⲙⲁ. A loanword from Greek γράμμα (cf. Förster 2002, 152–152), common in Greek medical authors but not paralleled to our knowledge in Coptic medical texts.

14/6 ⲁⲗⲗⲱⲏ. A loanword from Greek ἀλόη (cf. Förster 2002, 34). For the medicinal use of aloe in Coptic texts, see Till 1951a, 46–47 no. 4; Richter 2014, 162.

14/6–9. The avoidance of iron (blades) when gathering medicinal plants and a general preference for encountering such plants in a pristine and pure condition are commonplaces of Graeco-Roman herbological lore (see in general Delatte

1961 and the excursus to §31). The direction to avoid iron is applied to the gathering of an herb for the treatment of sciatica specifically in Marcellus Empiricus, *De medicamentis* 25.14 (see the note on p. 14/1–20 above).

14/9 ⲛ̄ⲅⲣⲉϫ̣. For the pendant conjunctive, possibly a sign of translation of a Greek participle, see the note on p. 9/5 above.

14/10–11 {ⲉⲩ} ⲉⲩⲗⲓⲕ. For the dittography over the line, compare at p. 14/15–16.

14/11 ⲛⲧⲁⲗⲁ̣ϥ̣. For ⲛⲅⲧⲁⲗⲁ̣ϥ̣, by a similar simplification as in ⲛ̄ⲥⲁϩⲧⲉ at p. 13/16–17 above.

14/13–14. For instructions to match the hand used in application and the side where the affliction appears, see the excursus to §31.

14/14 ⲉϣⲁⲥⲧⲁϩ̄ⲥ̄. Haplography for ⲉϣⲁⲥⲧⲁϩ̄ⲥ̄ⲥ.

14/15–16 ϣⲟⲙⲛ̄ⲧ̄ⲧⲉ. For the dittography over the line, compare at p. 14/10–11; apparently the scribe wrote the masculine form ϣⲟⲙⲛ̄ⲧ̄ and subsequently recalled that the following word, i.e. ⲟⲩϣⲏ, is feminine, adding the feminine ending -ⲧⲉ at the beginning of the following line—compare the correct orthography ϣⲟⲙⲧⲉ at p. 13/14.

14/16 ⲛ̄ⲛⲟⲩϣⲏ. Dittography of the attributive for ⲛ̄ⲟⲩϣⲏ.

ⲉⲅⲧⲱϩ. The spelling with ⲅ for ⲕ is rare in Coptic words: see *P.Bal.* I pp. 95–96 §71.

14/17 ⲙⲡ̄ⲅ̄-. S ⲙ̄ⲡⲉⲕ-: for the spelling with ⲅ for ⲕ, see the preceding note.

14/17–18. For the avoidance of speech, see the excursus to §31.

ⲉⲗⲁⲁⲩ. A fold-under obscures the second ⲁ, but the letter has been confirmed on the original.

14/18 ⲛ̄ⲅⲡⲓⲣⲟⲩⲧ. Apparently an anomalous use of the qualitative of ⲡⲉⲓⲣⲉ (in the II form, cf. *CD* 267a s.v.: S ⲡ(ⲉ)ⲣⲉⲓⲱⲟⲩ, B ⲫⲉⲣⲓⲱⲟⲩⲧ) in place of the infinitive to form the conjunctive; cf. the analogous use of ϩⲙⲟⲟⲥ and ⲁϩⲉ discussed by Till 1961, 125 §257. Writings of the qualitative with final /t/ are uncommon even in Demotic, and B is apparently the only dialect to express final /t/ in the qualitative form, cited above. The sense is taken here to be a rendering of the passive of the Greek ἀστρονομέω or ἐξαστρονομέω "catch the stars", as technical term in popular medical recipes for the exposure of medicinal substances or other ritual materials to astral influences at night to enhance their efficacy: for Byzantine examples, see Zellmann-Rohrer 2018, 136–137 (text D5 §2) with n. 54.

ⲉⲃ̣ⲟⲗ ⲅ̄. An alternate reading and division ⲉⲕ̣ⲟⲗⲅ̄ are possible (for S ⲉϭⲟⲗⲅ̄), but the sense "to twist yourself up" is less apt in context.

ⲟⲩⲧ̣ⲱ̣. A loanword from Greek οὕτω: see Förster 2002, 597.

14/19 ⲥⲟⲩⲧⲱⲛ̄ⲅ. The ⲥ is obscured on a fold-under but has been confirmed on the original.

ⲟ̣ⲩ-. In place of ⲟ, ⲁ is palaeographically possible, but some form of the indefinite article is required.

14/20 [ⲥ]ⲉ̣ⲟⲟⲩⲛ. For [ⲥ]ⲓ̣ⲟⲟⲩⲛ, cf. Sa ⲥⲉⲁⲩⲛⲉ (*CD* 369b). For directions involving the bath see p. 9/17 with the note.

§2 A Textual Amulet for Gout (p. 2/10–17) (MZR)

The recommended cure for gout proceeds by a combination of ritual and therapeutic means, the inscription of magical words on metal, presumably to be attached to the patient as an amulet, and the utterance of the same words while the feet are washed. A comparable remedy is found in *P.London-Leiden* verso, column 10, where a sequence of words written in Greek script—*Thembarathem ourembrenoutipe aiochthou semmarathemmou naioou* (θεμβαραθεμ ουρεμβρενουτιπε αιοχθου σεμμαραθεμμου ναιοου, 6–10)—is recommended for inscription on silver or tin, to be bound to the feet of the patient with deerskin, when the moon is in Leo. This astrological indication is paralleled in the Michigan recipe, where the healing is timed with the waning of the moon, apparently as analogy for the disappearance of the gout. A similar combination is found in a procedure prescribed by the early Byzantine medical author Alexander of Tralles, with an incantation including Egyptian features inscribed on a gold leaf.

> προφυλακτικὸν ποδάγρας· λαβὼν πέταλον χρυσοῦν σελήνης ληγούσης γράφε ἐν αὐτῷ τὰ ὑποκείμενα καὶ ἐνδήσας εἰς νεῦρα γεράνου, εἶτα ὅμοιον τῷ πετάλῳ σωληνάριον ποιήσας, κατάκλεισον καὶ φόρει περὶ τοὺς ἀστραγάλους· ‘μεὶ θρεὺ μὸρ φὸρ τεὺξ ζὰ ζὼν θὲ λοὺ χρὶ γὲ ζὲ ὤν. ὡς στερεοῦται ὁ ἥλιος ἐν τοῖς ὀνόμασι τούτοις καὶ ἀνακαινίζεται καθ’ ἑκάστην ἡμέραν, οὕτω στερεώσατε τοῦτο τὸ πλάσμα καθὼς ἦν τὸ πρίν, ἤδη ἤδη, ταχὺ ταχύ. ἰδοὺ γὰρ λέγω τὸ μέγα ὄνομα ἐν ᾧ ἀναπαυόμενα στερεοῦνται· ἴαζ ἀζὺφ ζύων θρὲγξ βαὶν χωώκ. στερεώσατε τὸ πλάσμα τοῦτο καθὼς ἦν τὸ πρῶτον, ἤδη ἤδη, ταχὺ ταχύ.’
>
> A prophylactic against gout: take a gold leaf when the moon is waning and write on it the (words) given below; bind it in crane sinews, then make a tube of the same size as the leaf and enclose it, and wear it about the ankles: “*Mei threu mor phor teux za zōn the lou chri ge ze ōn*. As the sun is made firm in these names and renewed each day, so do you (pl.), make firm this creature as it was before, now, now, quickly, quickly. For behold, I utter the great name in which what is at rest is made

> firm: *iaz azuph zuōn threngx bainchōōk*. Make firm this creature as it was before, now, now, quickly, quickly."[361]

The Egyptian influence makes itself felt in the formulaic closing expression of urgency, "now, now, quickly, quickly" (ἤδη ἤδη, ταχὺ ταχύ), encountered several times in Greek and Coptic transliteration in the Michigan codex (see the note on p. 8/4). For at least one of the magical words an Egyptian etymology is probable: *bain chōōk* (βαὶν χωώκ from *bꜣ n kk.w*) "Soul of the primeval god of darkness".[362]

The therapeutic approach in this recipe, of treatment with a bath of warm liquid, is on record in its turn in Dioscorides for olive-water and vinegar.[363] We have therefore a conjunction of pharmacological and ritual healing, in which powerful words are believed to enhance the healing capabilities already existing in a medicinal preparation.

§3 An Isiac Invocation for Disorders of the Uterus (pp. 2/17–3/15) (MZR)

A new section must have originally begun here, for which the rubric has fallen out in the copying, as the following invocation bears no relation to the preceding treatment of gout (§2). Worrell and subsequent translators have nevertheless assumed a continuous procedure, the invocation taken as the referent of τοῦτο at p. 2/16. The instructions at p. 3/13–14, to wet (βάψον) a flock of wool, in the absence of any further specification, perhaps suggest that the lost rubric contained some preliminary instruction to utter the invocation over a liquid, in which the wool would then be dipped.

The invocation begins in Greek, then shifts to a lengthy name of the goddess Isis with Egyptian elements and Coptic script characteristics (ⲧⲛ̄ⲧⲱⲣⲉⲱ "the great goddess"), before returning to Greek for the request itself. It is broadly comparable to an invocation of Isis, spoken in the person of Thoth, in a fourth-century Greek handbook on a papyrus bookroll (*PGM* VII), as recognized by van der Vliet.[364] After an aromatic burnt-offering directed towards the moon, Isis is invoked,

361 *Therapeutica* 12, 2:583 Puschmann (cf. Heim 1893, 535 no. 204). For this recipe as illustrative of the Graeco-Egyptian magical tradition see recently Bohak 2016, 367–369.

362 Quack 2019a, 245–246; see also the commentary to p. 3/3.

363 *De materia medica* 1.102.1, 5.13.2.

364 *PGM* VII.492–504; van der Vliet 1991, 228–231.

> ἐπικαλοῦμαί σε κυρία ᾿Ισι ᾗ συνεχώρησεν ὁ Ἀγαθὸς Δαίμων βασιλεύ⟨ειν⟩ [-ων pap.] ἐν τῷ τελείῳ μέλανι.
> I invoke you, lady Isis, to whom the Good Divinity has granted (the right) to rule in the perfect black.

There follows a recital of "your name" (τὸ ὄνομά σου), in fact a sequence of epithets mostly derived from Egyptian that parallel the Michigan text: "*Lou loulou batharthar tharēsibath atherneklēsich athernebouni ēichomō chomōthi Isis Sothis souēri Boubastis eurelibat chamari neboutos ouēri aiē ēoa ōai*" (λου: λουλου: βαθαρθαρ· θαρησιβαθ: αθερνεκλησιχ αθερνεβουνι: ηιχομω: χομωθι: ᾿Ισι Σῶθι: σουηρι· Βούβαστις· ευρελιβατ᾿: χαμαρι: νεβουτος: ουηρι: αϊη: ηοα· ωαι). Then comes a self-identification of the practitioner as Thoth and the point of the prayer itself, a request for general protection.

Van der Vliet, who was the first to point out the relation to the Michigan text, argued for an astral context for ἐν τῷ τελείῳ μέλανι here too, in which μέλαν refers to the "blackness" of the night sky, of which Isis is queen, where Preisendanz had translated the phrase in *PGM* VII as "im ganzen Schwarzland (Ägypten)". In the Hermetic Corpus, Isis speaks of having been honored τῷ τελείῳ μέλανι, in the context of revelation received via Kamephis and ultimately from Hermes "the recorder of all deeds" (ὁ πάντων ἔργων ὑπομνηματογράφος), and in a Greek hymn from Roman Oxyrhynchus (*P.Oxy*. XI 1380) she is praised twice in connection with writing (γραμματική, 3/48–49 and 6/123–124), and hailed in the probable Egyptian exemplar for various Greek acclamations as inventor of language,[365] so the interpretation as the substantive μέλαν, "ink" is therefore also possible,[366] and at least in the Michigan text the explicit link between Isis and the moon is lacking. More generally Isis is called μελανηφόρος in the Orphic Hymns (42.9), which would seem to refer to the wearing of black garments. In view of the concern of the invocation with the healing of inflammation and other disorders of the female womb (3/8–12), a connection with the euphemistic sense of μέλαν as "(dark-colored) pubic hair" or "pudendum" found in Graeco-Egyptian ritual texts (*Suppl.Mag*. II 71 fr. 5/2 with the note) is also attractive, as a naturally "perfect", that is, healthy, disposition is precisely what is sought for the womb here.

---

[365] Quack 2003, 338 (with 352) §31.

[366] *Corp. Herm*. fr. 23.32; Festugière and Nock 1945–1954, 3: clxvi–clxviii, however, prefer the interpretation of Preisendanz.

A parallel presentation of the two invocations (from the opening through the list of the goddess's names) may be useful, alongside a third, in a Coptic curse on a lead tablet of the sixth or seventh century CE,[367] also adduced by van der Vliet, which illustrates the continued circulation of vestiges of a similar invocation applied to aggressive magic, with no remaining connection to Isis:

PGM VII	Michigan Ms. 136	T.Köln inv. 35
ἐπικαλοῦμαί σε	ἐπικαλοῦμαί σε	
κυρία ʾΙσι	τὴν μεγίστην ʾΙσιν	
ἣ συνεχώρησεν ὁ	τὴν βασιλεύουσ̣α̣ν	
Ἀγαθὸς Δαίμων		
βασιλεύ⟨ειν⟩		
ἐν τῷ τελείῳ μέλανι·	ἐν τῷ τελείῳ μέλανι	
τὸ ὄνομά σου·	ἡ δέσποινα̣ θεῶν	
	οὐρανοῦ γένεσι·	
λου: λουλου:		
βαθαρθαρ·		
θαρησιβαθ:		(...)
αθερνεκλησιχ	ⲁⲑⲉⲣⲛⲉⲕⲗⲏⲥⲓⲁ·	ⲑⲉⲣⲛⲓⲕⲗⲏⲥⲓⲁ
αθερνεβουνι:	ⲁⲑⲉⲣⲛⲉⲃⲟⲩⲛⲓ·	ⲑⲉⲣⲛⲉⲙⲟⲛⲓ
	ⲗⲁⲃⲓⲥⲁⲭⲑⲓ·	ⲗⲁⲃⲏⲥⲁⲭⲑⲏ
ηιχομω: χομωθι:	ⲭⲱⲙⲟⲭⲟⲱⲭⲓ·	ⲭⲱⲙⲁⲭⲱ [c. 5]ⲱⲑ
ʾΙσι Σῶθι:	ⲓⲥⲓ· ⲥⲟⲩⲥⲏ·	
σουηρι:	ⲙⲟⲩⲛⲧⲏ· ⲧⲛ̄ⲧⲱⲣⲉⲱ·	ⲙⲱⲛⲟⲩⲥⲁ
Βουβαστις:	ⲓ̈ⲱⲃⲁⲥⲧ: ⲃⲁⲥⲧⲁⲓ̈·	
ευρελιβατ':	ⲣⲓⲃⲁⲧ: ⲭⲣⲓⲃⲁⲧ·	
	ⲑⲉⲣⲏⲥⲓⲃⲁⲧ·	ⲑⲁⲣ̣ⲥ̣ⲓⲃⲁⲑ ⲑⲁⲃⲁⲣⲓⲱⲑ (...)
χαμαρι: νεβουτος:	ⲭⲁⲙⲁⲣⲉⲓ· ⲭⲩⲣⲓⲑⲓⲃⲁⲑ·	
ουηρι:	ⲥⲟⲩⲉⲣⲏ·	
	ⲑⲁⲣⲑⲁⲑⲁⲃⲁⲁⲑⲑⲁ· ⲑⲁⲑ·	
	ⲃⲁⲑⲁⲑ· ⲗⲁⲑⲁⲓ̈· ⲁⲭⲣⲁ·	
αϊη: ηοα· ωαι	ⲁⲃⲁⲑⲁⲓ̈· ⲁⲏ·	

[βασιλεύειν corr. eds.; βασιλευων pap.]

[367] Published erroneously under T.Köln inv. 10 (*P.KölnÄgypt*. I 11) 1–9; the inventory number is actually T.Köln inv. 35: see Love fc. b. The invocation is referred to collectively as "these names of this powerful stele" (ⲛⲉⲓⲣⲁⲛ ⲛ̄ⲧⲉⲓⲛⲟϭ ⲛ̄ⲥⲧⲏⲗⲏ ⲉⲧϭⲙ̄ϭⲟⲙ).

PGM VII	Michigan Ms. 136	T.Köln inv. 35
I invoke you,	I invoke you,	
lady Isis,	greatest Isis,	
to whom the Good	who	
Divinity has granted		
to rule	rules	
in the perfect black.	in the perfect black,	
Your name:		
	the mistress of the gods,	
	origin of heaven,	
Lou loulou		
batharthar		
tharēsibath		
atherneklēsich	*atherneklēsia*	*therniklēsia*
athernebouni	*athernebouni*	*thernemoni*
	labisachthi	*labēsachthē*
ēichomō chomōthi	*chōmochoōchi*	*chōmachō ...ōth*
Isis, Sothis	*isi sousē*	
souēri	*mountē tentōreō*	*mōnousa*
Boubastis	*iōbast bastaï*	
eurelibat	*ribat chribat*	
	therēsibat	*tharsibath thabariōth*
chamari neboutos	*chamarei churithibath*	
ouēri	*souerē*	
	tharthathabaaththa thath	
	bathath lathaï achra	
	abathaï	
aïē ēoa ōai	*aē*	

A detailed discussion of the etymologies and proposals for semantic content of specific elements of the divine names in the Michigan text can be found in the line-commentary. Throughout, in addition to the Coptic grapheme adopted in ⲧⲛ̄ⲧⲱⲣⲉⲱ, the influence of traditional Egyptian religion is strongly in evidence. In this light, consideration should be given to the increasing number of Demotic hymns to Isis that are becoming known and published, discussed in **Transmitting Textual Traditions**. Greek versions of these, such as the extensive hymn from Roman Oxyrhynchus (*P.Oxy.* XI 1380),[368] would have provided already a ready gathering of motifs from which the epithets of §3 could have been drawn.

§6 A Cure for Fever via Homer and an Angel (p. 4/1–12) (MZR)

The recipe approaches fever via two ritual texts, the first drawing on Homer, *Iliad* 3.33–35, and the second a prayer to the angel Gabriel. The Homeric text appears to have been selected for its analogical relation to the scenario of treatment and its intended result.[369] The relevance is probably felt in the collocation of τρόμος, "trembling", corresponding to the literal "shivering" of the term used here for fever (ῥῖγος), and the verb ἀναχωρεῖν "withdraw". Inserted in the context of the healing scenario, the Homeric text comes to describe how the shivering brought on by the fever first takes hold of the body (ἔλλαβε γυῖα), then presumably abates after the speedy removal of the danger. The relation becomes even stronger if, out of the original epic context, ἀνεχώρησεν is construed with τρόμος as its subject instead of τις as required in the original, and the generic sense of the aorist is dropped, hence, "trembling has taken hold of the limbs, and has withdrawn," an analogy to the desired result in the case of this procedure.

As commentators have generally agreed, the fundamental mechanism in Homeric incantations is analogy, whether restricted to the individual verse selected, or to its larger narrative context. The *Iliad*, and to a lesser extent the *Odyssey*, appealed as divinely inspired poetry, providing a model for the order of the cosmos and an extensive repertory of analogies for afflictions and their successful resolution. That the Homeric poems themselves reflected a world in which incantations were both present and acknowledged as effective—witness the well-known episode of the staunching of the blood of Odysseus with an ἐπαοιδή, and the elaboration of the visit of Odysseus to the underworld in which he summoned the shades of the dead by another ἐπαοιδή, reported in the *Cesti* of Julius Africanus as including familiar "magical" divine names such as Αβλα-

[368] For this text, see now Nagel 2019, 600–645; 840–852, and for some Demotic hymns from Oxyrhynchus probably related to it, see recently Quack 2016a, 279; 2016b, 111. For a comprehensive study of the hymns to Isis known from temple texts, see now all the collated sources in Nagel 2019, §4, and for a collation of the papyrological sources, see Nagel 2019, §6.1.

[369] On the use of Homer for incantations in the Greek tradition the fundamental study remains Collins 2008, which is however in need of supplement, and a systematic catalogue of attestations following the preliminary collection of Heim (1893, 514–520 nos. 151–160) remains a desideratum, as does a more satisfactory treatment of the non-papyrological materials (e.g., the important witness of Marcellus Empiricus belongs to Late Antiquity, not the second century CE as Collins 2008, 211); see also recently Zellmann-Rohrer 2016 and 2019a, 284, and the commentary in *P.Philammon* pp. 128–129.

ναθω—can only have enhanced this appeal.[370] The extensive use of epic diction in Greek invocations in Egypt can be seen in the "hymns" collected and reconstructed in *PGM*. As a popular school text in Graeco-Roman Egypt,[371] the Homeric poems were likely to be broadly familiar, including among those also versed in traditional Egyptian religion who undertook to learn Greek. The presence of Homer and other Greek literary texts among the books read by Egyptian priests is probable in the case of the town of Tebtunis in the Fayum, the same region where the Michigan text was produced.[372]

The majority of the surviving attestations of Homeric incantations concern healing and protection. As such they are on record relatively early, as the Neoplatonist philosopher Iamblichus (ca. 245–325 CE) reports Pythagorean use of Homeric verses to promote health. In particular, the Sicilian philosopher Empedokles (fifth century BCE) is said to have recited the description of the drug by which queen Helen calmed her banquet guests (*Odyssey* 4.221), to calm a young man about to attack one of Empedokles' pupils.[373]

After this early attestation of the practice, albeit preserved in a much later author, the next reference comes in a second-century literary parody of Lucian of Samosata. In a dialogue between Hermes and the infernal ferryman Charon, Hermes offers to heal the latter's blindness by reciting a passage from the *Iliad* as an incantation (ἐπῳδή: *Charon* 7). In this selection, Athena promises to remove the mist from the eyes of Diomedes, allowing him to distinguish between men and gods in battle (*Iliad* 5.127–128).

The most substantial collection comes in the mid-fourth century CE, in a notebook codex belonging to Aurelius Philammon, a municipal official in the city of Hermopolis, three pages of which are devoted to recording magical recipes. Among these are at least seven single lines from the *Iliad* prescribed via utterance or inscription for medical purposes.[374] One of the seven was in independent circulation a century or two before its collection in the codex.[375] The fourth-century Paris magical codex (*PGM* IV) offers two prescriptions for the amuletic use of lines from the *Iliad*, one internally titled "three-verse assistant of Homer",

---

[370] Staunching blood: *Odyssey* 19.455–462 (see recently Zellmann-Rohrer 2020c, 310–311 n. 2). Incantation in the underworld: *Cesti* 18, from *P.Oxy*. III 412.

[371] Cribiore 1996, 46, 49.

[372] Hickey 2009; cf. also Litinas 2014, 335–337.

[373] *De vita Pythagorica* 25.113; cf. also 25.111, 29.164.

[374] P.Berl. inv. 9873 (ed. *P.Philammon*; cf. *PGM* XXIIa), pp. 22–23: *Iliad* 1.67 for headache; *Iliad* 1.60 for fever; *Iliad* 1.75 for hemorrhage plus *Iliad* 1.96 to coerce a patient who fails to pay via re-infliction of the illness; 2.548 for disorders of the breasts and uterus; *Iliad* 3.40 as a contraceptive; *Iliad* 4.141 for an uncertain indication. There are possibly three further, fragmentary recipes according to the most recent editors, but the readings are highly doubtful (p. 23/1–13).

[375] P.Harr. inv. 303a front, of the second or third century CE (ed. Zellmann-Rohrer 2016).

and the other specifically aiming to restrain anger.[376] The Michigan text is noteworthy for prescribing a longer text, of three continuous lines, in contrast to the preference for single lines in other formularies and medical authors (see below), or the Paris codex, which combines multiple discontinuous lines.

Outside of Egypt, the amuletic use of Homer can be noted across several medical authors of the late Roman and late ancient periods, roughly contemporary with the Michigan codex. The fourth book of the *Iliad* is recommended in its entirety, presumably in book-roll form, to be placed beneath (sc. the bed of) a patient to protect against malarial fever in the verse medical handbook of Quintus Serenus, composed between the late second and fourth centuries CE: the choice is likely again analogical, the number of the book, four, corresponding to the "quartan" type of fever, recurring every fourth day on the ancient counting.[377] An amulet on a pewter leaf from Roman London features hexameters in Homeric style similar to those said to have been issued by the serpent-deity Glykon and circulated by his prophet Alexander of Abonouteichos in Paphlagonia; the text, which refers to the protection of Apollo, was probably produced as a defense against plague in the mid-second century CE (*SEG* LXIII 832).

The medical collection of Marcellus Empiricus, of the early fifth century CE, though composed in Latin, offers two such recipes along with several other ritual texts in Greek. The first prescribes two lines from the *Odyssey* (11.634–635) to help dislodge a bone stuck in the throat, which can either be spoken in the patient's ear or written down as a textual amulet.[378] Besides the analogy, in which the obstruction is equated with the head of the Gorgon feared by Odysseus in the original text—a motif that circulated on its own in both Greek and Latin—,[379] the use of a longer passage of two lines is comparable to the Mich-

---

[376] The τρίστιχος Ὁμήρου πάρεδρος, *PGM* IV.2145–2151, prescribing *Iliad* 10.564, 10.521, 10.572 (cf. Pachoumi 2017, 42, 56, 101); and the θυμοκάτοχον πρὸς φίλους, *PGM* IV.467–474, with *Iliad* 8.424, 10.193, 10.564, 10.521, 10.572, 5.385.

[377] Quintus Serenus, *Liber medicinalis* 907 (cf. Heim 1893, 518), "Place the fourth (book) of the Maeonian *Iliad* beneath one who fears (quartan fever)" (*Maeoniae Iliados quartum suppone timenti*).

[378] Marcellus Empiricus, *De medicamentis* 15.108 (cf. Heim 1893, 490 no. 95; 516 no. 151), "For a bone or whatever else sticks in the throat, these verses are to be either spoken in the ear of the one who is choking or written on a sheet, which should be bound to his neck with thread—a remedy which nothing surpasses: 'Lest dread Persephone send from Hades the head of the Gorgon, that terrible monster'" (*ad os siue quid aliud haeserit faucibus hi uersus uel dicendi in aurem eius qui offocabitur uel scribendi in charta quae ad collum eius lino alligetur. quo remedio nihil est praestantius:* 'μή μοι Γοργείην κεφαλὴν δεινοῖο πελώρου ἐξ Ἄϊδος πέμψειεν ἐπαινὴ Περσεφόνεια.')

[379] The motif of equating the obstruction with a member of the Gorgon's body recurs in Marcellus Empiricus, *De medicamentis* 8.172 (cf. Heim 1893, 489–490 no. 94), a Latin incantation stating, "I kiss the mouth [or, bone] of the Gorgon" (*os Gorgonis basio*), recommended for foreign bodies both in the eyes and the throat; and similarly in the *Mulomedicina Chironis* 974, ed. Oder

igan codex, with three lines, against the preference for single lines elsewhere in the tradition. The second recipe, for a textual amulet on fresh papyrus, applies a slightly modified version of the epithet of the Sun as watcher and listener of all in *Odyssey* 11.109 (=12.323), apparently as an analogy for the clear sight of the patient that is supposed to be defended from ophthalmia.[380]

That such procedures were not only prescribed in manuals, but also applied in practice, is already indicated indirectly for earlier periods by the testimony of Iamblichus and the parody of Lucian discussed above. Likely contemporary with the Michigan codex are two amuletic gems of unknown provenance, on both of which the same line from the *Iliad* has been inscribed (5.291), apparently as protection against the evil eye. This identification is suggested both by the iconography of the "suffering eye" attacked by wild animals accompanying the inscription on one object, and the analogical connection of the line itself, in which the goddess Athena guides the spear of the warrior Diomedes such that it pierces the eye of a foe.[381] A third gem, whose purpose remains unclear, applies *Iliad* 8.69 (=22.209), which mentions the readying of a golden scale by Zeus (*SEG* LXIV 2063): the first editor considers an apotropaic function but finds it difficult to reconcile with the verse, and indeed a more proactive approach to success in battle, the immediate context of the verse, or commerce as suggested by the scales, might be considered. A less certain case is the inscription of five lines from the *Iliad* (24.171–175) accompanied by an alphabet on the plaster of a wall in a house at Rome, in a context dated to the second or third century CE. Al-

---

1901 (cf. Önnerfors 1993, 200–201), simply *os Gorgonis*; a Greek version involving the goddess Athena may survive in the medieval additions to the *Euporiston* of Theodore Priscianus, "Pallas has swallowed the Gorgon's bones" (Παλλὰς Γοργόνης ὀστᾶ κατέπιεν, interp. ad 1.25, ed. Rose 1894, 283; understand an original ὀστᾶ κατέπιεν in place of the garbled *ostan catepieni* of the printed edition).

[380] Marcellus Empiricus, *De medicamentis* 8.58 (cf. Heim 1893, 496 no. 105), "This remedy too will doubtless prevent ophthalmia, if you act ahead (of it), written on a fresh sheet [...] 'The Sun, which watches over all and hears all.' This should be hung on the neck of the patient with thread, but it also allays incipient and chronic bleariness, if ritual purity is maintained by both (patient and healer) in the making and receiving of the amulet" (*hoc etiam remedium indubitate impetus oculorum si praeuenias prohibebit scriptum in charta uirgine* +ΟΥΒΡC+ΠΟΠΕΙΡΑC Ἥλιος ὃς πάντ' ἐφορᾷ καὶ πάντ' ἐπακούει. *quod ad collum dolentis licio suspendi debet, sed et coeptam atque inueteratam lippitudinem sedat, si in faciendo ac suscipiendo praeligamine castimonia ab utroque seruetur*). The vexed ΟΥΒΡCΠΟΠΕΙΡΑC could perhaps be emended to εὗρον ἀπὸ πείρας, "I have discovered (this remedy) by experience"; in any case a garbled translation from a Greek precursor is certain. For the Homeric text cf. also the invocation of the Sun as witness to an oath at *Iliad* 3.277, "and (you), Sun, who watches over all and hears all" (Ἠέλιός θ' ὃς πάντ' ἐφορᾷς καὶ πάντ' ἐπακούεις).

[381] "Suffering eye": a chalcedony gem, ed. *SGG* I 390; on the iconography cf. Faraone 2013a, 104. The other object is in the Wiesbaden Museum, ed. Rumpf 1866, reprinted in *IG* XIV 2580 (2); cf. Heim 1893, 517 no. 157.

though a mantic function has been suggested, an apotropaic aim seems likelier; in context, the promise of divine protection by Iris, messenger of the gods, has obvious analogical appeal.[382]

A final applied case is especially interesting as it matches exactly the prescription of a formulary recipe. On a gold sheet, which was originally rolled for insertion in a tube to be suspended on the body, and which can be dated to the second or third century CE, was found *Iliad* 2.95, describing the quaking of the earth at the hasty dispersal of an assembly of the Greek host at Troy.[383] The same verse is recommended for inscription on a gold sheet, when the moon is in Libra, or preferably Leo, as an amulet for gout in the late sixth century medical collection of Alexander of Tralles.[384] Likely an analogy is once again at work, with the aim that the feet should be healed of gout so that the patient may stride vigorously over the ground just as the Homeric warriors did.

After the early Byzantine corpus of Alexander of Tralles, the amuletic use of Homer continued in later Greek texts, most notably in a collection of advice on farming (and medicine), the *Geoponica*, and a veterinary treatise.[385] These texts, which would repay closer study, generally show the opposite of the development witnessed by the Michigan text, as will be examined presently: that is, they tend to present the Homeric verses on their own, in isolation from Christian additions.

In the Michigan codex the Homeric incantation is combined with the ritual tying of seven knots, and a further invocation, pronounced while the user faces east, to the angel Gabriel. The latter is more direct, simply invoking the angel

---

382 Found in salvage excavations at Via S. Basilio, ed. pr. Pietrogrande and De Marco 1938, 422–425 (with photograph); cf. *BE* 1950 no. 233, with the suggestion of an apotropaic function, but the further proposal there that it may have been written following the use of an oracle (repeated by Collins 2008, 226–227) is improbable: the copying of a portion of the alphabet below (ι through ω in a square four letters to a side, proceeding in columns from top to bottom, then left to right) should not be confused with the numeric key to the "Homer Oracle" (Ὁμηρομαντεῖον) in *PGM* VII.1*–66*, 1–148a (similarly *P.Oxy.* LVI 3831; *Suppl.Mag.* II 77), especially since in a true oracle consultation the numbers returned should be in a random order. Rather, the alphabet could contribute to the apotropaic assemblage, as is already allowed in *BE*.

383 Washington, D.C., Dumbarton Oaks Museum, acc. BZ1953.12.52, ed. Ross 1965, 29 no. 29, "The assembly rushed about, and the earth groaned beneath" (τετρήχι δ' ἀγορή, ὑπὸ δὲ σ|τεναχίζετο γαῖα; notation of line break added from photograph); cf. Kotansky 1991, 118 and 134 n. 83; Collins 2008, 225–226.

384 Alexander of Tralles *Therapeutica* 12, 2:581 Puschmann (cf. Heim 1893, 516 no. 152), "They also say to write the Homeric verse, 'The assembly rushed about, and the earth groaned beneath,' on a gold sheet when the Moon is in Libra, and it is much better if it is in Leo" (λέγουσι δὲ καὶ τὸν Ὁμηρικὸν στίχον· 'τετρήχει δ' ἀγορή, ὑπὸ δ' ἐστοναχίζετο γαῖα' χρυσῷ πετάλῳ γράφειν αὐτὸν οὔσης σελήνης ἐν ζυγῷ, κάλλιον δὲ πολὺ ἐὰν ἐν λέοντι εὑρεθῇ).

385 *Geoponica* 7.31.2 (*Iliad* 8.170; cf. Heim 1893, 516 no. 153) and 10.87.6 (*Iliad* 5.387; cf. Heim 1893, 516 no. 154); *Hippiatrica Cantabrigiensia* 10.5, ed. Hoppe and Oder 1927 (*Iliad* 5.749 = 8.393). For two further Byzantine instances, see Zellmann-Rohrer 2016, 7.

three times as κύριος "lord", then requesting that he heal the patient (θεράπευσον τὸν πάσχοντα). Gabriel's presence is a sure sign of the influence Judaeo-Christian traditions, as at least partially informing this recipe. There is a broadly comparable adjuration of Gabriel alongside Oriel and Raphael in a later fragment of an iatromagical formulary, for healing from boils:

> ⲉⲧⲃⲉ ⲧⲡⲁⲓϣⲉ· ϯⲧⲁⲣⲕⲟ ⲙⲙⲟⲕ ⲡⲁⲅⲅⲉⲗⲟⲥ ⲉⲧϫⲓ ϩⲙⲟⲧ ϩⲓϫⲛ ϣⲱⲛⲉ ⲛⲓⲙ ⲛϣⲁϥⲉⲓ̈ ⲉϫⲛ ⲡⲣⲱⲙⲉ ⲙⲁⲗⲓⲥⲧⲁ ⲡⲉⲓϣⲱⲛⲉ ⲡⲁⲓ̈· ⲛϣⲁϥϥⲓ ⲙⲡⲣⲱⲙⲉ ϩⲙ ⲡⲉϥⲅⲉⲣⲟⲥ· ⲙⲁⲣⲉϯⲡⲁⲓϣⲉ ⲉ̅ⲓ ⲉⲃⲟⲗ ϩⲛ ⲇ̅ⲇ̅ ⲟⲣ̅ⲓ̅ⲏ̅ⲗ̅ ⲅⲁⲃ̅ⲣ̅ⲓ̅ⲏ̅ⲗ̅ ⲣⲁⲫ̅ⲁ̅ⲏ̅ⲗ̅· ⲡⲉⲧⲧⲱⲃ`ϩ´ ϣⲱⲛⲉ ⲛⲓⲙ : ⲙⲁⲣⲉϥⲗⲟ ⲛϭⲓ ⲛⲇ̅ⲇ̅ ⲛⲟϣⲡϥ ϩⲓ̈ ⲏⲣⲡ - - -
>
> For boils: "I adjure you, the angel who receives grace against every sickness that befalls mankind, especially (μάλιστα) this sickness that takes mankind in their old age (γῆρος). May these boils depart from so-and-so. Oriel, Gabriel, Raphael, the one who consoles <in?> every sickness, let so-and-so get relief". Cast (lit. blow) it over wine.[386]

That this adjuration derived from a Greek exemplar, perhaps ultimately related to the present text, is all but assured by the presence of the loanwords γῆρος and μάλιστα.

The Byzantine continuation of the amuletic use of Homer, discussed already, further indicates how it could be reconciled, if not directly combined, with the Christian dispensation. An instructive parallel is the even more widespread use of the poetry of Vergil, who composed on similar themes in the same meter (dactylic hexameter) adapted in Latin, in healing incantations in Latin texts in the medieval West. In late ancient medical recipes, we find a parallel for the use of epic text against fever, namely *Aeneid* 4.129 (=11.1) recommended as an amulet against the quartan variety,

> item: in charta scribis, Oceanum interea surgens Aurora reliquit
>
> Likewise. You write on papyrus, "Meanwhile the rising Dawn left behind Ocean",[387]

and this same verse is also offered to ease birth, written on the lintel of a door,

[386] *P.Borg.Copt.* 278 p. 241/7–12 (ed. pp. 626–627; the text has been adjusted based on a collation, kindly communicated by Korshi Dosoo, with a photograph of the parchment).

[387] [Pliny], *Physica*, from St. Gallen, Stiftsbibliothek cod. 751, 3.18 (cod. p. 272.15–16, ed. Önnerfors 2006, 1: 91; cf. Heim 1893, 502 no. 121 and 519–520 no. 160).

> item ut cito pariat mulier: scribes in limine superiore ostii, 'Oceanum interea surgens Aurora reliquit.'[388]
> Likewise, so that a woman may give birth quickly. You will write on the upper sill of the door, "Meanwhile the rising Dawn left behind Ocean",

a goal pursued in turn by yet another verse, *Eclogues* 4.10, written on papyrus and attached to the mother's thigh,

> de muliere quae tarde parit: scribes in charta pura de uua tincta 'casta faue Lucina, tuus iam regnat Apollo.' et de licio dextro femori alligabis, et cum enixa fuerit, statim solues
> For a woman who is slow to give birth. You will write on clean papyrus with grape-extract, "Show favor, chaste Lucina: now is the reign of your Apollo." You will attach with thread to the right thigh, and when she has given birth, you will untie it at once.[389]

An anonymous medieval collection of the eleventh century brings *Aeneid* 10.1 to bear on the same birthing crisis. In two different versions, now in combination with Christian incantation motifs, analogies are drawn between the healing scenario and the miraculous births of Mary by Anna and Christ by Mary and the raising of Lazarus,

> si mulier non potest parere: liga hoc ad dextrum crurem, 'panditur interea domus omnipot⟨ent⟩is Olympi. Anna genuit Mariam, Maria genuit Christum. Lazare ueni foras.'
> If a woman cannot give birth, bind this to (her) right leg, "Meanwhile the house of almighty Olympus is opened. Anna bore Mary, Mary bore Christ. Lazarus, come forth",

and,

> si mulier de partu laborat: sc⟨r⟩ibe hoc in charta, 'panditur interea domus omnipotentis Olympi. ex tonna propera, Christus rex te uocat ut uideas lumen huius saeculi.' hoc scriptum cum litio nouo ligare debes ad coxam mulieris dextram et cum exierit infans cito tolle ne sequatur matrix. probatum est.

---

[388] Epistolary treatise of Theodore Priscianus to his son Octavius (a later addition to the *Euporiston*), §4, ed. Rose 1894, 345 (with Önnerfors 1993, 210 no. 25).

[389] Ibid. §2, ed. Rose 1894, 340–341 (with Önnerfors 1993, 210 no. 23).

> If a woman has difficulty in birthing: write this on a sheet, "Meanwhile the house of almighty Olympus is opened. Hasten from the tomb: Christ the king calls you to see the light of this world." You should bind this writing with new thread to the right thigh of the woman, and when the infant comes out, remove it quickly, lest the womb follow. It is proven.[390]

Both versions continued to be copied, with variations, until the fifteenth century, in combination with other Vergilian borrowings as well as Christian motifs, hymns, and Psalms.[391]

A final verse, *Eclogues* 4.7, was turned to the same purpose in a fifteenth-century manuscript.[392] The selection, "Now a new offspring is sent down from lofty heaven" (*iam nova progenies caelo demittitur alto*) proves both analogically appropriate for a successful birth and appealingly easy to reconcile with the Christian project of retrojecting prophecies of Christ's birth into pre-Christian literature.

It is against that background of the medieval Christian continuation in both Greek and Latin texts of the use of epic verse in incantations that the application in the Michigan codex takes on additional interest. A relatively sophisticated adaptation of multiple continuous lines of Homer, despite flaws in the copying, it also shows an integration with Judaeo-Christian traditions with respect to angelology that will have prepared the way for the later uptake of Homeric and Vergilian incantations in a more thoroughly Christian milieu.

---

390 London, British Library Sloane Ms. 475, ff. 23r and 113v (both unpublished).

391 Examples include a twelfth-century medical manuscript once at Herten, cod. 192, f. 88r (ed. Sudhoff 1917, 304); the fourteenth-century Munich, Bayerische Staatsbibliothek clm 4350, f. 84r (ed. Schönbach 1893, 40) and ibid. clm 7021, f. 188v (cf. Franz 1909, 2:202), and the fifteenth-century Heidelberg, Universitätsbibliothek cod. Pal. germ. 369, f. 169v (ed. Schönbach 1893, 40); with *Aeneid* 4.129 (=11.1), the fifteenth-century Heidelberg, Universitätsbibliothek cod. Pal. germ. 213, f. 96v (ed. Schönbach 1893, 40), and similarly the codex excerpted by Franz 1909, 2:201; with the following verse, *Aen.* 10.2, the fifteenth-century medical commonplace book London, British Library Harley Ms. 2558, f. 117r (ed. Jones 2007, 105 n. 17, not recognizing the Vergilian citations); with *Aeneid* 4.129 (=11.1) and *Eclogues* 4.10, the fourteenth-century Munich, Bayerische Staatsbibliothek clm 7021, f. 160v (cf. Schönbach 1893, 39).

392 London, British Library Sloane Ms. 3564, ed. Hunt 1990, 92.

§§9 and 10 The "Voice" and "Cow" of Amun (EL)

As an introduction to the following two excurses to §§9 and 10, here the nature of recipes comprising "divine dramas" will be presented—also termed variously as "*historiolae*" or "charms"—, as opposed to the combination of ritual instructions, invocations, commands, and *voces magicae* that comprise the other recipes in the Michigan codex.[393]

I. Divine Dramas in Egyptian Tradition

§§9 and 10 each concern a "divine drama" that constitutes a mythological precedent for the desired outcome—the rationale—for which the recipe would have been practiced. In Egyptian ritual tradition, a divine drama comprises a mythological narrative concerning protagonists and ancillary characters, and direct, unmediated dialogue of and between them. In the practice of magical texts, the recitation of such mythological precedents—the narrative descriptions of the times, settings, characters, actions, and dialogue of their characters—, and the analogies between the divine protagonist in such mythological precedent and the practitioner or client in contemporary rituals, provide the efficacy through which the desired outcome is brought about.

In a divine drama, a protagonist interacts with other characters in a mythological landscape, presumably conceptualized as being set in mythological time, but often narrated with dialogue in the present. As such, this episode serves as a precedent to the ritual as undertaken in contemporary time. In certain spheres of Egyptian ritual practice,[394] the efficacy of the divine dramas embedded in mythological precedents was unlocked quite literally through re-enacting them—through dramatic performance.[395] In the context of temple rituals, the king's

[393] For this typology of these features in magical texts, and its related bibliographies, see Love 2016, 121–122 n. 36–39. There, "commands" are referred to as "invocations for task", but the former is now preferred.

[394] As in Love 2016, 120 n. 34, I treat the differentiation between ritual practices that were undertaken in the temple, in a funerary context, or in a personal context, as one primarily of *function* and not of *form*, i.e. a ritual practiced for the benefit of a deity/deities and/or thereby the king/Pharaoh is a temple ritual; that practiced for the benefit of a deceased individual is an afterlife ritual; that practiced for the benefit of a living individual to bring about a desired outcome in the lived experience of that individual is a magical ritual.

[395] The examples cited here are among those considered by Gillam as examples of "highly structured ritual routines" of drama (2009, 2, with the introductory bibliographies to each example,

coronation, the sed-festival ensuring his renewal upon the throne, and execration rituals that destroyed the king's enemies, saw practitioners—the king or priests as his proxies—performing the role of divine protagonists, principally Horus, by undertaking dramatized ritual practices that re-enacted mythological precedents. These mythological precedents, and their desired outcomes, e.g. the coronation and renewal of the king or the destruction of his enemies, were actualized by virtue of being re-enacted, their efficacy stemming from the analogy between mythological setting and contemporary time, divine protagonists and human practitioners. In the context of afterlife rituals, e.g. the ritual of *Mummification* or *Opening the Mouth*, the practitioners—such as lector priests—identified with the role of divine protagonists, such as Anubis in his role as the mummifier of Osiris's corpse who ensured his survival as a corporeal being or Horus in his role as the *stm*-priest of Osiris who revivified his corpse, respectively. Ritual practices in Egyptian tradition contain a plethora of mythological allusions and involve the identication of the practitioners with certain divine protagonists, yet this is mostly without the direct recitation of the narrative of those mythological precedents.

Nevertheless, that is not to say that such dramatized performances of mythological precedents are not attested. The cosmogonic *Conflict of Horus and Seth* over the throne of Osiris is a prime example, in which the king, royal children, priests, and court officials would all re-enact the roles of specific divine protagonists, for which stage settings and props are even attested.[396] *The Stanzas of the Festival of the Two Kites*, first practiced as part of the Khoiak festival of Osiris and later adapted into afterlife ritual texts, saw three roles being played, the first by a lector priest, and the other two by priestesses, who must be virgins—or at least women who have not yet borne any children—, be hairless, wear wigs, carry tambourines, and have the name of the goddess whom they are playing—either Isis or Nephthys—inscribed upon their arms. In dramatically performing the role of these two goddesses, the sisters and wives of Osiris, their "weeping and wailing actually help[ed] to revivify and transfigure" the deceased deity Osiris, or the Osiris of the deceased individual.[397] Of particular relevance to the divine drama of §9 is Sauneron's assessment of the textual sources for the *Mystery of the God's Birth* from the Temple of Neith at Esna, which he argues

---

summarizing the comprehensive study in Gillam 2005). For studies of drama in Ancient and Graeco-Roman Egypt, see the summary and bibliography in Gillam 2009, 4–6.

[396] As summarized recently by Gillam, extant textual sources for the dramatized re-enactment of the cosmogonic *Conflict of Horus and Seth* date from the late Middle Kingdom to Roman Period (2009, 2–3 with the bibliography there).

[397] Smith 2009, 98.

also preserve a composition that would have been undertaken as a dramatized performance.[398]

In other spheres of Egyptian ritual practice, principally in the context of magical rituals—i.e. rituals for the personal benefit of non-divine, non-royal living individuals—the efficacy of divine dramas was unlocked through recitation and the implicit analogies drawn between contemporary practitioner or client and divine protagonist, rather than dramatized performance of the type just described. Nevertheless, the analogies to be drawn behind this conceptualization of ritual, where mythological times, settings, characters, actions, and dialogues are not just alluded to but re-enacted or recited, underpin much of the tradition of Egyptian ritual, however the exact *form* of the practices themselves may vary. Whether re-enacted or recited, analogies were drawn between the role and actions of the contemporary practitioner and the divine protagonist in the mythological precedent, which underpins the efficacy of the ritual practices themselves. In doing so, an analogy was drawn between contemporary and mythological time. As the desired outcome was achieved in mythological time as preserved in the mythological precedent, so too will—through re-enactment or recitation of the ritual—the desired outcome be achieved for the practitioner or client in contemporary time.

It is through the use of the term "divine drama" that this study aims to draw into focus the ritual mechanism that underpinned so much of the tradition of Egyptian ritual practice—whether temple, afterlife, or magical; the process of analogy between contemporary ritual practices and the narration and dialogue of mythological precedents on the one hand, and contemporary practitioners and divine protagonists on the other. Indeed, although the term "*historiola*"—"short story"—has gained traction in the study of magical texts,[399] and the term "charm" has recently been introduced in the study of ancient ones, the term "divine drama" instead keeps the study of comparable textual traditions and ritual practices as attested in temple, afterlife, and magical texts within the terminology of the wider discourse within Egyptology, where neither "*historiola*" nor "charm" is current. For example, the dramatized re-enactment of mythological precedents evidenced in "dramatic texts" or the recitation of mythological precedents preserved from Ancient and Graeco-Roman Egypt,

[398] As summarized by Gillam (2009, 4), see the bibliography there.

[399] A principal objection to the use of this term will be clear from a reading of the excurses to §§9 and 10, where the supposed "story" is not so much a "story", but rather a drama that plays out through narration and direct, unmediated dialogue principally in the present, as well as in past, time. A reader does not experience being told a "story", but rather being witness to (fragments of) a "drama". Further objections include the unfortunate use of the Latin diminutive, striking the reader as somewhat derogatory, as well as its inaccuracy, in so far as many "divine dramas" in Egyptian tradition, including those utilized in magical practices, are in no way "short".

such as those noted above, are often referred to in Egyptological discourse as "cult"[400] or "ritual"[401] dramas of ritual practice that re-enact the "divine", "sacred",[402] "holy",[403] or "cosmic"[404] dramas of those mythological precedents.[405]

"Divine drama", then, encapsulates both the times, settings, actions, characters, and dialogues of mythological precedents *and* their re-enactment as part of a dramatized performance *or* recitation in contemporary time, where the role of the practitioner or client is analogous to that of the divine characters. These texts are often "narrative" in the sense that a mythological scene is set and the actions of its characters are narrated, but in Egyptian tradition these narratives are rarely exclusively narrative descriptions, because their characters often enter into a direct, unmediated dialogue, fundamental to the "dramatic" nature of these compositions. Thus, divine drama as a term unifies the *form* of this textual tradition among the *functions* for which it was employed in temple, funerary, and magical rituals, while also highlighting the importance of the analogy between the mythological times, settings, characters, actions, and dialogues and those of the contemporary ritual practiced. The re-enactment or recitation of a divine drama unlocks the efficacy of the mythological precedent, actualizing the outcome of the divine drama for the contemporary practitioner or client.

II. Divine Dramas in the Study of Magical Texts

The textual tradition of divine dramas in the specific context of magical texts and their accompanying ritual mechanics have long been identified as a subcategory of magical texts, termed variously as "*historiolae*"—"short stories"—or "charms", as proposed in a recent study that considered them part of a cross-

400 Assmann (2005) uses "cult drama" to refer to that dramatized performance of priests in afterlife rituals.

401 Teeter refers to the funerary procession in Egyptian tradition as a "ritual drama" (2011, 138). For a cross-cultural comparison of the "ritual drama" in the *Horus Myth of Edfu* with two other contexts, see the study by Podemann Sørensen 1986.

402 On the "sacred drama" of *The Triumph of Horus and Seth*, see Fairman 1974.

403 For the *Ramesseum Dramatic Papyrus* as a "holy drama", see Bleeker 1958, 7.

404 In the context of the *Daily Ritual*, a priest would re-enact the role of a deity in order to participate in the "cosmic drama of the battle between chaos and order", while the ritual of *Opening the Mouth* when practiced in an Egyptian temple on cult statues was also a "cosmic drama": so Dieleman 2005, 82; 182.

405 Although the present author utilized the term uncritically in Love 2016, the following study elucidates the reasoning for the favored term "divine drama". Principally, the term "divine drama" unifies the *form* of the textual tradition among the *functions* of the ritual traditions in which it was employed in temple, afterlife, and magical rituals, and contextualizes the study of "divine dramas" in magical texts among the wider discourse of "drama" in other ritual traditions from Ancient and Graeco-Roman Egypt, rather than drawing upon frameworks from fields concerned with distinct cultural and temporal frames.

cultural phenomenon.[406] The "theory", the mechanics behind the "narrative power" of such "*historiolae*"—as Frankfurter termed them—in magical texts was proposed in a formative and influential study by Frankfurter (1995). [407] In that study, Frankfurter drew from a discourse familiar within Egyptology about how performing—narrating—mythological precedents "situates or directs their 'narrative' power" into the ritual context, albeit while utilizing the term "*historiola*", rather than a term current in Egyptology.[408] "Charms", synonymous with ritual texts that comprise only "*historiolae*", was recently introduced as a term for the sub-category of magical texts that—mostly—lack invocations, commands, *voces magicae*, ritual instructions, or any of the other genre features of magical texts.[409] Frankfurter thus presents "*historiolae*" as efficacious in and of themselves.[410] This is because they contain "the *authoritative discourse of precedent* in a given region at a certain time".[411] The recitation or the inscription of their narrative actualizes their efficacy, whereby the latter "generally functioned to 'lock in' the power of the uttered words for ongoing effect"—although

[406] Most notably in Blumell and Dosoo 2018 and van der Vliet 2018. Blumell and Dosoo (2018, 222 n. 54) utilize the term "charm" in order "to distinguish the brief narrative charms from longer invocations with significant non-narrative content". In my judgement, however, a study of the divine dramas embedded within magical texts first within the broader context of the Egyptian ritual tradition, and the discourse thereon within Egyptology, would be a desirable first step, preceding the importing of a framework of analysis developed for the heuristic study of magical texts and traditions of ritual practice from entirely distinct cultural and temporal contexts, that of the study of medieval European Christian magic. Indeed, Blumell and Dosoo anachronistically apply the term "charm" to all examples of what they term "charms" from Pharaonic and Graeco-Roman Egypt (2018, 226–227; 241–245), thereby overwriting the terminology established in Egyptology, while also drawing together a vast corpus from entirely distinct cultural and temporal frames without engaging with the distinct discourses on these phenomena within, for example, medieval/early modern European studies and Egyptology, let alone the notable distinctions between the corpora (e.g. present time and direct, unmediated dialogue between characters).

[407] "*Historiolae*" are "the performative transmission of power from a mythic realm articulated in narrative to the human present" (Frankfurter 1995, 464). For a bibliography on the "*historiolae*" in the context of Egypt, see Love 2016, 121 n. 40. To that, add the two recent studies in the preceding footnote.

[408] Frankfurter 1995, 457; n. 2–3.

[409] The complications in the application of this term so defined, however, are illustrated by the fact that the assemblage of ostraca (O.BYU Mag.) that forms the centerpiece of the recent study of Coptic "charms" by Blumell and Dosoo (2018) in fact opens with a series of *voces magicae* inscribed before the narration of the divine drama begins. This demonstrates rather clearly that the above typology of the different components of magical texts and thereby the practiced rituals may well be a heuristic tool for modern scholars, but that such a typology does not seem to represent a categorization that would have been recognized by contemporary practitioners and clients.

[410] Whether this was the case for *PGM* IV.94–113, embedded in a composite recipe whose constituent elements make little sense when practiced on their own, has been treated at length in Love 2016, §5.

[411] Frankfurter 1995, 474.

they are generally conceived of as principally oral—recited, rather than inscribed—texts.[412] Frankfurter further applied speech-acts theory to identify the mechanism behind the efficacy of the "*historiolae*", in which "the utterance 'performs' the action desired",[413] mechanics common not only to traditional Egyptian ritual, but also traditions elsewhere in the Near East, including those which drew from Egyptian ritual practices.

The mythological precedent of a divine drama was presumably conceptualized as having occurred in mythological, deep time. Noteworthy, and often understated, however, is that the narration of, and direct, unmediated dialogue within, those divine dramas is often in the present tense. In the traditional Egyptian context, this appears to reflect the conceptualization of both linear (*ḏ.t*) and cyclical (*nḥḥ*) time. While the rising and setting of the sun is one episode that can be described linearly as beginning and ending, it also is a daily event that can be described cyclically as recurring. This is, then, quite distinct from the concept of the "*historiola*" as developed for the study of medieval European Christian magic.[414] There, the "*historiola*" referred to a "short story" where the characteristic reference is to *past* biblical events in the life of Christ or the patriarchs, among others, which only happened *once*. Consequently, from the perspective of their practitioners and clients, these could have been conceptualized less as mythological than historical.[415]

In divine dramas, action occurs not in the human but in the divine sphere, and it is between these spheres that analogies are drawn regarding the problem that requires a resolution—the rationale behind and the desired outcome of the ritual practice. Analogically, as the problem is resolved in the mythological precedent, so too shall the contemporary problem find resolution. Here, the divine dramas are distinct from other mechanics of ritual practice, such as invocations in the name of deities, commands to them, and identifying statements, often including coercion to compel the invoked and commanded deities. In this way, as Frankfurter highlighted, divine dramas are distinct from ritual practices whose speech

---

412 Frankfurter 1995, 463. On this, see the discussion on "Textual vs. Oral Transmission" (V) in **Transmitting Textual Traditions**.

413 Frankfurter 1995, 466.

414 A notable example is that from an "Anglo-Saxon charm" cited as a cross-cultural comparison by Blumell and Dosoo (2018, 256 n. 152), which is not only narrated in the past, but also lacks direct or unmediated dialogue to be recited in the present tense.

415 For example, in a group of procedures to stop bleeding, attested in medieval Greek, Latin, and Syriac, citing the lithification of the blood of Zacharias mentioned in the *Protevangelium of James*, e.g. "The prophet Zacharias was murdered in the temple. His blood congealed like a stone and will not be removed until his avenger comes", sometimes expanded with commands or wishes about the patient's blood, etc.: for the Zacharias type see in general Barb 1948; for Greek and Syriac, relevant witnesses will be published in the corpora currently in preparation by Zellmann-Rohrer for the respective languages; for an orientation to the Syriac corpus see id. 2021.

acts command and coerce, instead declaring a situation a *fait accompli*.[416] The authority and thereby efficacy of the practice rests in the narrative; the recitation itself only actualizes its desired outcome.

Developing this thesis, van der Vliet drew from literary criticism, introducing the typology of "voiced" as opposed to "oral" texts in order to explain the apparent dichotomy between magical texts which evidence an "essentially oral genre", where "poetic qualities provide the key to its efficacy in performance", and the fact that all magical texts from Egypt are the "product of scribal culture".[417] Given that "oral literary strategies and formats", while having a profound impact on *textual structure*, "are not themselves indicative of the oral origins of that text or even its oral transmission over time", texts can bear "the stamp of orality". That quality, however, comes not because they are "oral" texts, but because they are "voiced" texts—written texts whose efficacy depends on oral performance. Divine dramas are thereby the principal example of "voiced" texts in the genre of magical ritual and stand alongside the "voiced" hymns and liturgies of Egyptian temple and afterlife rituals.[418]

In addition to these considerations, Frankfurter makes two further important delineations in the *structure* of his "*historiolae*":[419] (i) those which are the sole constituents of magical texts, whose mechanics comprise only their narrative, can be typologized as "*historiolae* proper"; (ii) those in magical texts which include subsidiary invocations or commands—"directive utterances"—can be typologized as "clausal *historiolae*". As will be seen, both §§9 and 10 feature the mythological precedent of a divine drama, but conclude with commands that, while cited by a divine protagonist, provide the fundamental "clausal" element, i.e. the element that stipulates the desired outcome to be actualized by the recitation or inscription of the text. Thus, the practitioner identifies with the protagonist of the mythological precedent by reciting and thereby actualizing the resolution of the mythological precedent in the divine drama. In doing so, the practitioner acquires the authority and efficacy, through the authoritative and efficacious narrative and dialogue of the mythological precedent, that affect the contemporary practiced ritual, bringing about its desired outcome in the human sphere, exactly as had occurred in the divine sphere as narrated in the mythological precedent.

[416] Frankfurter 1995, 468.

[417] Van der Vliet 2018, 161. This is then contrary to the fundamental thesis of Blumell and Dosoo (2018), who argue for a principally oral, or at least mixed oral and textual transmission, as discussed and appraised at length in "Textual vs. Oral Transmission" (V) of **Transmitting Textual Traditions**.

[418] Discussed further in "Textual vs. Oral Transmission" (V) of **Transmitting Textual Traditions**.

[419] Frankfurter 1995, 469.

III. The Caveats to the Excurses to §§9 and 10

Before embarking on a close treatment of both §§9 and 10, caveats concerning the nature of the extant texts need to be raised. As discussed in the commentary to §§9 and 10, the extant form of both texts includes certain and possible mistakes, miscopyings, and issues of discontinuity which suggest that something may have been missed, lost, or confused during their histories of textual transmission.[420] However, given that both §§9 and 10 exist in this form in an extant source, the textual *structure* and *content* of these recipes are taken in these excurses as integral in and of themselves. Irrespective of any potential errors, and potential proposals as to how they should be emended by modern scholars, their form is, after all, the form in which they were copied into the Michigan codex. This was, then, the form in which they would have been practiced, and in which they would have served as a source text for any further copying of the recipes in subsequent textual transmission.

One final consideration is that in order to tease out the resonances of the divine dramas of both §§9 and 10, a wide range of sources will be drawn upon. In the context of Egypt, with its millennia of textual culture production, drawing diachronic parallels across vast temporal and spatial frames is not only possible, it is often seen as desirable given the sparsity of synchronically extant evidence, and the even more disjointed approach to their publication. Nevertheless, when the viability of textual transmission is not considered, this is an approach that—although fundamental to philology, especially in the editing of texts—must be undertaken with caution.[421] Therefore, although in certain cases informative parallels are only found in distinct temporal and spatial contexts to the Michigan codex, these excurses will nevertheless privilege sources from the Graeco-Roman Period, whose *content* could reasonably be considered to have been current in the textual, oral, and aural milieux of the *script communities* and *communities of practice* that existed in late Roman Egypt.[422]

---

[420] For example, in §9 there is an object missing in the expression "oil for bringing out of", leaving the extant text incomplete. This object could simply have been missed in the copying of the text over the page (p. 5 to p. 6) and could have been as simple as "the child", see the commentary to p. 5/20. Nevertheless, it demonstrates one specific scribal copying error, leaving open the possibility of copying errors elsewhere.

[421] See in particular the comments in Love 2018/19b, 114 with n. 30.

[422] See "Language and Script Communities, Domains, and Variety in the Roman Period" (I) in **Transmitting Textual Traditions**.

IV. The Structure of the Excurses to §§9 and 10

The following two excurses begin by providing a summary of the narrative and mechanics of the divine dramas that comprise each recipe. Following this, the divine dramas are treated section by section, with the Coptic text presented alongside an interlinear translation, visualizing and elucidating the *textual structure* clause by clause. This in turn allows a study of the shape and texture of the syntax and semantics of the clauses that make up each section, and thereby a detailed consideration of §§9 and 10 as "voiced" texts of oral production, recited (produced) by practitioners and heard (responded to) by clients through aural reception. The construction and reification of narrative momentum and the efficacy of the mythological precedent can thus be considered, while a consideration of the layers of (re)composition serves to elucidate the history of (re)composition and textual transmission.[423] The *textual content* of each of these sections is then treated, with emphasis on the mythological and cosmogonic resonances from traditional Egyptian cultural repertoires, as well as the treatment of both parallels and novelties. This will serve to contextualize §§9 and 10 within the complexities of textual traditions that make up the Graeco-Egyptian magical papyri (GEMP), in turn highlighting that the Michigan codex is to be contextualized at the nexus between these textual traditions and ritual practices and those of the later Coptic magical papyri (CMP) of Christian(ized) Egypt.

§9 The Voice of Amun (pp. 5/1–6/5) (EL)

Voice (or, sound) of wind (or, breath), when there is no wind.
Voice (or, sound) of wave (or, flood), when there is no wave.
Voice of Amun, the three gods.

"Amun, where is it that you are going in this form, in this manner?"

"It is with the south-wind that I am going, northwards between reed and rush, {between} I am going to Abydos between these two mountains of these two hills.
What I am mounted on is a white horse, a black horse was before me,
while the books of Thoth are with me, those of the Great-of-Five in my hands.
What I cause to give birth are the ones who are pregnant.
What I close up are those who miscarry.
What I cause to be fertile is every egg, except the infertile eggs."

[423] See further **Transmitting Textual Traditions**.

He was sent, Thoth. He came out before me.
"Amun, where is it that you are going?"

"The Three of Isis (or, the three Isises), today, it is for four days (or, times) that she is suffering (in labor). It is so-and-so many times that he releases the birth bricks."

"If you have not found me, have not found my name, have not found a little oil for bringing out of <...> and you should put it along the ridge of her back downwards, saying:
'Cease! Cease there! Prepare yourself! Prepare your womb! Serve your offspring! Produce milk for Horus your son through the power of the lord god!'"

I. Narrative and Mechanics

Through the recitation of §9, practitioner and client—or, indeed, physician and patient—are transported into mythological time. In the mythological scene setting that opens §9, there is a dissonance, a tension between existence and absence. As will be seen, the sound or voice of the wind or breath as well as that of the flood or wave are resonant of Amun as the primordial creator deity who was the wind that blew over the Primaeval Ocean before creation. Furthermore, the reference to either a divine triad or to Amun's tripartite nature as solar creator alludes to his role as the superordinate deity, who brought himself into being before bringing deities and humanity into being. This mythological scene is set through an unidentified narrator, where specifics are rare and characters are not introduced, but whose presence and absence, as well as identity, appear implicit. In the first scene, narration suddenly gives way to dialogue, whereby the central character, the protagonist Amun—implicit in the mythological scene setting—is introduced through a direct address.[424]

An unidentified, disembodied voice asks Amun where he is going, and why it is in such a particular form and manner—alluding to the wind and wave—that Amun is going. Amun answers, stressing that he is going with—indeed, in the form of—the south-wind, blowing northwards through the mythological landscape of riverbanks and marshes. The destination is specified as Abydos, and Amun is not only manifest in the south-wind, but also envisaged riding through this landscape in a corporeal form, mounted upon a white horse and bearing the Books of Thoth—an authoritative compilation of ritual texts in Egyptian tradition. With Amun's statements answering the questions of "where" and "in what form" posed by the unidentified, disembodied voice, Amun declares his motivation, the purpose of his form and thereby his journey, to ensure the successful

[424] In other divine dramas, passages concerning mythological scene setting sometimes narrate the actions of the character(s) in the third person.

delivery and suckling of a child. As discussed below, while presented in a reversed order with respect to the natural one, these roles are immediately reminiscent of those played by Amun in the ritual of the *God's Birth*, practiced in the cult of the child-god in the mammisis—"birth houses"—of Egyptian temples.[425]

In the following scene, having been sent by (an) unidentified agent(s),[426] Thoth presents himself to Amun—an act reminiscent of his role in the aforementioned ritual of the *God's Birth*. Stressing instead Amun's destination, Thoth again poses the question as to where Amun's journey is to take him. In the current form of the text,[427] Amun replies by explaining that at the moment of their dialogue "the Three of Isis" have been in labor for four days—"times"—a number that recalls the three midwives of the god's mother in that same ritual. Here, the temporal and spatial disjunction between the mythological precedent and contemporary practice are bridged, since the text in its current form offers a place in which the practitioner can specify the number of days—"times"—until the birth bricks are released, that is to say, safe delivery will be ensured because the lifetime of the child will have begun.

Amun's journey has thus concluded with him presenting the ritual instructions to be carried out and commands to be recited in his absence, lending them the authority and thereby efficacy of the mythological precedent;[428] as they served to bring Isis' labor to an end, so should they serve for the patient. An oil is to be put along the ridge of "her"—that is, Isis' and thereby the patient's—back, and certain imperatives are directed towards Isis and thereby the patient. These divinely-derived commands lead Isis, and thereby the patient, through the stages of safe delivery: firstly, by commanding Isis to "cease", i.e. her labor;[429] secondly, by ensuring that the womb is "prepared"—or, even, "secured"—for the delivery that concludes the labor; thirdly, to "serve" the newborn offspring through lactation and suckling—itself a matter of life and death for the newborn child. Lending further authority and thereby efficacy to the commands, they are identified not only as those given to Isis while she was in labor, but also as those that ensured the safe delivery and nourishment of Horus.

---

[425] For an introduction and bibliography to the mammisis, see Kockelmann 2011, as well as the discussion below.

[426] The Egyptian-Coptic uses the impersonal passive and does not introduce a postponed agent.

[427] Corruption may be suspected, but ultimately the text can be accepted as grammatically and syntactically integral in its extant form: see the commentary to p. 5/15, where some reconstructions are considered.

[428] In Frankfurter's typology, this statement "situates" the mythical precedent within the performative setting of the ritual by equating a substance from the former with a substance from the latter setting (1995, 470–471): see further the introduction to the excurses to §§9 and 10.

[429] Here the command is specified by the use of the imperative.

The divine source, and thereby authority and efficacy, of the commands is given in a final clause as "the lord god". Clearly a later interpolation into the composition, this closing statement is one common to the tradition of Coptic magical texts, but—as will be seen[430]—need not be taken in this context as one of an overtly Judaizing or Christianizing influence, and thereby copyist(s) and practitioner(s).[431] Nevertheless, the authoritative and efficacious mythological precedent of the divine drama, expressing reflexes of both the complexities of Egyptian cosmogonies and the ritual of the *God's Birth*, is anchored in the contemporary context of the Michigan codex by use of a closing formula resonant to the temporal frame of its production and use.[432] Here, then, the traditional alongside contemporary content of the composition approaches a metaphorical representation of juxtaposition of mythological precedent and contemporary practice inherent in the divine drama itself.

In what follows, a close reading of the *textual structure* and *content* will serve to elucidate the divine drama that unfolds in §9, the mythological and cosmogonic resonances from Egyptian tradition that are implicit in the narrative, the motifs drawn from them, and how these combine to give narrative momentum to the presentation of problem and resolution fundamental to the mechanics of this divine drama.

I.1. The Mythological Scene Setting

ϩⲣⲟⲩ ⲛ̄ⲧⲏ̣ⲟⲩ ⲉⲙ̄ⲛ̄ⲧⲏ[ⲟⲩ] "Voice (or, sound) of wind (or, breath), when there is no wind"
ḫrw n tw ỉw mn tw
ḫrw ṯ3w nn ṯ3w ỉm=f "Voice (or, sound) of wind, when there is no wind in it"[433]
ϩⲣⲟⲟⲩ ⲛ̄ϩⲟⲓ̈ⲙⲉ ⲉⲙ̄ⲛ̄ϩⲟⲓ̈ⲙⲉ· "Voice of wave (or, flood), (when) there is no wave"
ḫrw n hym ỉw mn hym

---

[430] In these excurses and also in **Transmitting Textual Traditions**. See also the following two footnotes.

[431] Contrary to the interpretations of Frankfurter, who refers to §§9 and 10 being "punctuated with references to the Christian God" (2018, 208), or "Christianizing accretions" (2009, 242), van der Vliet, who calls this particular invocation "a clear Christian insertion" (2018, 159), and Dosoo 2021. See also the following footnote.

[432] Indeed, given that this supplication comprises one clause added to the end of a substantial composition that does not contain anything that could be considered diagnostically Christian—as discussed more broadly in **Transmitting Textual Traditions**—this clause could be considered an appropriation of an efficacious invocation from Jewish or Judaeo-Christian magical texts into a pre- and thereby non-Christian recipe rather than syncretism of a "pagan" divine drama into a Christianized magical tradition—contrary to Frankfurter, van der Vliet, and Dosoo, see the preceding footnote. After all, and contrary to those prior opinions, during the Roman Period syncretism was not a one-way street from "pagan" to Christian: see "Syncretism in the Other Direction" (VI) in **Transmitting Textual Traditions**.

[433] (P.Chester Beatty VII 6/7).

ẖrw mw n ms.t ḥꜥpỉ “Voice (or, sound) of water, (when) the Nile has not been born”[434]
ϩⲣ´ⲟ`ⲟⲩ ⲛ̄ⲁⲙⲟⲩⲛ ⲡϣ̄ⲙ̄ⲛ̄ⲧ̄ⲛ̄ⲧⲏⲣ· “Voice of Amun, the three gods”
ẖrw n ỉmn pꜣ ẖmt nṯr.w
šꜣ=tw -st r wbn rꜥ.w r psḏ ỉtn r psḏ ỉtn r ḏd.t n pꜣ ntỉ m tpḥ.t=f “One should heed the rising of the sun, the shining of the disk, and what is said by he who is in his cavern”[435]

I.1.a. Textual Structure

The treatment of the mythological scene setting of §9 is brought into focus here by comparison to a partial parallel from the Egyptian magical tradition preserved in P.Chester Beatty VII, a bookroll of magical texts dating to the 19th Dynasty (1291–1191 BCE) from Deir el-Medina on the West Bank of Luxor[436]—that is, a millennium and a half before the Michigan codex was produced. In the case of the first two phrases, close semantic parallels are differentiated from one another only by the change in the syntax and lexicon of the Egyptian language over this vast temporal frame, serving to illustrate the complexity of creative considerations inherent in the apparently paradoxical mythological scene setting.

The tripartite structure of the mythological scene setting is clear from the layout of the text above, while each clause in this tripartite structure also comprises a pairing; each begins with ϩⲣⲟ(ⲟ)ⲩ “voice” or “sound”, stating their presence and thereby existence, before immediately contrasting this in the first two clauses with their absence and thereby non-existence.[437] The repetition of ⲧⲏⲟⲩ and ϩⲟïⲙⲉ, respectively, emphasizes this pairing, which then leads to a direct contrast in the following clause. Although the third clause does not exhibit the same parallelism of sentences expressing existence and non-existence joined together, the apposition of two nominal phrases as a pairing fulfills the same structure as the preceding two, rounding off the mythological scene setting.

434 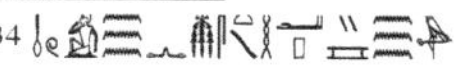 (P.Chester Beatty VII 6/7–8).

435 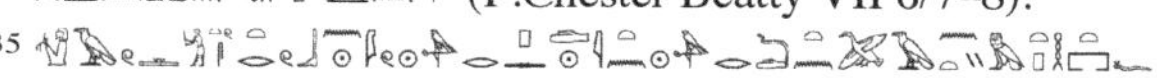 (P.Chester Beatty VII 6/8).

436 P.Brit.Mus. EA 10687, ed. Gardiner 1935, 1:55–56; 1935, 2: pls. 33–38.

437 As discussed below and in the commentary to p. 5/1–3, the syntax and thereby structure of these invocations are notably pre-Coptic, according more closely to the partial parallel in earlier Egyptian presented above than to the partial parallel in later Coptic presented below. Compare the partial parallel in the first two lines of P.Saqqara inv. F.17.10, discussed below and re-edited in the appendix, which has—by comparison—been syntactical updated so as to be grammatical Coptic: ⲟⲩⲛ̄ⲧⲏⲟⲩ ⲙ̣ⲛ̄ⲧⲏⲟⲩ ⲟⲩⲛ̄ϩⲱⲓⲙ ⲙⲛ̄ϩⲱⲓⲙ.

I.1.b. Textual Content: Amun and the Wind

In Egyptian tradition, "wind" or "breath"—Coptic ⲧⲏⲟⲩ, Egyptian *ṯ3w*—was analogous to, and in certain contexts thereby synonymous with, life. To "give wind (or, breath)" (*rḏi̓ ṯ3w*)—i.e. the "breath of life" (*ṯ3w n ʿnḫ*)—was a divine prerogative, the equivalent of giving life, while the absence of breath was the equivalent of death.[438] While it is the "breath of life" that keeps all beings alive,[439] the revivification of a deceased—their triumphing over death—served to give breath back to the corpse.[440] The juxtaposition, then, between the creative efficacy of *ṯ3w* "wind" or "breath" is apparent in the mythological scene setting of §9. While wind is present, life is possible, and while wind is absent, life is impossible—the scene setting is not only a juxtaposition, but also a tension between these states of existence. As will be seen, these resonances, which find their latest reflexes in the tradition of Coptic magical texts during the 10th or even 11th century CE, go back to the complexes that comprise Egyptian cosmogonies.[441]

A further juxtaposition prominent in the Egyptian tradition is the invisibility yet audibility of the wind. That is to say, the "wind" (*ṯ3w*) makes a "sound" (*ḫrw*), it has a "voice" (*ḫrw*),[442] and it is that "voice" or "sound" which can be "heard" (*sḏm*), yet neither can be "seen" (*m33*).[443] These qualities are then

[438] In a Demotic narrative: "She fell to the ground because there was no breath of life [coming into her flesh]" (*i̓:i̓ri̓⸗s h3y r p3 i̓tn r bn-i̓w ṯ3w[-n-ʿnḫ] i̓yi̓ [r-ḫn r n3y⸗s i̓wf.w]*) (P.Carlsberg 207 x+1/22–23), restored with parallels in x+1/20 and x+1/28–29, ed. Tait 1991, with corrections in Quack and Ryholt 2000.

[439] In a Demotic cosmology: "for [the] gods, [people], *sš*-beasts and the herds (?), the fish, the birds, the serpents, and the plants, the breath of life is what causes them to live" (*n [n3] nṯ[r.w n3 rmṯ.w] n3 sšm.w i̓rm n3 "... n3 lym.w n3 i̓pt.w n3 ḏ[tf.w] n3 sym.w p3 ṯ3 n p3 ʿ[n]ḫ p3 nti̓ [t]i̓ ʿnḫ⸗w*) (P.Carlsberg 302 verso group 1 fr. 13 2/10–12), ed. Smith 2002.

[440] The later title of the well-known ritual of *Opening the Mouth* (*wp.t-r3*) ritual is *Opening the Mouth for Breathing* (*wpy-r3 n snsn*), see Smith 2009, Texts 16–19. Consider also the later traditions of afterlife ritual texts such as the *First* and *Second Letter for Breathing* as well as *Letter for Breathing that Isis made for her brother Osiris*, see Smith 2009, Texts 25–33. In P.Rhind 1 (ed. Möller 1913; cf. Smith 2009, Text 14), the deceased is addressed: "May your nose breath the breath of life" (*snsn šy.ṯ⸗k ṯ3w n ʿnḫ*) (P.Rhind 1 6/d6), and, "May your nose breath the breath of life" (*snsn ḫnm.ti̓⸗k swḥ n ʿnḫ*) (P.Rhind 1 6/h7). The cosmogonic treatise *On the Primaeval Ocean* perhaps even attests a conception of the breath of life as the exhalation of the Primaeval Ocean (P.Carlsberg 302 verso group 1 fr. 13 2/5), see Smith 2002, 106; 113–115.

[441] There were numerous Egyptian creation myths in circulation contemporaneously, each stemming from their own regionalized traditions and increasing in entropy over time.

[442] As already noted by Sethe (1929, 96 n. 4), compare John 3:8: "The wind blows where it wishes, and you hear its sound, but you do not know where it comes from or where it goes. So it is with everyone who is born of the Spirit."

[443] This "voice" or "sound", then, is hardly that of Isis as "a mythical healer", as interpreted by van der Vliet (2018, 157).

transferred into the characteristics of Amun himself.[444] In the Temple of Munti at Medamud, a pun on Amun's name (*ỉmn*) and the wind (*ỉwn*) is found in the expression that "his name is wind" (*ỉwn rn⸗f*).[445] In a hymn to Amun-Shu from the Temple of Amun at Hibis in the el-Khargeh Oasis, Amun is described as one whose "voice is heard, (but) he is not seen, while he causes every throat to breath".[446] No matter how "high" (*ḳꜣỉ*), i.e. "loud", his "voice" (*ḫrw*) was, he could not be seen[447]—he was "the hidden one". Thus, both *like* and *as* the wind, Amun was invisible—*ỉmn* deriving from the root "to hide" and "to be hidden". Amun was, then, invisible and as "He whose name is hidden" (*ỉmn-rn⸗f*), unknowable and unassailable, for to know the names of deities was to have power over them. Here, the conceptualization of the wind, its voice or sound, and the deities which manifest as the wind accumulate around the identity of the protagonist of §9, Amun.

Amun was himself synonymous with the wind, as its creator[448], its controller[449], its conferrer,[450] and as one who could also take it away.[451] Indeed, in the ritual of the *God's Birth* discussed below, Amun is described thus: "It is you who gives wind (or, breath) between the earth and heaven and whose voice (or, sound) is heard without (it) being seen".[452] Here, then, there is a direct equation between the wind that blows between the heaven and earth, and its invisibility, manifest as the voice of Amun, which can be heard but not seen. Finally, the epithet of the "eldest wind" (*sms.w-nṯr*)[453] is resonant with Amun's assimilation to the role of Atum as the primordial creator deity, the wind that blew over the Primaeval Ocean before creation.[454] The association between the voices or sounds of the wind or wave and that of Amun illuminates a possible reference in §9 to creation itself.

---

444 See Morenz 1950, 83–94.

445 From the transcription cited in, and discussed by, Sethe 1929, 94 §198.

446 *sḏm.tw ḫrw⸗f | nn mꜣꜣ.tw⸗f ḥr srḳ ḥty.t -nb*, see Brugsch 1878, pl. 16 l. 38, as discussed in Morenz 1950, 90.

447 Amun-Re, King of the Gods, is designated elsewhere as "loud of voice, which cannot be seen" (*ḳꜣỉ ḫrw n mꜣꜣ.tw⸗f*), as transcribed and discussed in Sethe 1929, 97 §204.

448 "The god who created the wind" (*nṯr-ỉr-ṯꜣw*); "He who created wind" (*ỉr ṯꜣw*).

449 "Lord of the wind" (*nb ṯꜣw*). As noted by Sethe (1929, 90–91 §187) and Dieleman (2005, 159; 15 n. 36), the identity of the "lord of winds" is even specified in the demotic version of P.Rhind 1, where the epithet "lord of the wind" is glossed "who is Amun" (6/d3–4).

450 "The breath (i.e. wind) in the nose of the gods" (*ṯꜣw n fnd⸗sn*); "the breath of life in all things" (*ṯꜣw n ꜥnḫ m fnd n ḫ.wt -nb(.wt)*); "He who gives breath" (*ḏd-ṯꜣw*), see *LGG* 8, 54.

451 "When he removes it, their death comes" (*wꜣỉ⸗f ỉwỉ mwt⸗sn*). See Sethe 1929, 90–92 §185–193, with references

452 *ntk dd ṯꜣw ỉm.wtỉ p.t tꜣ | sḏm⸗tw ḫrw⸗f n mꜣꜣ.tw⸗f* (*Dendera Mammisi* 269.3–4); *ntk dd ṯꜣw ỉm.wtỉ p.t tꜣ | sḏm.tw⸗f n mꜣꜣ.tw⸗f* (*Edfu Mammisi* 171.1–2).

453 For this epithet, see *LGG* 6, 349.

454 See Sethe 1929, §151; 179; 193, with references.

Other reflections of these characterizations of Amun are also found in the Graeco-Roman Period in both afterlife and magical ritual texts. Commands in afterlife ritual texts declare that "Amun will give breath (*ṯꜣw*) to you" (P.Berl. inv. 8351 2)[455]; that "Amun is with you, giving breath (*ṯꜣw*) to you" (P.Louvre N 3284 1/20–21)[456]; or that "Amun will come to you with the breath of life (*ṯꜣw n ꜥnḫ*)", invoked to "give me sweet breezes (*ṯꜣw.w nḏm*) for my nose" (P.Louvre N 3148 6/10–11)[457]. Furthermore, in technical and ritual divinatory texts of the Roman Period, Amun is also described as bringing the child Horus "the breath of life" (*ṯꜣw ꜥnḫ*) (P.Vind. D 12006 recto 3/14).[458] References to Amun as a deity of the wind are also found in perhaps the earliest magical text in Demotic. P.Heid. inv. D 16,[459] dating to the 7th or 6th century BCE, which features a recipe titled "another spell" (*ky-rꜣ*) concerning "Amun-Re of Karnak", and in the line preceding this title, reference is found to a deity "whose face is in (or, as) (the) wind" (*ḥr=k m ṯꜣw*) (recto x+4). In the late Ptolemaic P.Mil. inv. D 5, in an erotic recipe for bringing a targeted woman to the practitioner through allegory with Isis and Osiris,[460] an identifying statement reads: "I am the wind (*ṯꜣw*) that blew first, in order to fertilize (?) the womb (*ꜣty(.t)*)" (x+1/x+13). As studied by Dieleman (2005, 159–160), the recipe for the consecration of a ring from the 2nd century CE P.Leiden I 384 verso[461] preserves later echoes of these manifestations and roles of Amun in an invocation: "Come to me, the one from the four winds, the almighty god, the one who blew into mortals breath for life, master of the beautiful things of the cosmos. Listen to me, lord, whose secret name is unutterable".[462] These three brief examples evidence the resonances of both the association of Amun and the wind, and the wind with creation, utilized in the Egyptian magical tradition, and go some way to bridging their transmission from the New Kingdom P.Chester Beatty VII, through the Late and Ptolemaic Period, into the early to late Roman Period.

455 Ed. Smith 1993, 23–29 no. B pls. 1–4.

456 Ed. Herbin 1994, 25–27; 510–513 no. N pls. 29–31; cf. Smith 2009, Text 25.

457 Ed. Pierret 1873, 42–79.

458 Ed. Stadler 2004; cf. Quack 2008, 362–376; Nagel 2019, 785–790.

459 This manuscript is to be published by Joachim Quack, who is thanked for providing a working edition.

460 This manuscript is to be published by Joachim Quack, who is thanked for providing a working edition—aspects of this manuscript were also discussed in Love 2016, 43 n. 141; 163.

461 *PGM* XII.201–269, see Dieleman 2005, 145–170.

462 δεῦρό μοι, ὁ ἐκ τῶν δ̅ ἀν[έ]μων, ὁ παντοκράτωρ θεός, ὁ ἐνφυσήσας πνεύματα ἀνθρώποις εἰς ζωήν, δέσποτα τῶν ἐν κόσμῳ καλῶν, ἐπάκουσόν μου, κύριε, οὗ ἐστιν τὸ κρυπτὸν ὄνομα ἄρρητον (*PGM* XII.238–240 = P.Leiden I 384 verso 10/27–29, where col. 10 = Greek-language col. 7).

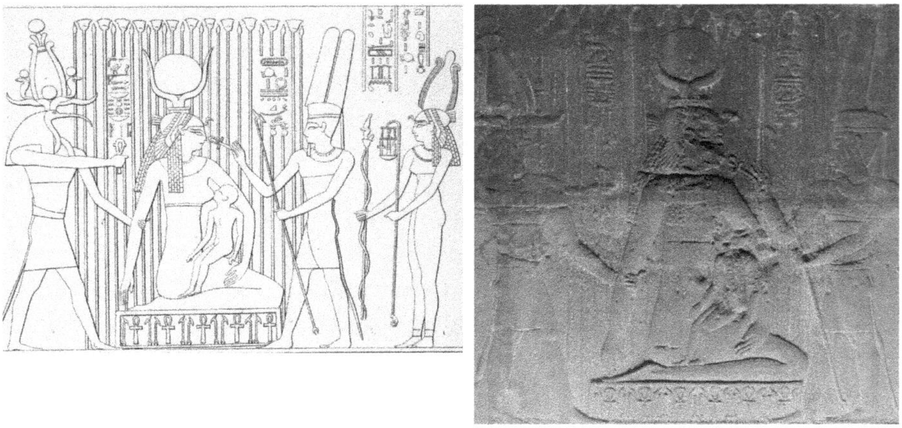

Isis in the papyrus thicket of Khemmis, suckling the child-god Horus and being given life by Amun[463] (*Monuments* I, pl. LXXIX.1; photo: Aidan McRae Thomson)

I.1.c. Textual Content: Amun and the Wave

As the "wind" was analogous to and synonymous with life, the connotations of the semantic range of Demotic *hym*, from Egyptian *hꜣn.w*, are similar—although attested comparably infrequently. In a copy of the *Great Hymn to the Sun* from the tomb of Ay at Amarna,[464] the wave is described as the equivalent of rain, that is, life-giving, a gift of the solar creator—as the Nile (*ḥꜥpy*) is given to the sky (*p.t*) as rain, the sea (*wꜣḏ-wr*) makes waves or floods (*h(ꜣ)n.w*) against the mountains (*ḏw.w*) in order to irrigate (*tẖb*) the fields (*ꜣḥ.wt*).[465] The role that the "wave" or "flood" plays is therefore one of irrigation, of linear and cyclical life-giving—once, *every* year. Indeed, the absence of the "irrigational", "immersive" (*tẖb*) qualities of the "wave" or "flood" causes fish to drown,[466] while the "wave" or "flood" also has the capacity to "fight" (*ꜥḥꜣ*) the "desert" (*mr.w*)[467]—bringing cultivation, and thereby life.

[463] See now also *Philä* II, 12. As noted by Stadler (2004, 220), this motif—Amun bearing the *ꜥnḫ* while approaching Isis who suckles her child—is described in P.Vind. inv. D 12006: "Amun approaches (as) the breath of life" (*ẖne.n=f ỉmn* (*n*) *ṯꜣw ꜥnḫ*) (recto 3/14).

[464] Ed.pr. Davies 1908, 29–32; pls. XXVII and XLI.

[465] Davies 1908, pl. XXVII ll. 9–10.

[466] In a magical text from P.Brit.Mus. EA 10042 (P.Harris 501) (7/8–11), ed. Lange 1927; Leitz 1999, 31–50, as Isis flaps her wings, she seals the opening of the river, leaving the fish in the mud (*ḏỉ=s sḏr pꜣ rm ḥr ḥꜣy.t*), without a wave to wet (or, immerse) them (*bw tẖb.n -sw hꜣn.w*) (7/9), resulting in their drowning.

[467] In a Hymn to the Nile, "the waves are fighting the desert" (*h(ꜣ)n.w (ḥr) ꜥḥꜣ mr.w*) (O.DeM 1675 recto l. 4), ed. Posener 1980, 99 pl. 81–84.

Amun's association with the creative efficacy of the flood is evidenced in his epithets as "the very great Inundation" (*ḥʿpy-ꜥꜣ-wr*), "He who inundates the Two Lands" (*bʿḥ-tꜣ.wi*), "the sustenance of the Nile" (*kꜣw-ḥʿpy*), and, in turn, "He whose wife is the field" (*ḥm.t=f-ꜣḫ.t*) and "He whose semen is grain" (*mtw.t=f-ḫ.t-n-ʿnḫ*).[468] Indeed, there is little to separate the associations between Amun's first role as primordial creator during the primordial time (*pꜣw.t*) and his perpetual role as the guarantor of the flood, harvest, and thereby nourishment of the people of Egypt, which in turn facilitates the maintenance of his cult.

I.1.d. Textual Content: Amun and the Three Gods

It is notable, then, that the partial parallel from the New Kingdom in P.Chester Beatty VII to the motifs expressed in the mythological scene setting of §9 diverges in the third passage. In that partial parallel no mention of Amun is made, rather one is instructed to heed the rising of the sun, the shining of the disk. The totality that the opening three passages of the partial parallel express is that which unifies the three elemental powers which, in the Egyptian conceptualization of the cosmos, could bring about direct effects in the human sphere: (i) air from the wind; (ii) water from the Nile or Primaeval Ocean; (iii) fire from the light of the sun.[469] The reference to Amun in §9, then, is perhaps more of a conceptual parallel than at first it seems. Once elevated during the New Kingdom to his position as the assimilated solar creator—the superordinate deity—Amun was also conceptualized as unifying these three elemental powers. Thus, he becomes not only the "noble Ba who came into being first, who created heaven, earth, and the mountains", but also he who "created life (*ʿnḫ*) from wind (*ṯꜣw*), light (*ḥꜣy*), the Nile (*ḥʿpy*), and fire (*ʿnḫ.t*), from whose work everything lives".[470] Perhaps it is not only because Amun is the protagonist in §9 that he is invoked here, but also because Amun is resonant of "the rising of the sun" and—particularly as Amun-Re—"the shining of the disk", through his multiplicity of creative associations which are found in the partial parallel in P.Chester Beatty VII.

The "voice" or "sound" of Amun that is introduced is accompanied by an apparent epithet of Amun, "the three gods". As an identification for Amun, this epithet can also be traced back to the New Kingdom, during which Amun, Re, and Ptah—the three principal deities of that time—were conceptualized as both a trinity and a unity. In the 300th verse (*ḥw.t*) of a Hymn to Amun dating to the New Kingdom, this very concept is found:[471] "All (the) gods are three. Amun,

---

[468] *LGG* 8, 57.

[469] Discussed with references in Sethe 1929, 96 §202.

[470] Note the pun on *ʿnḫ.t* "fire" and *ʿnḫ* "life"; from TT1, as cited in Sethe 1929, 96 §202.

[471] As discussed in Gardiner 1905, 35–36; Zandee 1947, 141. As noted also in the commentary to p. 5/2–3, Korshi Dosoo is thanked for highlighting this possibility.

Ra, and Ptah, there is none like them. Hiding (*ỉmn*) is his name as Amun. He is Ra as the face. His body is Ptah."[472] That is to say, the unity has three manifestations: hidden, visible, and corporeal. This tripartite nature of the divine is reflected in the three principal sites of Egypt at that time: "Their cities are upon the earth, established forever: Thebes, Heliopolis, and Memphis for eternity".[473] Together, these deities and their associated toponyms express the process by which divine ordinances are transmitted from the divine to the human sphere; elsewhere in the 300th verse it is specified that divine messages come from heaven, are heard in Heliopolis, i.e. by Re, repeated to Ptah in Memphis, and then sent to Thebes, i.e. the city of Amun, via Thoth,[474] where they are answered, that is, decided. The verse closes with reference to the three gods once again, "Amun together with Re … totaling three".[475]

The persistence of the conceptualization of a unity comprising a trinity is, to a modern reader, perhaps at first most obvious from Christian conceptualizations of the divine. However, this is also found in Egyptian tradition among various formulae that identify particular gods to be "one and the same together with other gods".[476] Amun's tripartite nature has already been discussed with regards to the air (from the wind), water (from the Nile or Nun), and light (from the sun), each of which is reflected in the partial parallel from P.Chester Beatty VII. There, the "rising of the sun" is the sun-god's creative agency—its emergence from being hidden—, manifest as Amun, the "shining of the disk" is the sun-god's visible manifestation as Re—that is, the sun—, while "he who is in his cavern" relates to another epithet of the sun-god in his evening (set) form, with a complex of creative associations.[477] Thus, all three of these aspects seem resonant in the mythological scene setting of §9 in both the composition of the three passages, and the reference to Amun as "the three gods".

Nevertheless, the only direct parallel to this expression in Egyptian is in Demotic *pꜣ ḫmt nṯr.w* "the three gods" [478] (P.Krall 8/9; 8/16), where it refers instead to Apis, Mnevis, and Pharaoh. Furthermore, where references to "the three gods" persist in the tradition of Coptic magical texts, this is with reference

---

[472] *ḫmt.w -pw nṯr.w -nb.w · ỉmn rʿ ptḥ nn sn.nw⸗sn · ỉmn rn⸗f m ỉmn · ntf rʿ m ḥr ḏ.t⸗f ptḥ* (P.Leiden I 350 4/21–22), ed. Gardiner 1905; Zandee 1947.

[473] *n.wt⸗sn ḥr tꜣ smn r nḥḥ · wꜣs.t ỉwn.w ḥw.t-kꜣ-ptḥ r ḏ.t* (P.Leiden I 350 4/22).

[474] Note again the role of Thoth as divine intermediary.

[475] *ỉmn ḥnʿ rʿ · … dmḏ ḫmt.w* (P.Leiden I 350 4/25–26)—Ptah is presumably lost in the lacuna.

[476] Assmann 1998, 143.

[477] Compare *ḳrr.tỉ* and *pꜣ-ntỉ-ẖn-tꜣy⸗f-tpḥ.t*, see *LGG* 7, 223, as well as the associations with the cavern being the place from which Hapi, i.e. the (god of the) flood, flowed forth, see Smith 2009, 645 n. 123, with references.

[478] Erroneous listed as **nṯr.w-ḫmt* in *LGG* 4, 536, which is not attested—thus reported erroneously by van der Vliet (2018, 156 n. 28).

to a triad of named gods.[479] That reference to a triad of deities was once made in a source text but has been lost from §9 during its history of textual tradition might therefore be considered. Nevertheless, an interpretation which would fit with the consideration of Amun's role in the ritual of the *God's Birth* is considered below.[480]

I.1.e. Textual Content: Amun and the Egg

Further on in the divine drama, Amun declares to the unidentified, disembodied voice that he is the one who causes "every egg" (ⲥⲟⲟⲩϩⲉ ⲛⲓⲙ) to be fertile. The intervening dialogue of the divine drama will be taken up later in this excursus. At this point, now that Amun's role as the creator and manifestation of the wind, flood, and light has been considered, it is important to highlight a pun fundamental to certain Egyptian conceptualizations of creation that has been lost in the course of the lexical evolution of the Egyptian language from the Pharaonic to Roman Period.[481] The "egg" (*swḥ.t*) in Egyptian tradition was conceptualized as the female counterpart of the "wind" (*swḥ*)—a synonym of *ṯ3w*, but one with particular creative resonances.[482] In the Hermopolitan Cosmogony, the egg was a mode of creation, appearing on the primaeval mound—in some traditions, created by the Hermopolitan Ogdoad who were born "when there was no egg" (*n wn swḥ.t*), in others, laid by a bird, having emerged from a primaeval lotus, or fashioned or produced by the sun-god himself—and hatching to reveal the sun as the first god.[483] These associations further demonstrate, as argued above, that the mythological scene setting is resonant of the primordial time, the time of tension and juxtaposition between presence and absence, that is, existence and the non-existence preceding it.

In a study of the treatise *On the Primaeval Ocean*, Smith identified Amun as the deity personified by virtue of never being named, the deity which is itself the identification of the wind. In that cosmogony, the "four winds of the sky", i.e. stemming from the four cardinal points,[484] merge into a single high wind which brings about creation by separating the sky from the earth and then forming or

---

[479] See the commentary to p. 5/2–3.

[480] In the context of the ritual of the *God's Birth*, discussed below, consider the obvious trinities of Amun, Hathor, and Khonsu or Amun-Re, Hathor, and Khnum—all prominent in Scene II of the ritual of the *God's Birth*, see Daumas 1959, 395–403.

[481] Punning is found throughout mythological and cosmogonic as well as ritual texts, see the examples in Morenz 1950, 98.

[482] As studied by Morenz 1950, 74–83, see also 89–101.

[483] Smith 2002, 60 n. 209–213.

[484] Smith 2002, 63. Resonances are even found among the GEMP, consider "These four winds which are outside, bring the light into me!" (*p3y=y fdw ṯ3w nti n-bl r:iny p3 wyn n=i r-ẖn*) (*P.London-Leiden* recto 2/6).

fertilizing an egg from which the sun—manifest as Pshai—emerged.[485] As such, Amun is "the wind (*swḥ*) that endures in all things" and—familiarly—the "giver of breath (*ṯ3w*) to the one who is in the egg (*swḥ.t*)".[486] In the context of the ritual of the *God's Birth*, "the one who is in the egg" is applied to the unborn child-god.[487] Other such puns on the "wind" (*swḥ*) and "egg" (*swḥ.t*) provide an important complement, for example, in the characterization of the Theban Nome at the Temple of Montu at Karnak as "the egg which came forth from the wind" (*swḥ.t prỉ m swḥ*).[488]

In association with such cosmogonic traditions, Amun was identified as "He who created the egg" (*sḫpr-swḥ.t*), and correspondingly addressed in hymns, albeit often paradoxically: "You appeared in the flood within the hidden egg"[489] and "He who formed his own egg",[490] expressing the paradox that Amun was both the creator of the solar egg and the deity—the sun-god—that emerged from it.[491] In the aforementioned Hymn to Amun-Shu from the Temple of Hibis in the el-Khargeh Oasis, the physical form of Amun is described: "his body is the wind (*swḥ*), the sky is his head".[492] The extension of the semantic range of the root *swḥ* was such that it is also attested with creative associations as a verb, for example with the god Khnum as subject and "the water" (*mw*, i.e. semen) as object, he "who forms in the womb, in order to cause the egg (*sw(ḥ.t)*) to come into being (*sḫpr*)"—a pun on the process of the fertilization of the egg and the Egyptian word for "egg".[493] Although such direct punning has been lost through the lexical evolution of the Egyptian language, these resonances were nevertheless inherent in the composition of §9, and perhaps still consciously in circu-

---

[485] Smith 2002, 62.

[486] As discussed in Smith 2002, 63.

[487] At Edfu, Hathor is announced: "It is the Lady of Dendera who gives the breath of life to the nose of her son, who is (still) in his egg." (*wnn nb(.t) ỉwn.t ḥr ḏỉ.t ṯ3w n ꜥnḫ r fnḏ n s3=s ḫnt.ỉ swḥ.t=f*) (*Edfu Mammisi* 17.8). (Dagmar Budde is thanked for highlighting this passage in a personal communication.)

[488] As discussed in Smith 2002, 61; Morenz 1950, 99–100.

[489] *ḫꜥ=k m n.t m swḥ.t ỉmn.t* (Smith 2002, 63, with references). This relates to Amun being "He who hid himself in the pupil" (*ỉmn -sw m ḏf*), in which the "pupil" refers to the solar eye, i.e. sun disk, itself equated with the primordial egg that contained the sun-god (Smith 2002, 63–64).

[490] *nbw swḥ.t=f ḏs=f* (Smith 2002, 54 with n. 246).

[491] A related paradox is that whereby Pshai is both the descendent and predecessor of Amun, literally "elder than the one who created him" (Smith 2002, 63).

[492] *ḥꜥ.w=f m swḥ ṯ3p.t ḥr-tp=f* (ed. Brugsch 1878, pl. 25 col. 5–6), as identified and discussed by Morenz (1950, 91).

[493] Accompanying a relief of Tiberius worshipping before Khnum in the portico of the mammisi at Philae (northern relief in the second register from the top of the eastern wall), see *Philä* II, 180–181. This, and the semantic range of *swḥ*, is treated in Morenz 1950, 90–91, while the punning of "wind" and "egg" is discussed especially ibid. 99–103.

lation within the milieux in which the source texts were compiled and redacted, from which §9 was ultimately drawn.[494]

I.2. Parallels to the Mythological Scene Setting

The conclusion of the mythological scene setting in §9 provides an opportunity to consider its motifs alongside the three most obvious partial parallels. The recipe against poison in the aforementioned P.Chester Beatty VII provides the earliest partial parallel identified. But those motifs are also found in a recipe to ensure menstruation in a Demotic text on an ostracon (O.Stras. D 1338), dating to the early Roman Period (i.e. 1st or 2nd century CE), unprovenanced but acquired in Luxor. The gap in time between this example is, then, the smallest to §9. Finally, the latest reflex of those motifs is found in an amulet for healing through unblocking in P.Saqqara inv. F.17.10, dating to the second half of the 10th or 11th century CE and excavated at Saqqara.

P.Chester Beatty VII comprises a papyrus bookroll formulary containing numerous recipes for banishing scorpions from a place or their poison from a body. Divine dramas feature commonly, either with protagonists and the dialogue of their divine dramas, or simply with the mythological scene setting—as in the following example—, while compositions comprising direct invocations and commands are also found. Featured in a series of recipes to bring out the poison from the body of a patient, the recipe with partial parallels to the motifs of §9 is titled "Another" (*k.t*), and reads:

"Voice (or, sound) of wind, (when) there is no wind in it. Voice (or, sound) of water, (when) the Nile has not been born. One should heed the rising of the sun, the shining of the disk and what is said by him who is in his cavern. Oh poison, come (forth) upon the earth from the limbs of NN (m.), born of NN (f.)."[495]

Here, following the discussion above, the resonance of the tension between presence and absence, existence and non-existence, is clear. There is an evident comparison between the "bringing out" of a poison from the body of a patient, and the "bringing out" of the child from the woman suffering a protracted labor in §9. The analogical efficacy of the recipe lies not only in the analogy between the association of the mythological scene setting with the primordial time, but also the reference to the solar cycle as discussed above, whereby the manifestations of the sun-god as rising (just visible), shining (visible), and set in a cavern (invisible) express both a creative efficacy and a perpetual cyclical reality. As these phenomena occur, so should the poison come out of the patient.

---

[494] See further **Transmitting Textual Traditions**.

[495] *k.t ḫrw ṯꜣw nn ṯꜣw im=f · ḫrw mw n ms.t ḥꜥpi · šꜣ=tw -st r wbn rꜥ.w · r psḏ itn r ḏd.t n pꜣ nti m tpḥ.t=f · mtw.t mi ḥr tꜣ · m ḥꜥ.w n mn msi̯ n mn.t* (P.Chester-Beatty VII 6/7–7/1).

The partial parallel in Demotic on the ostracon (O.Stras. D 1338),[496] currently being re-edited by Joachim Quack,[497] appears to comprise a single copy of a recipe—perhaps once held among several loose leaves in a collection of numerous recipes—, and reads:

"Spell of causing that the blood of a woman falls every month (?). Oh heaven, do not create wind (or, breath)! Oh sea, do not create wave (or, flood)! Make *hik* (*ḥyḳ*) for me (?)! Oh great noble god who rejoices in truth! Oh heaven, do not … me! Search after these things that I have said today, after that which I have said as *hik* (*ḥyḳ*) with the voice (*ḫrw*) of Isis, the great, the mother of the god, when she searched for the great god in Kush, saying: 'Come to me, oh gods of the south, north, east, (and) west, through the voice (*ḫrw*) of Amun, the great god, lord of Thebes. Come to me, oh great Ennead, oh small Ennead! Do not hide yourselves from me today! Do what I have said to you (pl.)! Oh divine influence (*ḫyṱ*) of him who is upon this bark of millions … divine influence (*ḫyṱ*) of Ptah-Tatenen, the father of the gods, the great Shai, the Nun (Primaeval Ocean) who is under the earth! Oh divine influence (*ḫyṱ*) of the two sisters, Isis and Nephthys, these two goddesses which Kematef, the great Shai, has created! Oh divine influence (*ḫyṱ*) of every god and goddess of Upper and Lower Egypt! Have … NN (f.) before him who … […] … […]'".[498]

Besides evidencing an otherwise apparently unparalleled myth of Isis searching for Osiris in Kush,[499] the mythological associations presented in this recipe are beyond those of any of the other texts featuring partial parallels to the mythological scene setting of §9. Although the reading "every month" (*ꜣbd -nb*) is uncertain, the desired outcome of the recipe is evidently that to bring about menstruation—conceptualized as an unblocking. As highlighted by Ritner, the "natural order is to be halted" until the desired outcome is brought about.[500] Van der Vliet emphasized further that the utilization of the motifs is therefore not directly comparable to §9, because the commands are explicitly that the wind and the flood should cease,[501] and by extension, not that they are present and absent. Consequently, as the creative efficacy of the wind and flood are to cease, so too are the perpetual cycles of life, until the desired outcome of the recipe is brought about. Instead of providing direct analogies, here the motifs have been repurposed in the Demotic text as a compulsion of the invoked and commanded

[496] Spiegelberg 1911, 34–37; pl. 6 no. 1; Thissen 1991, 374; Ritner 1995, 3343–3344; van der Vliet 2018, 156–157; Nagel 2019, 802–803.

[497] Who is thanked for sharing his re-edition of the text ahead of its publication, the re-readings from which are incorporated here in English translation.

[498] *ỉ tꜣ p.t m-ỉrỉ̯ ỉrỉ̯ ṯꜣw | ỉ pꜣ ym m-ỉrỉ̯ ỉrỉ̯ ḥym* (O.Stras. D 1338 l. 2).

[499] Thissen 1991, 374.

[500] Ritner 1995, 3343.

[501] Van der Vliet 2018, 157.

deities. This fits well within the composition, because those deities are then elaborated through various theonyms, epithets, and associations. Furthermore, as discussed above, since the associations of the compulsion are those of the primordial time and creative efficacy, the motifs were evidently conceptualized as being potent enough to coerce, to compel the invoked deities to heed the commands recited by the practitioner.

While the partially paralleled motifs here are repurposed as commands of compulsion, the mythological allusions inherent in the further invocations and commands of the recipe are clearly related to the aforementioned cosmogonic associations of those motifs to the primordial time and creative efficacy. Isis' searching for Osiris recalls a pivotal moment in Egyptian mythological time, as the reconstitution of Osiris, the conception of Horus, and the latter's ascension to the throne mark the end of the era of Seth and the beginning of the reign of the Horus kings—the reign of the kings of Upper and Lower Egypt as worldly incarnations of Horus. This, then, serves as the authoritative and thereby efficacious mythological precedent for the ritual practice. Notably, it is Isis' invocations and commands that are repurposed at the end of the divine drama. It is the "voice" (*ḫrw*) of Isis that is cited, yet the efficacy of the command is nonetheless specified as coming "through the voice (*ḫrw*) of Amun". Indeed, reference to Amun follows that to the four deities of the cardinal points, themselves manifestations of the winds that blow from those points, and thereby to the host of associations of creative efficacy discussed above. The Heliopolitan Cosmogony is then alluded to by reference to the "Great Ennead"—an alternative name for the Heliopolitan Ennead with Atum, and thereby sometimes Amun, at its head—, while the "Lesser Ennead" alludes to the deities attending on Osiris. The "divine influence" (*ḫyṯ*) of certain deities, expressing both their beneficent and malignant efficacy, is invoked and commanded in the second section of direct commands, following the practitioner's declaration: "Do what I have said to you (pl.)!". Through this particular efficacy, then, the desired outcome for the female patient will be brought about.

P.Saqqara inv. F.17.10 comprises a paper strip inscribed with one recipe. The presence of a placeholder for the personal name of a patient suggests a formulary, but—given the format and folding—the manuscript could also have been used as an amulet.[502] Excavated at Saqqara among the debris from a shaft tomb (F17), built into the mastaba of Akhetep, the amulet's findspot was only a short distance from the ruins of the Monastery of Apa Jeremiah, as has been

502 This parallel was first identified by Zellmann-Rohrer based on the presentation of the document in Ziegler 2013 during his own work on the Michigan codex; the Saqqara text has since been independently discussed by Müller 2017 and re-edited by van der Vliet 2018, with different readings and interpretations from those proposed here. A re-edition of the text is therefore provided in the appendix.

highlighted by van der Vliet.[503] Dated by van der Vliet to the 10th or 11th century CE, but by Müller more specifically to the second half of the 10th century CE,[504] this manuscript was produced within a considerably different cultural and religious milieu from that of Pharaonic, early, and late Roman Egypt of the previous partial parallels. Reflecting the fact that dialect and idiom are indexes of place, as opposed to time, however, a relatively standard Sahidic is complemented with the substitution of ω for ο, exhibiting some of the same variances—albeit with different orthographic conventions—of Hand 1 of the Michigan codex. Indeed, such variances may be understood as reflecting a Mesokemic influence,[505] despite lacking the distinct orthographic conventions of that literary dialect. The brief text, re-edited in the appendix, reads:

"There is wind, there is no wind; there is wave, there is no wave; the seven voices of the snake heads, they came up from the sea (or, Fayum) to release everything that is bound in (the) knot, for nothing is bound, no wood shall be sharp in (the) knot, for the snake that is unbound has completed another for you here (and) today. It is Iao who loosens you. It is Adonai who releases you. It is Eloi who gives (a) path for you to save (or, preserve) yourself, immediately, (oh) NN."

Stripped of the "voice" or "sound" of both the wind and wave, written at a point in the evolution of the Egyptian-Coptic lexicon where the latter really only meant "wave"—as opposed to "flood"—, syntactically updated to be grammatical Coptic, and divorced from the cultural and religious context in which such motifs would have had clear resonance, the latest reflexes of the motifs in the mythological scene setting in §9 are heavily reduced. Nevertheless, this presence is notable in and of itself. Despite the fact that all of the subsequent narration is distinct in content and resonance, these motifs were still used centuries later in a mythological scene setting to frame a divine drama. The divine drama that unfolds in the one brief passage that follows is the reference to the "seven voices of the snake heads", and then the emergence of these heads from the water, which then establish the precedent of unblocking through "releasing" (ⲃⲟⲗ). The analogous ritual mechanics in the mythological precedent are clear. How the authority and thereby efficacy of the recipe relates to the "snake heads", however, is less so,[506] as is the specific body part that is to be

---

[503] Van der Vliet 2018, 146.

[504] Van der Vliet 2018, 146; Müller 2017, 130.

[505] Müller expressed a similar view (2017, 131), while noting that literary Mesokemic would have ⲙⲙⲁⲕ not ⲙⲙⲱⲕ.

[506] Van der Vliet (2018, 153) remarked that the emerging of snakes from the sea "defies interpretation in terms of Christian models", suggesting tentatively instead "avatars of the Egyptian snake god Shai-Agathos Daimon" (2018, 157). Van der Vliet's claim that this "gains some likelihood from the popular veneration of Shai as a domestic protective deity", who is "attested till well in the fifth century", citing Quaegebeur 1975, 160–166 and Frankfurter 1998,

unblocked.[507] Following these commands, a tripartite set of invocations specify the means through which the desired outcome is brought about—the "loosening", "releasing", and "path-making" of Iao, Adonai, and Eloi, respectively.[508]

It is important to stress, however, as van der Vliet has done,[509] that there is nothing diagnostically Christian about these names, nor this recipe—with Müller even highlighting the absence of any cross or staurogram.[510] Van der Vliet does consider that these names are more likely to be interpreted as features of the Christianization of the text, but he draws upon overtly Christianized divine dramas as parallels to make this case, stating that the closing supplication of §9 is also "a clear Christian insertion", which—as will be seen—has been assumed rather than demonstrated.[511] Thus, as discussed at length in **Transmitting Textual Traditions**, this does not constitute diagnostic Christianization, with the extant pattern of evidence instead suggesting a discontinuity between the motifs of the "wind" and "wave" and the larger set of Christian(ized) motifs utilized in mythological scene setting and divine dramas.

In summary, each recipe in which the motifs from the mythological scene setting of §9 are partially paralleled exhibits the pairing of blockage and its resolution in unblocking. In all but the latter case of the Saqqara text, this association is also reflected explicitly in the desired outcome of the practices, where unblocking results in healing (from poison, from a lack of menstrual flow, or from a difficult labor). The interpretation of the creative resonances of these motifs as discussed above entails here an expression of the tension between existence (of a poison or a blockage in the body) and absence (of menstrual flow or delivery), between creation (the life-giving associations of menstruation and childbirth) and its opposite (death from poison or an illness caused by blockage),

---

63–64, is not based upon historical evidence, but on extrapolations from hagiographical sources—see the argumentation against the use of hagiographies in this way in Love 2016, §7.4.3.3 and Smith 2017, §7.1.5–7.1.13, esp. §7.1.8, the latter also deconstructing the thesis of the domestic—"miniaturization" of the—worship of Pshai. Albeit without citing any of these, or any other, criticisms, counter-argumentations, and refutations of his thesis, Frankfurter has gone from appraising the hagiographic episode central to his original argument as a "priceless picture, authentic in many details, of persisting Egyptian religion and perhaps even of the historical cult of Shai" (2007, 188) to reappraising it as "a legend", "fictional, yet filtering local monastic memories of charismatic holy men", "a Christian scribe's view of domestic ritual in a village that had so far retained its traditional cult" (2018, 45; 77; 26).

[507] See further the discussion in the appendix.

[508] Also discussed in van der Vliet 2018, 159.

[509] Van der Vliet 2018, 154; 158.

[510] Müller 2017, 130.

[511] Van der Vliet (2018, 159–160), who notes that "the original evocation of a snake-shaped healing power" is "at odds" with "names of the biblical God". However, if the text has been Christianized—as van der Vliet argues—, this apparent problem has rather been resolved by the very co-existence of these entities in a Christian(ized) text.

as well as explicitly in some cases between sealing and the releasing of such sealing. The result, in all cases, involves bringing something out of the body. To apply these insights to the mythological scene setting of §9, it should be noted that the wind is a "hypostasis" of Amun: Amun both provides and embodies the wind, while the wind also "symbolizes freedom of movement, since the impossibility of confining or obstructing it is proverbial".[512] This consideration, then, allows the associations and roles of Amun discussed so far to be contextualized even more clearly within motifs that relate to ritual practices for blocking and unblocking. How these motifs relate specifically to the divine drama that unfolds in §9, and their resonances with the ritual of the *God's Birth* and Amun's role therein, will be considered after a treatment of the dialogue that follows the mythological scene setting.

II. Divine Dialogue

ⲁⲙⲟⲩⲛ ⲉⲕⲛⲏⲩ ⲧⲱⲛ ⲙ̅ⲡⲉⲓ̈ⲥⲙⲟⲧ ⲙ̅ⲡⲉⲓ̈ⲣⲏⲣⲉ·
ỉmn ỉ:ỉri̯=k nꜥ(y) tn n pꜣy smt n pꜣy rt.ṱ
"Amun, where is it that you are going in this form, in this manner?"
ⲉⲓ̈ⲛⲏⲩ ⲙ̅ⲡⲧⲟⲩⲣⲏⲥ ⲉϩⲏⲧ ⲟⲩⲧⲉ ⲕⲁϣ· ⲟⲩⲧⲉ ⲕⲁⲙ· {ⲟⲩⲧⲉ}
ỉ:ỉri̯=ỉ nꜥ(y) n pꜣ tw-rsy r ẖt ỉwṱ ḳš/gš ỉwṱ ḳm ỉwṱ
"It is with the south-wind that I am going, northwards between reed and rush, {between}
ⲧⲓⲛⲁⲉⲃⲱⲧ· ⲟⲩⲧⲉ ⲡⲁⲓ̈ⲧⲟⲟⲩ ⲥⲛⲁⲩ· ⲛ̅ⲧⲉ ⲧⲉⲓ̈ⲥⲓⲃⲓⲧ ⲥ̅ⲛ̅ⲧⲉ·
tw=ỉ nꜥ(y) (r) ỉbt ỉwṱ pꜣy tw sn.nw ntỉ tꜣy sbt.t sn.ty
I am going to Abydos between these two mountains of these two hills.
ⲉⲓ̈ⲧⲁⲗⲏⲩ ⲉϩⲧⲟ ϩⲁⲧ: ϩⲧⲟ ⲕⲁⲙ ⲉⲛⲉϥϩⲁⲣⲟⲓ̈· ⲉⲣⲉⲛ̅ϫⲱⲱⲙⲉ ⲛ̅ⲑⲟⲟⲩⲧ ⲛ̅ⲧⲟⲧ: ⲛⲁⲡⲟⲣ†ⲟⲩ ϩ̅ⲛ̅ ⲛⲁϭⲓϫ·
ỉ:ỉri̯=ỉ tỉ.t-ꜥl r (wꜥ) ḥtr ḥt (wꜥ) ḥtr km | ỉw wn-nꜣ.w=f ẖr-rꜣ=ỉ | ỉw nꜣ ḏmꜥ.w n tḥw.tỉ n-tr.ṱ=ỉ na pꜣ wr-tỉw ẖn nꜣy=ỉ gyḏ(.t)
What I am mounted on is a white horse, a black horse was before me, while the books of Thoth are with me, those of the Great-of-Five in my hands.
ⲉⲓ̈ⲧⲙⲁⲥⲓ̈ⲟ ⲛ̅ⲛⲉⲧⲉⲉⲧ
ỉ:ỉri̯=ỉ tỉ.t-msi̯ nꜣ ntỉ ỉwr.ṱ
What I cause to give birth are the ones who are pregnant.
ⲉⲓ̈ⲱ̅ⲧ̅ⲡ ⲛ̅ⲛⲉⲧϣⲓⲧ:
ỉ:ỉri̯=ỉ ꜣtp nꜣ ntỉ štỉ
What I close up are those who miscarry.
ⲉⲓ̈ⲧⲣⲉⲥⲟⲟⲩϩⲉ ⲛⲓⲙ ⲣ̅ϣⲁⲩ· ϣⲁⲧ̅ⲛ̅ⲥⲟⲟⲩϩⲉ ⲛ̅ⲁϭⲣⲏⲛ·
ỉ:ỉri̯=ỉ tỉ.t-ỉri̯ swḥ.t -nb ỉri̯-šw šꜥṱ n swḥ.t n ꜣkrn
What I cause to be fertile is every egg, except the infertile eggs."

[512] Smith 2009, 633.

II.1. Textual Structure

This section opens with a question posed by an unidentified, disembodied voice. Question and answer appear as a pairing, call and response: the question is posed as ⲉⲕⲛⲏⲩ "that you are going", followed by an interrogative, which is then paired and syntactically paralleled in Amun's answer as ⲉⲓ̈ⲛⲏⲩ "that I am going", followed by the adverbial element expressing both form and location. It is not that Amun "will go", but that he "is going"; that is to say, the movement is ongoing, and therefore the progress of the story actualizes the actions being narrated, providing narrative momentum and moving them from an ongoing present into a sense that their actions are already behind the narrative as it progresses. Pairings are found in the appropriate juxtaposition of "south" and "north", with repetition and further resonance in Amun's manifestation as the south-wind, that is, the wind that blows northwards. The syntactical structure ⲟⲩⲧⲉ ⲕⲁϣ and ⲟⲩⲧⲉ ⲕⲁⲙ presents a further pairing, differing in just one consonant and representing, as discussed below, a motif common to such divine dramas—pairings that implicitly encompass a totality. Although the syntax changes, the pairing of clauses is retained, with the verb ⲛⲁ expressing another form of "going" in the ongoing present that relates back to ⲛⲏⲩ. Here, the extant form of the text does not provide parallelism in the use of ⲟⲩⲧⲉ,[513] but instead in the juxtaposition of ⲟⲩⲧⲉ and ⲛ̄ⲧⲉ—itself a pairing that forms a pair with the preceding ⲟⲩⲧⲉ ⲕⲁϣ and ⲟⲩⲧⲉ ⲕⲁⲙ. This appears purposeful, however, because no juxtaposition of a pairing is required—the clause itself concerns pairs. That is to say, "reed" and "rush" concern two singularities, where ⲡⲁⲓ̈ⲧⲟⲟⲩ ⲥⲛⲁⲩ "these two mountains" and ⲧⲉⲓ̈ⲥⲓⲃⲓⲧ ⲥ̄ⲛ̄ⲧⲉ "these two hills" are two pairs, combined in a pairing of pairs, which then connects with the pairing of two singularities.

Such pairings continue in the reference to a "white" and a "black" horse[514], which encompasses a plurality and totality of the spectrum of color. These are each in turn paired with the "books of Thoth" and "those of the Great-of-Five", a pairing which actually describes the same referent, thereby comprising the entirety of the revered textual culture associated with Thoth. This section closes with Amun's declaration of his intent, manifesting his capacity to bring about the desired outcome for which he was sent, consequently also actualizing that outcome. Comparable to the opening mythological scene setting, the clauses are tripartite instead of bipartite, and the stressed syntax of the repeated ⲉⲓ̈- emphasizes that it is *only for* a particular purpose that Amun does what he does. Again, comparable to the three clauses of the mythological scene setting, the first two are a duality in syntactical structure and what they communicate—

[513] For the possibilities of what could be missing, see the commentary to p. 5/5.

[514] Notably in compounds evidencing pre-Coptic grammar, see the commentary to p. 5/7–8 and 5/8 and **Linguistic and Orthographic Features**.

Amun as the protagonist (subject), both immediate action and ongoing intent (verb), and a nominalized relative in the plural specifying the patients (object). The exception comes again in the third clause, where a syntactical pairing is found in the repetition of ⲥⲟⲟⲩϩⲉ "egg", the third "I" clause in fact being paired not with the preceding two, but with a following adverbial clause. Such nesting of syntactical and semantic pairings within one another is a motif that is particularly prominent throughout this section, and in turn resonates with the preceding section of mythological scene setting. Thus, even in the extant form of the text, the totalities expressed—through both syntactical and semantic pairings—evidence and lend a purposeful sense of structure and thus narrative momentum leading to its resolution, in a pattern fundamental to the mechanics of such divine dramas.

II.2. Textual Content

As described above, an unidentified, disembodied voice asks Amun where he is going, and particular stress is given in the syntax of the Egyptian-Coptic as to why it is in such a particular form and manner that Amun is going. Such rhetorical questions, whose answers are in principle known by the divine questioner but which by the act of being answered actualize their outcome in both the divine and human spheres, mythological and contemporary time, are known from the earliest to latest attested Egyptian mythological and ritual texts, spanning two and a half millennia.[515] More specifically, these interrogative motifs are maintained in the magical tradition in Egypt: appearing in Egyptian, Demotic, Greek, and ultimately Coptic magical texts.

When Amun answers, he does so stressing in a similar use of syntax that it is with—indeed, in the form of—the south-wind that he is going, blowing northwards through the mythological landscape of marshes and riverbanks. The claim that the divine protagonists and thereby also the practitioner *know* the name, form, and/or manner of a deity is a motif of ritual practice that is most instantly recognizable as part of the knowledge necessary for the deceased in their journey through the underworld in the *Book of the Dead*. In that complex of ritual texts, the deceased have to demonstrate that they *know* the names of the guardians through declarative utterances of their names: the deceased recites "I know you (pl.), (because) I know your (pl.) names."[516] In *naming* the guardians,

---

[515] Compare the 2,500 year spectrum of *PT* 470 from the Pyramid of Pepi I (c. second half of the 24th century BCE), in which Pepi is asked by the Bull of Offering who is instructed to let the king pass—"Where is he (i.e. Pepi) going?" (*sḏꜣ=f ṯnỉ*) (§914c)—with a divine dialogue from the copy of the *Myth of the Sun's Eye* in P.Leiden I 384 recto (c.101–150 CE), ed. Spiegelberg 1917a, in which the Nubian Cat asks her conversation partner—"where are you entering and where are going?" (*mtw=k ꜥḳ r tn mtw=k šmỉ r tn*) (9/19).

[516] *ỉw=ỉ rḫ.kw -tn rḫ.kw rn=tn* (*BD* 125 310Aa).

the deceased gains power over them, resulting in a response from the guardians: “You know us. Pass, then, through us.”[517] This motif is utilized in a plethora of contexts and is maintained until the latest pre-Coptic Egyptian magical texts, namely, those in Demotic. In the vessel inquiry of Khonsu in *P.London-Leiden* recto 9/1–10/22,[518] Khonsu is invoked with a series of epithets, including the one “whose name (*rn*) cannot be known, whose manner (*ky*) cannot be known, whose form (*smt*) cannot be known”.[519] And yet, of course, the practitioner then declares: “I know your name (*rn*), I know your manner (*ky*), I [know] your form (*smt*)”,[520] following up with a list of theonyms and manifestations of Khnum. In doing so, the practitioner acquires the efficacy through which to bring about the desired outcome of the ritual. Thus, in specifying the “form” (ϲⲙⲟⲧ < *smt*) and “manner” (ⲣⲏⲧⲉ < *rd.wi.ṱ*) in which he is coming[521]—clearly resonant of the wind and breath of creative efficacy discussed at length above—Amun is facilitating the practice by further actualizing what is *not known* as what is *known*.

In doing so, Amun specifies that he is traveling with the south-wind. From the earliest Egyptian ritual texts, the south-wind had associations of creative efficacy and childbirth. In *PT* 669, an afterlife ritual text for the benefit of king Pepi Neferkare inscribed upon the pyramid of Pepi II (c. middle of the 23rd century BCE), Pepi is described as “knotted” (*ṯ(ꜣ)š*), and it is said that “the egg (*swḥ.t*) has been broken open (*sḏ*) for him”, allowing him to fly forth. As a consequence of this (re)creative act as a new-(re)born Pepi, Neferkare requires care, and his *ꜣṯw.t*-wet-nurse and *mnꜥ.t*-wet-nurse are identified with the south-wind (*rs.w*) and north-wind (*mḥ.yt*) respectively. In *CT* 162, an afterlife ritual text for the benefit of a deceased individual entitled *Having power over the four winds of the sky*,[522] the south-wind is described as “a native of the south, which brings water, growth, and life; the south-wind is the breath of life; and that which it has granted to me is that which I may live through it”.[523] Elsewhere in the same recipe, those four winds are described as “the bulls of the sky” who came into being (*ḫpr*) before men were born (*n msy.t rmṯ.w*) and before gods existed (*n*

[517] *ỉw=k rḫ.tỉ -ns swꜣ -ỉrf ḥr=n* (*BD* 125 328b).

[518] *PDM* xiv.239–295.

[519] *ntỉ-ỉw bw-ỉrỉ rḫ=w rn=f bw-ỉrỉ rḫ=w ky=f bw rḫ=w smt=f* (*P.London-Leiden* recto 9/4).

[520] *tw=y ỉrỉ-rḫ.w rn=k tw=y ỉrỉ-rḫ.w ky=k tw=y [ỉrỉ rḫ.w] smt=k* (*P.London-Leiden* recto 9/4–5).

[521] Here, however, a lexically updated synonym has been substituted for the older *ky*/*gy*: *gy*, by comparison, survives in Coptic only in lexicalized ϭⲓⲛ- (< *gy n* “manner of”). The Inaros/Petubastis cycle, however, provides a predecessor for this use of ⲣⲏⲧⲉ < *rd.wi.ṱ*, in which the question is posed “What is the manner of the gods?” (*[rꜣ] nṯr.w ntỉ-ỉw rd.wi.ṱ=w pꜣy*) (P.Spiegelberg G/11), ed. Hoffmann 1995, 30–39.

[522] *sḫm m ṯꜣw.w fdw n.w p.t*. The creative efficacy of the four winds has been discussed above. For more on the four winds, see the bibliography in Smith 2002, 57 n. 188.

[523] *rs.w -pw rs.w m nḥs(.ỉ) rsw.t | ỉnn mw srd ꜥnḫ | ṯꜣw -pw ꜥnḫ rs.w | rḏt.n=f n=ỉ ꜥnḫ=ỉ ỉm=f* (de Buck, *CT* II, 397c–398d).

ḫpr.t nṯr.w). These examples highlight that the presence or absence of wind marks creation and the primordial time preceding creation as well as the cosmogonic associations of Amun manifesting as, and thereby traveling with or in, the south-wind. Indeed, the south-wind is credited with facilitating the Nile's flow from its source, increasing its yield, bringing livestock to the deceased, strengthening the eggs of the pregnant, lifting the Bas of the gods to the sky, and killing Apophis—the archenemy of the sun-god Re.[524] These attributes in turn link back to Amun as the "hidden one", the *unknowable*, particularly in his manifestations as "he with incomprehensible form as the four winds of the sky", whose "limbs are the wind".[525]

As the south-wind blows, and thus Amun journeys, he describes to the unidentified, disembodied voice not only that he is going with and thereby as the south-wind, but that this journey takes him northwards—"between reed and rush". This setting could be seen as reminiscent of the Edfu Cosmogony, in which a reed thicket was stirred by the creative power of the wind that blew through it.[526] The apposition of "reed" and "rush" also recalls an epithet of Egypt—"the two bushes"—referring to the reed of Upper Egypt and papyrus of Lower Egypt,[527] and perhaps therefore suggests that this duality represents the totality of Egypt. The specific terms utilized also offer another apposition for interpretation. The "reed" (ⲕⲁϣ < *gꜣš*) is described in the *Late Egyptian Miscellanies* as that growing on the banks of the Nile,[528] while a letter dating to the 21st Dynasty describes the "rush" (ⲕⲁⲙ < *ḳmꜣ*) as that to be removed from the land in order to cultivate it.[529] There are further mythological resonances, however, in the fact that the peripteros mammisis of the Graeco-Roman Period featured columns supporting floral capitals that served to imitate the papyrus

[524] See Kurth 1986, 1267 with n. 56–61. That is not to say that the south-wind is exclusively beneficent, however. The latest reference in pre-Coptic Egyptian comes again in *P.London-Leiden*, where Horus complains, "A fever has seized me. A south-wind has touched me." (*r wʿ g-ʿ-w-m-* ʿFl-Kr *ṯꜣi̯.ṯ(=i) | r wʿ ṯꜣw rsy ti̓.t-ʿḥʿ=i*) (verso 33/4).

[525] *twt ḏsr ḫpr.w m fdw ṯꜣw n p.t* and *ḥʿ.w=f m swḥ*, from a Hymn to the ten Bas of Amun from the aforementioned Temple of Amun at Hibis, see the discussion in Smith 2002, 57 n. 191 and 59 n. 200. Indeed, at Hibis Amun was also worshipped as Amun-Shu, see Morenz 1960, 89 with n. 2 for references to the corpus.

[526] See Smith 2002, 60. Consider also the above figure, depicting Isis as the god's mother suckling Horus in the papyrus thicket of Khemmis.

[527] *biꜣ.wi̓* (*bꜣ.ti̓*): see the discussion in Wilson 1997, 305.

[528] "The bushes of rushes are on the other side of the riverbank" (*tꜣ bꜣ.t gꜣš ḥr mrw*): P.Brit.Mus. EA 10249 (P.Anastasi IV recto 1a 13/3–4), ed. Gardiner 1937, xiv–xv; 35–36; Caminos 1954, 126–131.

[529] "And you should remove its reeds and plough it, and you shall make an arura of arable land of vegetables" (*mtw=k iṯꜣ pꜣy=s.t ḳm mtk sꜣk=s.t | mtw=k iri̯.t wʿ sṯꜣ.t ꜣḥ.t wꜣḏ*): P.Berl. inv. 8523 ll. 14–17, ed. Spiegelberg 1917b, 107–111.

swamps where the young Horus hid himself in Khemmis.[530] The passage is thus set in even closer relation to the narrative of the successful conception, gestation, birth, and suckling of the child-god Horus which features in the ritual of the *God's Birth*, treated below, and depicted in the above figure.

Following this mythological journey as currently extant, Amun names the specific toponym of Abydos as one destination, although it is possible that the source text to §9 contained further place-names lost in its history of textual transmission.[531] Given the association of Abydos with Osiris, and by extension the divine royal triad of him, Isis, and Horus, Abydos features prominently in the divine dramas of temple, afterlife, and magical ritual texts. Indeed, in such cases the instruction for deities to travel or to be prevented from traveling is often manipulated, expressing the tension and juxtaposition of movement and activity, with stillness and inactivity—further comparable to the presence and absence of the wind and wave. Unlike in the divine drama of an erotic recipe from the contemporary *PGM* IV, where the divine protagonist Isis is instructed to "go south of Thebes (and) to the north of Abydos",[532] journeying the totality of Egypt, i.e. everything north of Abydos and south of Thebes,[533] until she finds the character Belf, the extant texts here suggests that Amun is clear in his direction.

The potential resonances of journeying across all Egypt, however, are not limited to the "reed" and "rush" already discussed, nor to the potential that Amun was—at least in a source text—traveling elsewhere as well as to Abydos. His travels are also said to extend between two hills. The clearest parallel for these are the "two hills" (*ỉꜣ.tỉ*) of earlier Egyptian tradition, expressing both a

---

530 See Kocklemann 2011, 3.

531 Either an erroneous ⲟⲩⲧⲉ "between" has been added, or something is missing, with the former being much more likely—see the commentary to p. 5/5.

532 [ⲧⲉ]ϭ[ⲉ]ï ⲉⲣⲏ́ⲥ ⲛⲛⲉ́ ⲉ̀ⲡⲉⲙⲓⲧ ·ⲛⲛⲁⲃⲱⲧ (*PGM* IV.107), edited in Love 2016, §1.5 and discussed in Love 2016, §5.1. Dosoo 2021 states that "since Thebes is south of Abydos, this command is impossible", but this does not take into account the possibility that Isis is instructed to travel the totality of Egypt *until* Belf is found—consider also the following footnote.

533 §10 has "Make (for) the north of Abydos, make (for) the south (of) Thinis", a command which sees the divine protagonist meet themselves in the middle (Thinis being c. 25km north of Abydos). Therefore, it seems more likely that the traveling in *PGM* IV is to reflect the totality of Egypt rather than a juxtaposition of impossibilities, given that Abydos is north of Thebes—contrary to Dosoo 2021. After all, there is no need to assume that these divine dramas always direct their protagonists to journey to a particular place—traveling also relates to the passing of time. Indeed, these references to "north" and "south" could simply reflect the earlier resonances of traveling "downstream" and "upstream", which are instead to be found in the divine dramas of Egyptian magical texts. For example, in a recipe for "driving away (*sḥrỉ*) an enemy (*ḫft.ỉ*)" in P.Chester Beatty VIII (P.Brit.Mus. EA 10688), verso 4/1–7/5 no. 4 (Gardiner 1935, 1:72–74; 2: pls. 45–46), the question is posed "Does Osiris know its name?" (*nn rḫ wsỉr rn≠f*), because, if he does not, "I will not let him travel downstream to Busiris, I will not let him travel upstream to Abydos" (*bn-ỉw≠ỉ r ḏỉ.t ḫdỉ≠f r ḏd.w* | *bn-ỉw≠ỉ r ḏỉ.t ḫntỉ≠f r ꜣbḏ.w*) (verso 4/7–8).

particular domain dedicated to funerary deities and Osiris, or the apposition of north and south, and thereby again the totality of Egypt.[534]

In a departure from the vivid image of Amun traveling in and as the wind, he suddenly manifests in—presumably—corporeal form, stating: "What I am mounted on is a white horse, a black horse was before me", stressing the importance of his steeds in both cases through the syntax of this pairing of utterances. As first identified by Crum,[535] this statement is paralleled by that made by Horus in the aforementioned healing recipe of *P.London-Leiden* verso 33/1–9 (*PDM* xiv.1219–1227). In the commands closing the divine drama constituting that recipe, Horus heads up to the desert plateau at midday during the summer (*ꜣḫ.t*), but does so "mounted on a white horse, [...] a black horse"[536]—apparently not riding one horse that is being led by another, but those two horses in another combination, showing slight but important semantic differences. Besides the apposition and opposition of the colors expressing a spectrum, however, and thus perhaps a totality, this image has no direct resonance with obvious earlier mythological motifs. As an animal not indigenous to Egypt, it seems that the horse did not penetrate the Egyptian pantheon and Egyptian mythology, making the origin of this motif, at least to the present author, unclear, as well as its incorporation into §9 and the partial parallel of *P.London-Leiden*, suggestive of a much later composition than, for example, the mythological scene setting of §9.

The partial parallel with *P.London-Leiden* continues, as Amun adds in §9 that "the bookrolls of Thoth are with me, those of the Great of Five are in my hands", which is also expressed by Horus in that partial parallel, but with significant semantic differences.[537] The "Great of Five" is a long-established epithet for Thoth that, importantly for questions of transmission (whether textual or oral), appears to be exclusive to the Egyptian-language tradition. Thus, "those of the Great of Five" are synonymous with "the bookrolls of Thoth", another instance in which the text utilizes a pairing to encompass and thereby express a unity. On a previous occasion, I have discussed at length the appearance of the "bookrolls of Thoth" and "those of the Great of Five" in both of these magical texts alongside their appearance elsewhere in Egyptian literature and magical and other ritual texts.[538] To summarize the considerations in that study, as tomes of

[534] Discussed in *GDG* I, 22–23.

[535] Crum Notebook 87, 36—demonstrating that, while a specialist in Coptic, Crum was au fait with all stages and scripts of the Egyptian language, partly thanks to his colleague Sir Herbert Thompson, who worked with him on *A Coptic Dictionary*.

[536] *ỉw⸗f ḏị.t-/tỉ.t-ꜥỉꜥyṯ r wꜥ ḥtr ḥḏ* [...] *r wꜥ ḥtr km* (*P.London-Leiden* verso 33/1)—the lacuna does not appear sufficient to restore *ỉw⸗f ḏị.t/-tỉt-ꜥỉꜥyṯ*.

[537] "The bookrolls [of Thoth being] on him, those of the Great of Five in his breast" (*ỉw nꜣ ḏmꜥ [n ḏḥw.tỉ ḥr-ꜣ].ṯ⸗f nꜣe pꜣ wr-tỉw ẖn ḳn⸗f*) (*P.London-Leiden* verso 33/2).

[538] Love 2020, §5.3.

"textual authority",[539] the bookrolls "which Thoth wrote with his own hand", manuscripts full of ritual texts, were—as narrated in Egyptian literature—conceptualized as paradigms of efficacious ritual practices. While their appearance with Horus in the aforementioned divine drama of *P.London-Leiden* does not appear to lend him any efficacy in healing his fever,[540] the resonance in §9 seems instead to be that Amun is prepared with all the media required to hasten Isis' birth and bring her labor at last to an end.[541] The possibility remains, although not expressed in the text itself, that "the bookrolls of Thoth" were—as in Egyptian literary tradition[542]—conceptualized as the authoritative and thereby efficacious source of the invocations and commands utilized by Amun later in §9.

Amun's response closes with a tripartite statement featuring a particular stress in the syntax that he is to facilitate the birth of those who are pregnant, to close up those who miscarry, and to ensure the fertility of all eggs except those which are infertile. The significance of these statements has already been seen in the study of the associations of Amun as the "wind" (*swḥ*), the male counterpart of the "egg" (*swḥ.t*), as well as Amun's other associations of creative efficacy.[543] Indeed, in the aforementioned hymn to Amun-Shu from the Temple of Amun at Hibis, Amun is not only described as one whose "voice is heard, (but) he is not seen, while he causes every throat to breathe", but also as he "who strengthens the hearts of those who are (or have become) pregnant (*bkꜣ*) and those who give birth (*msi̯*), who gives life to those who come forth from her".[544] Below, the treatment of Amun's role in the ritual of the *God's Birth* highlights further resonances in these statements with the divine drama that unfolded in the mammisis—"birth houses"—of temples to celebrate, perform, and thereby actualize the conception, gestation, delivery, and suckling of the child-gods of those temples. Thus, these statements of both Amun's intention and efficacy are made not only in order that the practitioner identify with Amun and thereby acquire the efficacy to hasten the birth of the contemporary patient in labor—analogous to the mythological Isis in labor—but also to access that agency through the resonances of these statements with the host of associations with Amun's creative efficacy.

---

539 See Love 2020, §5–6, developing Love 2016, §7.6.3–7.7.

540 Suggesting that in the composition or compilation of such texts stock motifs could be utilized and adopted without them having any specific resonance in the target text.

541 In the Demotic tale of *Setne II*, the protagonist Hor-son-of-Paneshe is invited by Thoth to access the textual authority contained within the papyrus "which Thoth wrote with his own hand" for his own magical practices: see Love 2020, §5.3.2.

542 As studied in Love 2020, §5–6.

543 As discussed in Morenz 1950, 99.

544 *smn ỉb n bkꜣ ḥr msi̯.w sꜥnḫ pꜣ pri̯ ỉm=s* (Brugsch 1878, pl. 16 col. 38).

The journey that Amun takes across the mythological landscape described in the divine dialogue recalls in turn another of his roles. As Amun journeys towards the mother Isis who is struggling in her labor, his hastening is evocative of his role as the one who "hastens birth" (*sḫꜣḫ msi̯*). In the famous birth story in *P.Westcar*,[545] this is an epithet of the goddess Heqet,[546] one of the three midwives whose resonance with the "three of Isis" mentioned in §9 is discussed below. Invocations and epithets of Amun contained within the inscriptions upon the Temple of Opet at Karnak refer to many of the characteristics of Amun discussed already, from the creator[547] and manifestation[548] to the distributor[549] of wind, and thereby breath and life. Of particular note is that Amun is also given the epithets "he who hastens births and who gives the north-wind to the bones and flesh inside the womb",[550] as well as "he who comes forth hastening as the north-wind, who causes birth when his name is uttered".[551] After all, just as "one calls to him on the ocean" when sailors and their crews are at risk, "one calls to him in the mammisi" when mothers and their unborn children are at risk.[552] At Edfu, Amun is invoked to come, and describes himself as coming, in haste, in order to give the breath of life to his daughter.[553] This journeying resonates with Amun's hurrying to "hasten birth" just as one must hasten to rescue those in peril at sea. Amun is the deity who responds to liminal situations in which the distinctions between life and death are finely drawn.

Beyond the general resemblance in role, the specific turn of phrase is exactly that found in recipes to "hasten birth" (*sḫꜣḫ msw.t*) in the Egyptian magical and

---

[545] P.Berl. inv. 3033, ed. Lepper 2008.

[546] *ḥḳ.t ḥr sḫꜣḫ msw.t* (P.Westcar 10/8; 10/15; 10/23).

[547] "He who creates wind" (*ỉr(r) ṯꜣw*) (*Opet* 24; 166; 183.2).

[548] "He is the breath that dwells in all things, by which we live forever." (*swḥ -pw mn m ỉḫ.t -nb(.t) ꜥnḫ.tỉ ỉm⸗f ḏ.t*) (*Opet* 143).

[549] "He who gives the breath of life to every nose" (*ḏḏ ṯꜣw n ꜥnḫ r fnḏ -nb*) (*Opet* 157) or simply "He who gives breath to every nose" (*ḏḏ ṯꜣw r fnḏ -nb*) (*Opet* 117).

[550] *sḫꜣḫ ms(w.t) ḏḏ ṯꜣw mḥ(.tỉ) r ḳs ỉwf m-ẖnw n ḥm.wt* (*Opet* 123).

[551] *prr šš n (i.e. ḫꜣḫ m) mḥ.yt | ḏḏ ỉwr.t r tꜣ (i.e. ỉw tw) ḥr tm (i.e. dm) rn⸗f* (*Edfu Mammisi* 25.12). (Dagmar Budde is thanked for highlighting this passage in a personal communication.) The unmorphemic—unetymological—orthographies in this particular passage are numerous and notable, suggesting that this section was composed at a significantly late date after which several sound shifts had occurred. Similar epithets of Amun are found in the hymn to that god elsewhere in the Edfu Mammisi, cf. *Edfu Mammisi* 132.15–133.2.

[552] *nỉs⸗tw n⸗f m wꜣḏ-wr ꜥš⸗tw n⸗f m pr-msi̯* (*Opet* 123), compare "He whom one wishes to see, who hears when one calls to him from the mammisi, whose Ka is worshipped upon the ocean" (*nḥi̯ dgỉ sḏm ꜥš⸗tw n⸗f n pr-msi̯ ḏwi̯ kꜣ⸗f ḫnt wꜣḏ-wr*) (*Opet* 166).

[553] Amun speaks: "I hear what you have said, I hear your request" (*sḏm(⸗ỉ) ḏ(d.t)⸗ṯ | ndb(⸗ỉ) nḥ{t}⸗ṯ*) (*Edfu Mammisi* 152.8–9) and Neith commands Amun: "Hasten in satisfaction to the place where your daughter is, oh hastener, lord of the <sweet> wind" (*ỉś (i.e. ꜣs) m ḥtp r bw ẖ(r) sꜣ.t=k | p(ꜣ) šrš (i.e. ḫꜣḫ) nb ṯꜣw <nḏm>*) (*Edfu Mammisi* 152.11–12). (Dagmer Budde is thanked for highlighting these passages in a personal communication.)

medical tradition. For example, among the recipes in the papyrus bookroll P.Leiden I 348,[554] unprovenanced and dating to the 19th Dynasty, three recipes utilize this phrase to express their desired outcome. The first, the 28th recipe (recto 13/9–11) of the entire bookroll,[555] is titled "another (*k.t*) spell (*rꜣ*) for hastening (*sḫ.t*) the birth (*msw(.t)*)". In this recipe, the practitioner commands, "open (*wn*) for me", specifying that the outcome is "to cause that she, Hathor, the Lady of Dendera, be she who gives birth".[556] The second, the 33rd recipe (verso 12/11–11/2),[557] is titled simply "another" (*k.t*), but again concerns "hastening (*sḫ.t*) the birth (*msw.t*)". The third, the 34th recipe (verso 11/2–11/8)[558] is given the fullest title: "a spell (*rꜣ*) for hastening (*sḫ.t*) the birth (*msw.t*) of Isis". Isis, as in §9, and as Hathor in the preceding example, serves as the paradigmatic mother in childbirth—as it occurred and reoccurs in the divine sphere in mythological time, so shall it too in the human sphere in contemporary time. Developing the mythological precedent in detail, this recipe addresses first Re and his disk, and then the deities of the sky and of the land: "See! Isis is suffering (in) her back as a pregnant one, although her months are fulfilled, according to those required of pregnancy, with her son, Horus".[559] Those invoked deities are to "be astounded (*ggwi̯*)" if Isis were to spend any more time pregnant, that is, without giving birth.[560] The motif of presence as opposed to absence is then applied in a way that is directly evocative of the mythological scene setting of §9, with the practitioner then coercing the invoked deities: "For then there will be no heaven, for then there will be no earth, for then there will be no five epagomenal days, for then there will be no more offerings to the gods, the lords of Heliopolis, for then there will be weariness in the southern sky and there will be a storm coming out from the northern sky and cries of woe inside the shrine, sunlight will not rise, the Nile will not flood when it should emerge in its time!"[561] But the practitioner then manipulates the coercion of the invoked deities to specify, "It is not I who said it, it is not I who repeated it, it is Isis who said it, it is she who repeated it to you (pl.). For she has spent time without her

[554] Ed. Borghouts 1971.

[555] Borghouts 1971, 28, with commentary.

[556] *r ḏi̯.t=s ḥw.t-ḥr nb(.t) ỉwn.t ntỉ ḥr ms.t* (P.Leiden I 348 recto 13/10).

[557] Ed.pr. in Borghouts 1971, 30, with commentary.

[558] Ed.pr. in Borghouts 1971, 30–31, with commentary.

[559] *ỉst ꜣs.t ḥr mn.t pḥ.wi=s.t m ỉwr(.t) mḥ ꜣbd=s.t ⸢r-rḫ.t⸣ m ỉwr.t m šꜣ=s.t ḥr.w* (P.Leiden I 348 verso 11/4).

[560] "If she were to spend her time without giving birth" (*[ỉ]⸢r ỉry=s.t⸣[tꜣy=s]⸢.t⸣ ỉꜣd.t nn ms.wt*) (P.Leiden I 348 verso 11/4–5).

[561] *ḫr nn wn.w p.t | ḫr nn wn.w tꜣ | nn wn.w hrw 5 ḥr.i{w} rnp.t | ḫr nn wn.w wdn.w n nṯr.w nb.w ỉwn | ḫpr bꜣgꜣ m p.t rs.ỉ | prỉ ẖnn.w m p.t mḥ.tt | ꜥn.w m-ẖnw kꜣr | nn wbn šw | nn ḥwi̯ ḥꜥpỉ | bśy=f r tr=f* (P.Leiden I 348 verso 11/6–7).

son Horus, avenger of his father, being born",[562] redirecting the mythological precedent to Isis and—finally—to the contemporary patient: "Guard the birth of NN, daughter of NN, likewise!"[563] Thus, the divine drama draws its mythological precedent and paradigmatic authority, and thereby efficacy, not only from Amun's hastened movement throughout Egypt, but also from his role in both the mythological and magical traditions as a deity of "hastening birth", and more specifically as the one responsible for the hastening of Isis' birth, itself a motif attested centuries before its appearance in §9.

III. Amun in the Ritual of the *God's Birth*

ⲁⲩⲟⲩⲱⲧ̄ϥ ⲑⲟⲟⲩⲧ
i͗ri̯⸗w w(ꜣ)t⸗f tḥw.ti͗
He was sent, Thoth.
ⲁϥⲉⲓ ⲉⲃⲟⲗ ϩⲏⲧ:
i͗ri̯⸗f i͗yi̯ r-bl ḥꜣ.ṯ⸗i͗
He came out before me.
ⲁⲙⲟⲩⲛ ⲉⲕⲛⲏⲩ ⲧⲱⲛ·
i͗mn i͗:i͗ri̯⸗k nꜥ(y) tn
"Amun, where is it that you are going?"

III.1. Textual Structure

The divine dialogue transitions with the embodiment and identification of a divine questioner in Thoth, who is described as having been sent, and coming out before Amun—interrupting his journey. In doing so, he poses to Amun the same question asked by the unidentified, disembodied voice: "Amun, where it is that you are going?". This "going" (ⲛⲏⲩ) is the same as that featured in the preceding dialogue, recalling the earlier narrative structure in both syntax and semantics. The importance of the "I" expressed in that earlier narrative body is once again connected, whereby the protagonist, and thereby practitioner, describes Thoth as coming out in front of "me"—providing a spatial immediacy that helps again to *locate* the mythological precedent in the contemporary time of the practitioner. This should be compared directly to the comparable use of this motif in the divine drama of *PGM* IV.94–113, but there the phrase "Thoth, [(the) great], came in before her (and) asked her" is instead narrated in the third person in past, mythological time—thereby *not* locating the divine drama in a way that could serve as analogous to the practitioner, rather more to the client. Amun then answers this question in turn, transitioning from describing his form and manner of travel—not addressed in Thoth's questioning—and revealing that

---

[562] *nn i͗nk i͗:ḏd -sw | ḫr nn i͗nk i͗:wḥm -st | i͗n ꜣs.t i͗:ḏd -sw | nts{t} wḥm -s.t i͗w(r)⸗ṯn | r-nti͗ i͗ry⸗s.t i͗ꜣd.t | nn msi̯ šꜣ⸗s ḥr.w nḏ-i͗t⸗f* (P.Leiden I 348 verso 11/7–8).

[563] *šꜣu̯ msw.t ḏw msi̯.n p.t m-mi͗.ti͗t* (P.Leiden I 348 verso 11/8).

he is specifically traveling to Isis, the paradigmatic mother. Here, as the divine drama develops, Amun's role in the aforementioned ritual of the *God's Birth* and its significant resonances in §9 can be considered.

III.2 Textual Content

The practice of rituals that brings together Amun's creative associations with the air and egg is to be seen most clearly in the ritual of the *God's Birth* (*msw.t-nṯr*), that is, the rituals undertaken in the mammisis—"birth houses"—of temples to perform and thereby actualize the conception, gestation, delivery, and suckling of a child-god.[564] Traceable from the temple of Hatshepsut at Deir el-Bahari, dating—like the aforementioned Hymns to Amun—to the New Kingdom, the principal extant mammisis belong to the temples of the Graeco-Roman Period, during which the ritual of the *God's Birth* appears to have reached its most celebrated attested form.

The ritual of the *God's Birth* was first studied in totality and divided into scenes of divine drama by Daumas (1958), who undertook a synoptic study of the six principal versions of the relevant texts as preserved upon the walls of the mammisis of the New Kingdom at Deir-el Bahari and Luxor, of the Late Period at Dendera (reign of Nectanebo), of the Ptolemaic Period at Edfu and Philae, and of the Roman Period at Dendera (reign of Trajan). Although no manuscript copies of the liturgies that were recited as part of the divine drama of the conception, gestation, delivery, and suckling of the child-god are preserved, the cult of each mammisi must have been maintained through such copies, which would have been the preserve of the priestly *communities of practice* and *script communities* described in **Transmitting Textual Traditions**. Delineating the ritual into 16 scenes, Daumas was able to interpret the often illogical order in which the texts relating to the *God's Birth* appear upon the walls of the extant mammisis, in order to narrate the unfolding of the divine drama. A dialogue between Amun and the Ennead of Karnak as well as Thoth in Scene I frames the entire ritual by expressing the desired outcome from the outset: that of the conception, gestation, delivery, and suckling of an heir for Amun and thereby a successor upon his throne.[565] The child-god, in mythological time, is thereby analogous to the king, in contemporary time. Immediately, then, the correspondence between the ritual of the *God's Birth* and the desired outcome of §9 is clear, and it is these apparent associations that warrant discussion in greater detail.

---

[564] For a study of the mammisis, see Daumas 1958; 1977, for an introduction and bibliography, see Kockelmann 2011. For the concept of child deities, see Brunner 1977; Budde 2010a; 2011.

[565] Daumas (1958, 394) highlights the paradox of the Ennead bringing offerings for a child not yet conceived and explains this temporal disjunction as stemming from the fact that Amun's conceptualization of the child-god brings about his actualization.

The arrival of Thoth in Scene I,[566] in some traditions following the Ennead, is immediately reminiscent of the passage in the divine drama of §9 where Thoth was sent to Amun.[567] It is in this very first scene that the associations of Amun with the mythological scene setting presented above and the associations of Amun in the ritual of the *God's Birth* are clear. The role of Amun is described, and thereby actualized: "He gives every breath of life",[568] or he describes and thereby actualizes his own role when addressing the child-god: "I will give the breath of life to you, to your nose".[569] The child-god is then directly associated with the "egg", i.e. the origin of the first god—as discussed above.[570] In Scene II,[571] a dialogue between Amun and Hathor ensues (in the version at Dendera, also involving Khnum), where at Edfu Amun is described as he "who listens to pleas in every place … giving the breath of life to his son, he in perfection, hearing the pleas of millions, immediately, he who comes to the one who calls him"[572]—accompanying a depiction of Amun giving the hieroglyphic sign *ꜥnḫ* "life" to Hathor upon her birthing bed.[573] At Dendera, this is complemented by the description of Amun as he who "is coming, hastening in satisfaction so that my breath is at your (f.) nose, my life at your (f.) nostrils, I establishing your (f.) heart at its place".[574] The description of both Amun's role—life-giving—and his actions—hastening—has direct resonance with the textual content and narrative momentum in the divine drama of §9.

Scene III comprises an exchange between Amun and Khnum,[575] before Ihy is added in Scene IV,[576] where the coming and going of different deities in dialogue—each introduced with the formula *ḏd-mdw ỉn* "Words spoken by" and thereby recited by attendant priests—is resonant of the structure of the divine drama of §9, albeit with considerably more characters. The role of Thoth in Scene V at Dendera,[577] in place of that as interlocutor in §9, is to announce that Hathor is to be the mother of the child-god, and by announcing that Hathor "will

[566] Daumas 1958, 388–393.

[567] A direct address by Thoth to Amun, however, is not found (as Dagmar Budde is thanked for highlighting in a personal communication).

[568] *ḏi̯=f ṯꜣw n ꜥnḫ -nb* (*Edfu Mammisi* 8.10).

[569] *rḏi̯(=ỉ) n=k ṯꜣw n ꜥnḫ r fnḏ=k* (*Dendera Mammisi* 125.8 and 125.15).

[570] Nephthys is described as "She who gives health to the egg, who feeds its/her offspring as a young boy" (*swꜣḏ=s (r) swḥ.t rr nn.w=s m ḥwn*) (*Dendera Mammisi* 126.15).

[571] Daumas 1958, 395–403.

[572] *sḏm śpr.w wbꜣ ꜥnḫ.w n bw -nb … ḥr rḏi̯.t ṯꜣw n ꜥnḫ n sꜣ=f -sw m nfr ḥr sḏm śpr.w n ḥḥ ꜣs | ỉyi̯ n ꜥš n=f* (*Edfu Mammisi* 28.7–9).

[573] As discussed in Daumas 1958, 398.

[574] *ỉyi̯.tw n.t sṯꜣ.tw m ḥtp ṯꜣw(=ỉ) r fnḏ=t ꜥnḫ=ỉ r šr.ti=t smn=ỉ ỉb=t ḥr s.t=f* (*Dendera Mammisi* 131.10–11), as discussed in Daumas 1958, 399.

[575] Daumas 1958, 403–407.

[576] Daumas 1958, 408–421.

[577] Daumas 1958, 422–423.

see your son and your heart will be happy",[578] he actualizes this desired outcome. The sudden appearance and disappearance of deities is also common in the reconstruction of the ritual of the *God's Birth*, and, although there is no dialogue, Thoth is replaced by Khnum in Scene VI.[579]

It is in Scene VII that the first substantial hymns to Amun appear, which Daumas suggests were sung in the offering hall while the God's Birth itself was being dramatized in the sanctuary at Dendera.[580] These then lead to the return of Amun in Scene VIII.[581] In that substantial hymn,[582] Amun is invoked to "come to Hathor", that is, to the mother of the child-god at Dendera, because "It is you who gives breath to every nostril, who gives life to those in need, you are the sweet wind"[583] and because "It is you who enlivens the offspring in his egg, who joins the semen with the bones".[584] Elsewhere at Dendera, this is extended to refer to Amun's creative efficacy: "Come Amun! ... You are come, having returned in satisfaction. May <you> give the breath of life to deities and humanity!"[585]

Amun is not only invoked because of his creative associations, but also because "It is you who is called in the midst of trouble",[586] "It is you who listens to the requests of every face, whose ears are open to everyone",[587] and because "You are the Lord of life, who gives it to the one he loves".[588] Amun is the deity "who hears the petitions of the gods",[589] in his capacity as "lord of the sweet breath, who gives it to whom he loves",[590] and who also "hears the petitions of every man with open ears".[591] When responding, Amun replies, "I hear what you

---

[578] *mꜣꜣ⸗t sꜣ⸗t nfr ỉb* (*Dendera Mammisi* 18.8), as discussed in Daumas 1958, 422.

[579] Daumas 1958, 423–425.

[580] Daumas 1958, 434.

[581] Daumas 1958, 435–437.

[582] Partially paralleled at Edfu, see *Edfu Mammisi* 47–48. Budde locates this and other hymns within their contexts upon the inside faces of the portico, see Budde 2021, fig. 1 and 19. At Dendera, by comparison, the hymn is inscribed upon the walls of the offering hall, within the temple itself. For a bibliography to this hymn, see Budde 2021, n. 59, and for a bibliography on the research on hymns in Egyptology, see Budde 2021, n. 1–4.

[583] *ntk ḏd ṯꜣw r fnḏ -nb | sꜥnḫ m gꜣ.w | ntk ṯꜣw nḏm* (*Dendera Mammisi* 31.1–2).

[584] *ntk sꜥnḫ ṯꜣ m-ẖnw n štꜣ.t⸗f | ṯś mw m ḳ(ꜣ)ś.w* (*Dendera Mammisi* 31.4–5). At Edfu, this potency is ascribed to Khnum (*Edfu* V, 185.1). For *štꜣ.t* "egg" as a synonym for "womb", see Budde 2010b, 6–9.

[585] *mỉ ỉmn ... ỉw⸗k ỉyi̯.tw sṯꜣ.tw m ḥtp | ḏi̯<⸗k> ṯꜣw n ꜥnḫ n nṯr.w rmṯ.w* (*Dendera Mammisi* 267.3–4).

[586] *ntk nỉs n⸗f m-ẖnw n ḳsn.t* (*Dendera Mammisi* 31.5).

[587] *ntk sḏm śrp.w n ḥr -nb | wbꜣ ꜥnḫ.wỉ [n] ⸢bw -nb⸣* (*Dendera Mammisi* 31.6–7).

[588] *ntk nb ꜥnḫ ḏd n mry⸗f* (*Dendera Mammisi* 31.5).

[589] *sḏm śpr.w n nṯr* (*Dendera Mammisi* 127.5–6).

[590] *nb ṯꜣw nḏm ḏd n mri̯(.w)⸗f* (*Dendera Mammisi* 127.6).

[591] *sḏm śrp.w n ḥr(.w) -nb.w wbꜣ ꜥnḫ.wỉ* (*Dendera Mammisi* 127.8).

have said, I hear your request".[592] In such a capacity, Amun is commanded to "come to the King of Upper and Lower Egypt", i.e. the child-god Horus, implying a journey described by Amun in §9 when he is met en route by Thoth. In the Edfu Mammisi, this journey is explicitly referenced, with Amun given two alternative directions: "If you are on earth, reach the birth-house (i.e. mammisi)",[593] whereas "If you are in (or, as) the breezes of the air … may you enter the enclosure of the bed".[594] Here, then, there is further resonance with the reference in §9 to Amun traveling with the south-wind northwards, and with his destination that of the god's mother in labor.

Further resonances from §9 of Amun informing Thoth of Isis' labor appear in the Hymn to Amun from the ritual of the *God's Birth* where Amun is informed of the labor of Hathor, the mother of the child-god at Dendera: "Your daughter is pregnant; she has completed her total; her eyes are towards your coming. Come! Every haste! Not any delay!"[595] Subsequently, Amun is commanded to "give breath to your daughter"[596] because "the pregnant one speaks to you, her heart seeking, asking [you for] the breath together with what is in her womb",[597] and the culmination of that seeking is "so that you may make the sweet breath ascend to her with your fist so that she may [give birth]".[598] This need is directly comparable to the role of Amun as "he who gives breath to the nose(s) of those who are pregnant",[599] itself recalling Amun's tripartite declaration of intention and thereby efficacy earlier in §9.

In order that these invocations and commands be actualized, the hymn concludes with the final command to Amun: "Come to Hathor, the great (or, Lady of Dendera), coming and hastening in satisfaction!".[600] This in itself catalyzes the birth, allowing "his daughter", i.e. Hathor, also to "come in satisfaction". The hymn then closes with phrases that resonate with §9: "May you (f.) give nourishment to Horsematway, the child, son of Hathor".[601] Such nourish-

---

[592] *sḏm(=ỉ) ḏ(d.t)=ṯ ndb(=ỉ) nḥ{t}=ṯ* (*Edfu Mammisi* 152.8–9).

[593] *ỉn ỉw=k [ḥr tꜣ] śpr ḥw.t-wtṯ* (*Edfu Mammisi* 47.5).

[594] *ỉn ỉw=k m ỉr.w=k m ỉs-nꜣw … ꜥḳ=k [ḥw.t]-mśš (msẖn.t)* (*Edfu Mammisi* 47.6); *ỉn ỉw=k m ỉr.w=k m ỉs-nꜣw … ỉw=k m dwꜣ.t* etc. *ꜥḳ=k ḥw.t-sḏr* (*Dendera Mammisi* 27.6–7).

[595] *sꜣ.t=k ỉwr.t mḥ=s dmḏ=s | ỉr.wỉ=s m-sꜣ n ỉyi̯=k | mỉ | ꜣs -nb | m-ỉrw ḏf -nb* (*Edfu Mammisi* 47.8–9); *[sꜣ.t] ỉwr.t mḥ=s dmḏ=s | ỉr.wỉ=s m-sꜣ n ỉyi̯=k | mỉ ꜣs.tw m-ỉrw ḏf -nb* "Come, hastening, not any delay!" (*Dendera Mammisi* 27.8–9).

[596] *ỉmi̯ ṯꜣw n sꜣ.t=k* (*Edfu Mammisi* 47.10).

[597] *ḫr n=k ỉwr.t | ỉb=s ḥḥ.tw ḥr nḥi̯[=k r/n] ṯꜣw ḥnꜥ ỉm.ỉ ẖ.t=s* (*Edfu Mammisi* 47.14–48.1).

[598] *sꜥr=k n=s -rf ṯꜣw nḏm m-ꜥ (?) ꜣmm=k ḏi̯=s [msi̯ (?)]* (*Edfu Mammisi* 48.1); *[sꜥr=k n=s] -ỉrf ṯꜣw nḏm m-ꜥ ꜣmm=k ḏi̯=s [msi̯ (?)]* (*Dendera Mammisi* 28.4).

[599] *dḏ(.w) ṯꜣw ỉw fnḏ n bꜣḳ(.w)* (*Dendera* II, 125.13).

[600] *ỉmn mỉ n ḥw.t-ḥr wr | ỉw=k ỉyi̯.t ꜣs.t m ḥtp sp-sn* (*Edfu Mammisi* 48.3); *ỉmn mỉ n ḥw.t-ḥr nb(.t) ỉwn.t | ỉw=k ỉyi̯.tỉ ꜣs.tw m ḥtp sp-sn* (*Dendera Mammisi* 28.4–5).

[601] *dỉ=ṯ sꜥnḫ n ḥr.w-smꜣ-tꜣ.wỉ p(ꜣ) ẖrd sꜣ ḥw.t-ḥr* (*Edfu Mammisi* 48.4).

ment refers not only to the creative efficacy of a mother, but also tangibly to the sustenance that her son acquires from being suckled.

The divine drama of the ritual of the *God's Birth* continues in Scene IX with the actual birth of the child-god, and the recognition of the child-god by his father, i.e. Amun, in Scene X.[602] From this point, Amun's role is principally that of the predecessor of the ascendant king, the child-god Horus. Here, the resonances with §9 switch from being those with Amun to those with Hathor as the mother of the child-god—as Isis in §9. In the first of these two scenes Amun addresses Hathor, instructing her to "raise your beloved son, and he will fulfill his royal office"[603]—referring to successful delivery and ascension to the throne. After this, Hathor replies to Amun: "I have suckled your son, your beloved, with the milk which comes forth from my body; may it enter him as all life and power",[604] and "I suckle you with the milk which comes forth from (my) body."[605] Here, the importance of suckling as the final of four stages in the ritual of the *God's Birth* is reminiscent of the commands that Amun gives to Isis at the end of §9—to produce milk for her son Horus. This outcome is not only actualized through the performance of the divine drama in Graeco-Roman mammisis—including the recitations that form part of such a performance—, but also through the iconography that accompanies their monumental inscription upon their walls.

Three goddesses, immediately recalling the "three of Isis" or "three Isises" who appear in §9, are depicted delivering or suckling the child-god. At Armant, three divine wet-nurses are depicted and named by their epithets: "midwife" (*sms.yt*), "wet-nurse" (*mnʿ.t*), and "nurse" (*ḫnm.t*).[606] At Dendera, the three divine wet-nurses are Isis,[607] Wadjet, and Nekhbet.[608] There, Isis declares: "I suckle my young man to avenge his father. I feed him as a sovereign";[609] Wadjet: "I am the fine warder of the excellent child, the guardian of the august child. I am behind your head, surrounding your body";[610] and Nekhbet: "I am the perfect suckler, who suckles her son without tiring myself".[611] Indeed, at a further mythological level, the act of suckling by the mother of the child-god is crucial

---

[602] Daumas 1958, 437–449 and 449–460 respectively.

[603] *ỉw ꜥḥꜥ n⸗t sꜣ⸗t mr.t | ỉw⸗f r irị̂ ỉꜣw.t* (*Dendera Mammisi* 7.1–2)

[604] *rr.n(⸗ỉ) sꜣ⸗k mr⸗k m ỉrṯ.t pr(r.t) m ḥꜥ.w{t}(⸗ỉ) | ꜥḳ⸗s{n} n⸗f m ꜥnḫ wsr -nb* (*Dendera Mammisi* 7.3–4).

[605] *snḳ(⸗ỉ) -k m ỉrṯ.t pr(r.t) m ḥꜥ.w(⸗ỉ)* (*Dendera Mammisi* 104.6–7).

[606] As discussed in Daumas 1958, 444.

[607] As noted, Hathor is the mother of the child-god at Dendera.

[608] As discussed in Daumas 1958, 454–455.

[609] *mnꜥ(⸗ỉ) n ḫy⸗ỉ r nḏ ỉt⸗f | rr(⸗ỉ) -s m ỉty* (*Dendera Mammisi* 128.7–8).

[610] *ỉnk ḫnm.t nfr.t n.t ẖrd ỉḳr | nḥ.t n.t nn.w šps | wn⸗ỉ ḥꜣ tp⸗t ṅr sḫb ḥꜥ.w⸗t* (*Dendera Mammisi* 128.9–10).

[611] *ỉnk mnꜥ.t nfr.t mnꜥ.t sꜣ⸗s n wrḏ⸗ỉ* (*Dendera Mammisi* 128.11–12).

for the recognition of his legitimacy as successor to his father and imbues him with both royal and divine faculties.[612] The more deities do so, the more efficacious the ruler—indeed, seven goddesses—the "seven Hathors"—are depicted suckling the child-god at Edfu.[613] Scene XI in turn concerns the suckling of the child-god by the divine wet-nurses.[614] At Dendera, Nekhbet is the only goddess who speaks as she kneels behind and supports Hathor, while Hesat and Sekhat-Hor, the two other wet-nurses, are also depicted upon the bed holding and suckling the child-god in bovine-headed anthropomorphic forms and under the bed in fully bovine forms suckling a kneeling child-god.[615] One final notable resonance between the divine drama of the ritual of the *God's Birth* with §9 is that found in the specification of suckling. As the ritual of the *God's Birth* served to actualize four desired outcomes—the conception, gestation, delivery, and suckling of the child-god—the ritual of §9 aimed at two outcomes comparable to the latter two: the delivery and suckling of the patient's child.

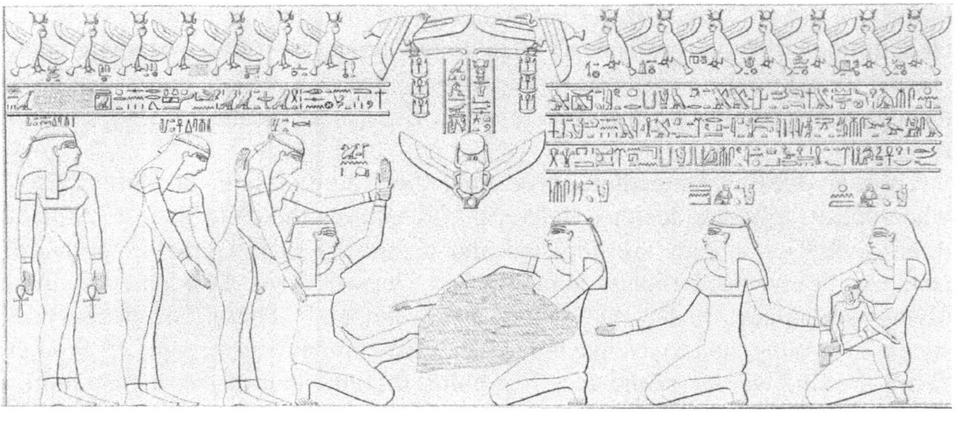

In the Temple of Armant, the delivery and suckling of the child-king of "the god's mother of Re" by the three goddesses—named by their epithets "midwife" (*sms.yt*), "wet-nurse" (*mnʿ.t*), and "nurse" (*ḫnm.t*)—is depicted (*LD* IV Plates, pl. 60a).

[612] Daumas 1958, 456, 461.
[613] *Edfu Mammisi* pl. 15: north wall of sanctuary A, third register from the bottom.
[614] Daumas 1958, 460–463.
[615] *Dendera Mammisi* 6 and 108, discussed in Daumas 1958, 460–461.

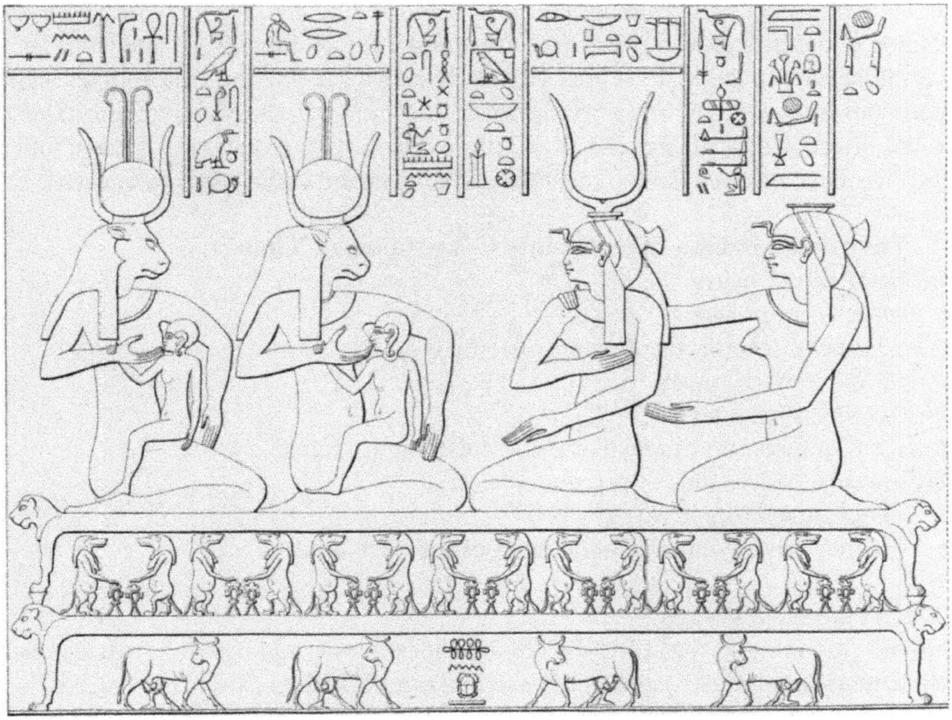

In the Dendera Mammisi, bovine-headed anthropomorphs Hesat and Sekhat-Hor are depicted holding and suckling the child-god, while anthropomorphic Nekhbet supports Isis. Four bovine manifestations are depicted below the bed (likely Hesat and Sekhat-Hor twice each), each of which suckles a kneeling child-god (compare the relief from Armant) (*LD* IV Plates, pl. 82b).

While the latter scenes of the ritual of the *God's Birth* do not exhibit comparable resonances with §9,[616] some of the invocations of, and epithets identifying, the deities involved are worth noting. Amun's role as the bringer of breath, and thereby life, is repeated and elaborated in Scene XV, and the reason why he in particular is called to come to the birth are specified: "You are he to whom those in trouble call".[617] The identification of the mother and the commands given by Amun are reminiscent of Hathor's identificatory statements in the last scene (XVI), where she states: "I am your mother, who made you as a youth. May you

[616] Scene XII concerns the enthronement of the child-god before the Great Ennead (Daumas 1958, 463–472) and the last four dialogues between different combinations of deities describing the divine and royal faculties of the child-god and the role that he will play. For these latter scenes, see Daumas 1958, 472–487.

[617] *ntk nis n≠f m-ẖnw ḳsn* (*Dendera Mammisi* 31.5); *nti≠k nis n≠f m-ẖnw ḳsn* (*Dendera Mammisi* 268.1–2); *ntk nis n≠f m-ẖnw ḳsn* (*Edfu Mammisi* 170.3–4).

suckle from (my) milk; may it enter you with life and stability",[618] coupled with Hathor's identification as "the fine wet-nurse, fat of breasts"[619] and "the fine wet-nurse, fat of milk".[620] Thus, Hathor declares: "I am the fine mother who feeds her son without tiring".[621] Here, at the close of the ritual of the *God's Birth*, resonances with the end of §9 are evident; as the delivery of the child(-god) has been ensured, so too must the suckling of the child(-god) be ensured.

IV. The Divine Drama Directed into Contemporary Time

ⲡϣⲟⲙ̄ⲛ̄ⲧ̄ ⲛ̄ⲏⲥ̄ⲉ̄: ⲡⲟⲟⲩ
pꜣ ḫmt n ꜣs.t (n) pꜣ-(h)rw
"The Three of Isis (or, the three Isises), today,
ⲉⲥϯⲛⲁⲁⲕⲉ· ϥⲧⲟⲟⲩ ⲛ̄ⲥⲟⲩ
iri̯=s ti͗.t nhḳ (r) ft.w n sw
it is for four days (or, times) that she is suffering (in labor).
(ⲟⲩ)ⲏⲣ ⲙⲉⲛ ⲟⲩ' ⲧⲉ ϥⲡⲟⲗ̄ϭ̄ ⲉⲛⲧⲱⲃⲉ ⲉⲙⲓⲥⲉ
wr irm wr tꜣy iw=f plg nꜣ tby(.t) n msi̯
It is so-and-so many times that he releases the birth bricks."

IV.1. Textual Structure

Amun's monologue that follows Thoth's questioning again utilizes syntactical and semantic pairings—even in the extant form of the text. The "three of Isis"—whose potential resonance with the midwives of the god's mother and wet-nurses of the child-god has been discussed above—open Amun's answer, whereby the numbers "three" and "four" are paired,[622] with each of the two clauses ending in -ⲟⲩ. The *action* of labor is then paired with the *place* of labor, that is, the birth bricks upon which the mother squats. This in turn draws the tripartite structure of three clauses together, because there is a reference to *time* in all three—the first, "today", the second "four days (or, times)", and the third "so-and-so many times". This brings all three within a temporal frame of both past and present—ongoing and thereby immediate—time. The ongoing problem, framed through *action*, *place*, and *time* is manifest in the description of them, and then drawn into direct analogy to the contemporary situation of the practitioner and patient by description, rather than direction.

---

[618] *i͗nk mw.t=k sḫpr.w m ḥwn | snḳ=k m i͗rṯ.t(=i͗) | ʿḳ=s n=k m ʿnḫ wsr* (*Dendera Mammisi* 19.13–14).
[619] *mnʿ.t nfr.t ḫpn i͗rṯ.t* (*Dendera Mammisi* 130.7).
[620] *mnʿ.t nfr.t ḫpn mn.ti͗* (*Dendera Mammisi* 130.2).
[621] *i͗nk mw.t nfr.t rr(r.t) sꜣ=s n wrḏ=i͗* (*Dendera Mammisi* 130.8)
[622] Notably, unlike in the mythological scene setting, both are expressed in their *absolute* rather than *construct* forms, emphasizing their pairing here.

IV.2. Textual Content

As discussed in the opening of this section, both §§9 and 10 feature the mythological precedent of a divine drama, but conclude with commands that, while cited by a character in that divine drama, direct the divine drama into contemporary time by stipulating the desired outcome to be actualized by the recitation or inscription of the text.[623] Thus, the practitioner first identifies with the protagonist of the mythological precedent through the recitation of the divine drama, and in doing so cites the authoritative, efficacious commands which that protagonist acquires in the narrative, which in turn affect the contemporary context of the practiced ritual, bringing about its desired outcome. In response to Thoth's questioning, Amun describes the mythological paradigm that has been unfolding in his absence, and to which he has been hastening. He is going to "the three of Isis today", because "it is for four days (or, times) that she is suffering". The paradigmatic number of days or times in which Isis, perhaps alongside her three midwives and/or wet-nurses, has been suffering in labor is thereby specified. Perhaps, then, the reference to "four" is instead derived from a source text, which was itself applied; that is to say, in the practice of the ritual this number could be replaced by the number of days or times on or in which the contemporary patient had already been in labor.[624] As discussed above, in the scenes of the ritual of *God's Birth*, the concept of the time of labor coming to completion is found throughout the mammisi texts. In a hymn to Amun in the Edfu Mammisi, that god is commanded to come because: "the pregnant one is bloated, she has fulfilled her time in which she must suffer, she has reached her time. ... Amun, her time (*św* > ⲥⲟⲩ) of searching for you has been reached!"[625]

At this point, an enigmatic phrase that has caused constant trouble in the interpretation of §9 appears.[626] Amun specifies, "It is so-and-so many times that he releases the birth bricks". In Egyptian tradition, attested from the 6th Dynasty (from the 24th century BCE) to early modern times,[627] birth bricks were those upon which women would squat, supported by other women, during labor:[628] the

---

[623] This is the "clausal" element in Frankfurter's typology of "*historiolae*"—see further the introduction to the excurses to §§9 and 10.

[624] For discussion and justification of these readings, see the commentary to p. 5/16, 5/17, and 5/16–17.

[625] *tꜣ iwrt ḫn.ti | mḥ=s dmḏ=s | i(w)=s ḳsn.ti | pḥ tr=s | ... | imn pḥ p(ꜣy)=s św n wḫꜣ=k* (*Edfu Mammisi* 132.17–18). (Dagmar Budde is thanked for highlighting this passage in a personal communication.)

[626] See the commentary to p. 5/17–18.

[627] See the sources discussed in Roth and Roehrig 2002, 129–131.

[628] In the Demotic tale of *Setne II*, ed. Griffith 1900, 142–207 (recent bibliography in Love 2020, §2.1), the gestation and birth of the character Siousire by his mother Mehusekhet is described in three stages: "She made her [10] months [of] pregnancy" (*iri̯<=s> pꜣy=s ꜣbd [10 n] iwr*); "She spread herself on the [birth] bricks" (*pš=s ⸢r tby⸣ ⸢n msi̯⸣*); "She bore a male child"

bricks aided both the act of delivery and the role of the midwife. In Egyptian tradition these were identified with particular goddesses,[629] but even in the tradition of Coptic magical texts they were given names.[630] Although the identity of the releaser is not made explicit,[631] the meaning of this otherwise enigmatic idiom "releasing the birth bricks" is clarified by the use of the verb *plg*/*plk* in direct association with bricks (*tby* < *ḏbꜣ.t*) in *P.Harkness*, dating to 61 CE. At the very beginning of this composition of afterlife texts for the benefit of a deceased woman named Tanaweruow, the text reads: "You will board (i.e. the bark). It is Isis who has rescued [you]. It is Neith who has given you a bark. It is the great gods of your town who have released (*plg*) your brick (*tby*)" (1/2). This last phrase is interpreted by Smith as referring directly to the "birth brick" (*tby msi̱*) upon which an individual's lifespan would be inscribed—as paralleled in other afterlife texts in hieratic (*msẖn.t*) and Demotic (*tby msi̱*).[632] As a result, as noted by Smith, the birth brick itself is also used to refer figuratively to both labor and childbirth.[633] Indeed, birth bricks were also found deposited in elite and royal tombs from the New Kingdom, serving analogously in the rebirth of the deceased after death as they served in the birth of the living after gestation.[634]

Thus, while in *P.Harkness* the reference is to the deceased's rebirth, where "releasing the birth brick" could signify the deceased being "released" from her fate,[635] in §9 the reference to "releasing the birth bricks" refers to facilitating the birth of living offspring—where *tby msi̱* (ⲧⲱ(ⲱ)ⲃⲉ ⲛⲙⲓⲥⲉ) translates earlier Egyptian (and hieratic) *msẖn.t* "birth brick", a term whose etymology literally means the "place of alighting". In this context, a traditional epithet of Isis as "the great goddess on her birth brick" takes on added significance.[636] The "releasing" of the "birth brick" thereby marks the beginning of the lifetime of the child,[637] its

(*⸢msi̱⸣⸗s ⸢wꜥ⸣ ẖm-⸢ẖ⸣l [ḥw].ṯ*) (P.Brit.Mus. EA 10822 verso 1/8–9). The most recent study of childbirth in Ancient Egypt is Marshall 2015. For the observation and description of childbirth in the Egyptian tradition, see Töpfer 2014.

[629] See the discussion in Roth and Roehrig 2002, 130–131.

[630] See Crum 1942.

[631] Given his role in determining the lifetime and fate of the newborn, discussed below, Thoth seems the most likely contender.

[632] See Smith 2005, 89.

[633] Smith 2005, 89. See further Roth 1992, 146.

[634] As studied by Roth and Roehrig 2002.

[635] Smith 2009, 278 n. 44.

[636] *nṯr.t ꜥꜣ.t ḥr msẖn.t⸗s*: P.Boulaq 3 x+6/15, ed. Mariette 1871, pls. 6–14: see Smith 2009, 235; Töpfer 2015.

[637] In the Edfu Mammisi, birth is also described as beginning upon a brick: "His (i.e. the child-god's) birth was begun upon a brick of gold, upon a floor of red jasper" (*ỉw ỉr.w mśw.t=f r ḏb.t n nb r śꜣ-tꜣ (i.e. śꜣt(.w)) n šnm (i.e. ẖnm.t)*) (*Edfu Mammisi* 204.13). (Dagmar Budde is thanked for highlighting this passage in a personal communication.)

admission into the lived sphere, and, in Egyptian tradition, the moment at which its fate is decided.[638]

In some Egyptian texts, the lifetime of a child is described has having been written at birth by Thoth upon the birth brick.[639] This resonance is also found in the aforementioned Temple of Opet at Karnak—itself called the "mansion of the birth brick"[640] —, where the god is described as having been "distinguished upon the birth brick from the day of his birth".[641] The concept remains relevant even in the latest mythological text in Demotic of the 2nd century CE, with the *Myth of the Sun's Eye* mentioning that one's lifetime begins with one's being placed upon the birth brick.[642] Perhaps most significant, given the resonances of §9 with the ritual of the *God's Birth*, is that in the mammisi at Philae, Thoth is both depicted and described as "he who calculates lifetime, who calculates a long lifetime for the son of Isis".[643] Thus, it seems that the "he" who is responsible for "releasing the birth bricks" in §9 is implicitly Thoth, who has already figured in the divine drama. In parallel with the preceding phrase, either the length of the patient's—as Isis'—labor, or the number of times the patient—or Isis—has been in labor, is to be brought into consideration alongside the number of times the birth bricks have been released, that is to say, the number of lifetimes of her children that have begun.

---

638 As discussed by Roth and Roehrig (2002, 137), this is evidenced up until the Roman Period. In the tale of *Setne II* (as cited above), the lifetime of a deceased man is described as "his lifetime which Thoth wrote for him in order to give it (?) to him (and) with regards to his fortune on earth (*pꜣy⸗f ꜥḥꜥ n ꜥnḫ r:sẖꜣ ḏḥw.tỉ r-r⸗f r tỉ.ṯ⸗f (?) n⸗f r-ꜥ.wỉ pꜣy⸗f ꜥw n ỉr.t ḥr pꜣ ⸢tꜣ⸣*) (P.Brit.Mus. EA 10822 2/11). The parallels to this in P.Rhind 1 and P.Rhind 2 have been noted by Griffith (1900, 48–49 n. l. 11); see also the following footnote.

639 As noted by Griffith (1900, 48–49 n. l. 11): "up to the end of his lifetime which Thoth wrote for him on his birth brick" (*r pḥw n pꜣy⸗f ꜥḥꜥ r:sẖꜣ n⸗f ḏḥw.tỉ ḥr tꜣy⸗f tby-msi̯*) (P.Rhind 1 1/d7); "it happened after it was written upon his birth brick" (*ḫpr⸗s r sẖꜣ⸗w -s ḥr tꜣy⸗k tby-msi̯*) (P.Rhind 1 2/d1–d2). Note that in the hieratic versions of the afterlife ritual texts of P.Rhind 2, "birth brick" is written *msḫn.t*. To those, add: "You (f.) entered the embalming place at the end of your (f.) lifespan which Thoth wrote for you" (*ꜥḳ⸗t r tꜣ wꜥbꜣ.t m pḥw n pꜣy⸗t ꜥḥꜥ r:sẖꜣ n⸗t ḏḥw.tỉ*) (i.e. upon the birth brick) (P.Rhind 2 3/d1–2), see Smith 2009, 342 with n. 41.

640 The "mansion of the birth brick" was also a generic term for mammisis.

641 *ṯnỉ.tw⸗f ḥr msḫn.t ḏr hrw msw.t⸗f* (*Opet* 41). Consider also "Shai (i.e. fate) distinguished him [upon (?)] the birth brick" (*ṯni̯ -s(w) šꜣw [ḥr (?)] msḫn.t*) (*Opet* 264) and "he (i.e. the king) brought your Shai (i.e. fate) upon your birth brick" (*ỉni̯⸗f šꜣw tp msḫn.t⸗k*) (*Opet* 222).

642 "They have been put at their place upon their birth brick in Upper Egypt again" (*ḫꜣꜥ⸗w n⸗w tꜣy⸗w s.t ḥr tꜣy⸗w tby.t n msi̯ n tꜣ-šmꜣy ꜥn*) (P.Leiden I 384 recto 5/14).

643 *ḥsb ꜥḥꜥ.w | ḥsb ꜥḥꜥ.w ꜣw n sꜣ ỉs.t* (*Philä* II, 361.16–17).

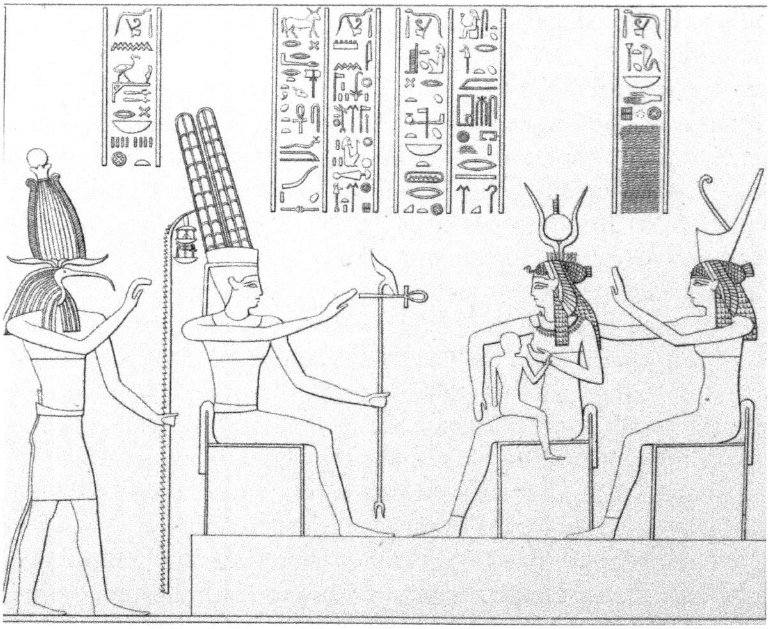

Thoth calculates the lifetime of the child-god immediately following his birth, while Amun is depicted presenting life (*ꜥnḫ*), which is one more described as "giving wind (i.e. breath) (*ṯꜣw*) to the nose"[644] (*Monuments* I, pl. LXXVI.2).

V. Amun's Instructions: Ritual Action

ⲉⲥⲧⲱ
ꞽw⸗s tꞽ.ṱ
"If
ⲙ̄ⲡⲉⲕϭⲛ̄ⲧ̄
bn-pw⸗k gmi̭.ṱ⸗ꞽ
you have not found me,
ⲙ̄ⲡⲉⲕϭⲓⲛⲉ ⲙ̄ⲡⲁⲣⲁⲛ·
bn-pw⸗k gmꞽ̭ n pꜣy⸗ꞽ rn
have not found my name,
ⲙ̄ⲡⲉⲕϭⲓⲛⲉ ⲛ̄ⲟⲩϣⲏⲙ ⲛ̄ⲛⲉϩ ⲛ̄ⲉⲓⲛⲉ ⲉⲃⲟⲗ ϩ̄ⲙ̄
bn-pw⸗k gmꞽ̭ n wꜥ ḫm n nḥ n ꞽnꞽ̭ r-bl ẖn
have not found a little oil for bringing out of <...>
ⲛ̄ⲅ̄ⲧⲁⲁϥ ⲟⲩⲧⲉ̣ ⲡⲗⲉⲃⲉⲛ ⲛ̄ⲧⲉⲥϫⲓⲥⲉ ⲉⲡⲉⲥⲏⲧ ⲛ̄ⲕ̄ϫⲟⲟⲥ
*mtw⸗k tꞽ.t⸗f ꞽwṱ pꜣ *lbn n tꜣy⸗s ṯse(.t) r pꜣ ꜣsṱ | mtw⸗k ḏd⸗s*
you should put it along the ridge of her back downwards

[644] For the text see now *Philä* II, 380–381: *ḏd ṯꜣw r fnḏ* (here l. 13).

V.1. Textual Structure

The semantic and syntactical pairings that have been discussed above as both evidencing and providing textual structure and narrative momentum are seen again in Amun's ritual instructions—above—and commands—below. In a tripartite structure, three clauses, common to both the mythological scene setting with ϩⲣⲟ(ⲟ)ⲩ and Amun's proactive monologue ⲉⲓ̈- "that I", begin ⲙ̄ⲡⲉⲕ-, followed by forms of the same verb ϭⲓⲛⲉ "to find". The object of that verb is expanded each time in a crescendo of length, beginning simply with "me" (a pronominal object), building through "my name" (a nominal object), and climaxing with "a little oil for bringing out ..." (a nominal phrase). Here, repetition and syntactical development go hand in hand. Thus, the juxtaposition of what has not been found by the protagonist being communicated in the narrative provides momentum towards its conclusion, and thereby resolution. A duality of movement of ⲉⲓⲛⲉ ⲉⲃⲟⲗ "bringing out" and ⲧⲓ ⲉⲡⲉⲥⲏⲧ "putting down(wards)" is also found in the pairing of *what* the oil will achieve, and *where* the oil should be applied.[645] That is, the *how* connecting the *what* and *where*—causality linking *action*, *place*, and thereby also *time*. The textual content of this section is analyzed collectively with that of the following section, below.

VI. Amun's Commands: Ritual Utterance

ϫⲉ
ḏd
saying:
ⲁⲗⲟ ⲁⲗⲟ ⲙ̄ⲙⲁⲩ
r:rwỉ r:rwỉ n-ỉm=w
"Cease! Cease there!
ⲥⲙ̄ⲛ̄ⲧⲉ· ⲥⲙ̄ⲛ̄ⲧⲟⲩⲟⲟⲧⲉ·
smn.ṯ=t smn tȝy=t ȝty.t
Prepare yourself! Prepare your womb!
ϣⲙ̄ϣⲉ ⲙ̄ⲡⲟⲩⲙⲁⲥ
smšỉ̭ n pȝy=t ms
Serve your offspring!
ⲣ̄ⲉⲣⲱⲧⲉ ⲛ̄ϩⲱⲣ ⲡⲟⲩϣⲏⲣⲉ
irỉ̭ ỉrte n ḥr pȝy=t šrỉ
Produce milk for Horus your son,

[645] In the ancient Mesopotamian incantation *A Cow of Sîn*, discussed in the excursus to §10, the "oil from a jar" (*šaman pūri*) that aids the delivery of the calf is a direct pun on "heaven" (*šamû*) and "calf" (*būru*)—resonating with the fact that the "Milk Calf" thereby born is the offspring of divine parents.

ϩⲛ̄ ⲧϭⲟⲙ ⲙ̄ⲡϫⲟⲉⲓⲥ ⲡⲛⲟⲩⲧⲉ·
ḫn tꜣ gm n pꜣ ṯs(ỉꜣ) pꜣ nṯr
through the power of the lord god!"

VI.1. Textual Structure

Amun's ritual instructions concerning oil, beginning with ⲉⲥⲧⲱ and continuing through the following commands, are again framed with ϫⲉ. Pairings feature once again through repetition and syntactical development. A simple imperative ⲁⲗⲟ "Cease!" is developed into an imperative that specifies *place*, ⲁⲗⲟ ⲙ̄ⲙⲁⲩ "Cease there!" A simple imperative ⲥⲙ̄ⲛ̄ⲧⲉ "Prepare yourself!"—also constructed with the particular second person singular feminine object—then opens a pairing, followed by an imperative ⲥⲙ̄ⲛ̄ⲧ- that specifies an expanded (nominal) object "your (f.) womb". This development is taken forward to the third imperative, itself not repeated or paired, but a pairing is instead seen between ⲧⲟⲩ-ⲟⲟⲧⲉ "your (f.) womb" and ⲡⲟⲩ-ⲙⲁⲥ "your (f.) offspring" in the object of this imperative, and the preceding. Here, the specification of two objects also expresses *time*—before and after—and *place*, inside and outside of the womb. This schema is extended to the fourth imperative ⲣ̄ⲉⲣⲱⲧⲉ "Produce milk!", where the object is again developed: the act benefits ⲡⲟⲩ-ϣⲏⲣⲉ "your (f.) son". Thus, this pattern also resonates with, and perhaps even actualizes, the process from "womb" (gestation and labor) to "offspring" (delivery) to "your son" (suckling). This structure is rounded off by an interpolation that describes the agent of the commands, as such falling not just outside of the preceding patterns, but also outside of the conceptualizations that underpin the preceding commands.

V.2 & VI.2. Textual Content

The final invocations and commands closing the divine drama follow. The juxtaposition between *knowing* and *not knowing* that is common to Egyptian ritual tradition again appears.[646] Here, however, the evolution of the Egyptian language over millennia has resulted in lexical updating,[647] whereby it is not a matter of *knowing* (*rḫ*) a name, but *finding* (*gmi̯*) a name, which—by extension of "finding out"—comes to mean "to know".[648] As an expression, this is, however, already

[646] For an example see below. This motif is so ubiquitous in Egyptian temple, afterlife, and magical ritual texts as to make further citations redundant.

[647] See further the discussion of this in "Transcribing and Translating Textual Traditions in the late Roman Period (3rd – 4th centuries CE)" (III) of **Transmitting Textual Traditions**.

[648] Note that in Coptic the descendant of Egyptian *rḫ* exists only as the auxiliary verb ϣ- "to be able to", and that the semantic range "to know" comes to be inhabited by Egyptian *gmi̯*, Coptic ϭⲓⲛⲉ.

found in pre-Coptic Egyptian magical texts.[649] The situation in which the protagonists, and thereby practitioners, declare that they *do not know* is immediately resolved when they go on to state what it is that they *do not know*, actualizing the *knowing*. Thus, in the mythological precedent the protagonists of divine dramas in the divine sphere present what needs to be known, allowing for it to be known, and for it to be utilized in the human sphere, despite the absence of those divine protagonists. In §9, although not specified, it appears that it is Amun who is speaking. He is, after all, the deity who has journeyed to Isis, armed with the "bookrolls of Thoth", and those final commands also reveal the desired outcome of the practice: the delivery and suckling of the child. Amun proceeds to explain to Thoth what could have been done had Thoth "not found" Amun, i.e. acquired the authoritative commands, and had "not found" his name, i.e. acquired the efficacy to utilize those commands. As common to such rhetorical statements in the dialogues of divine dramas, Amun then proceeds to provide the ritual instructions to be followed—to apply "a little oil for bringing out <...>", "downwards along the ridge of her back"—and the commands to be recited: "Cease! Cease there! Prepare yourself! Prepare your womb! Serve your offspring. Produce milk for Horus your son through the power of the lord god!"

Such a structure is paralleled in many magical texts comprising principally divine dramas in which a dialogue between characters provides the ritual instructions and commands that are authoritative by nature of originating in the mythological precedent of the divine sphere, but which—in the *absence* of that deity—can be utilized in contemporary rituals in the human sphere. Perhaps the clearest parallel is in P.Schmidt 1 (ed. Kropp *AKZ* 1, 11–12 A; *AKZ* 2, 3–6 no. 1),[650] a papyrus of the 6th or 7th century CE with the structure of a formulary but folded into a square as if produced as an amulet. This manuscript is inscribed exclusively with a divine drama of Horus and Isis,[651] but one utilizing Old Testament apocrypha in conjunction with angels and cherubim deriving from a Jewish or Judaeo-Christian cultural repertoire. In the divine dialogue of this example, Horus is apparently complaining of sleeplessness on account of his desire for seven maidens. There, Isis responds with this motif in a comparable

---

[649] Alongside the lexically older passages relating to *knowing* the name (*rn*), manner (*ky*), and form (*smṯ*) in the vessel inquiry of Khonsu in *P.London-Leiden* recto 9/1–10/22 (*PDM* xiv. 239–295 = *GEMF* 17 ix/1–x/22), discussed above, one passage has the practitioner state: "when I have not done it through the delay, when I have not found your name" (*ỉw bn-pw=ỉ ỉrỉ͗=f ẖr pꜣ ꜣsḳ ỉw bn-pw=ỉ gmỉ͗ rn.y=k*) (*P.London-Leiden* recto 9/11).

[650] See also Martín Hernández and Torallas Tovar 2012 as well as the treatment of this example among the corpus of "*historiolae*" in Frankfurter 2009 and "charms" in Blumell and Dosoo 2018.

[651] This is one of what Blumell and Dosoo (2018) termed the "Horus-Isis charms". The value of this term, typology, and the nature of the divine dramas contained in that corpus have been discussed in the introduction to the excurses to §§9 and 10 as well as in **Transmitting Textual Traditions**.

structure: "Even <if> you had not found me, and had not found my name; take a cup [and] a little water, whether a little breath or a breath of your mouth or a breath of your nose, and call down over them, 'Oh cher[ubim (?) also (?)], oh two angels who placed sleep upon Abimelech for 72 [years], place sleep on NN!'"[652] Thus, Isis provides Horus with ritual instructions and commands to be invoked in order that as she used them to "place sleep upon Abimelech for 72 [years]", so too will the invoked powers "place sleep on NN", i.e. the client of the practice. The motif and mechanism of this particular sub-category of magical texts have recently been studied comprehensively by Blumell and Dosoo,[653] who provide a formative theory of the workings of the "Horus-Isis charms"—all of which are treated. They highlight that the rhetorical responses given in such "*historiolae*"—as they term them—"serve as a paradigm for help in future cases in which the original source of power is absent"; "even without access to the deity, the actions listed afterwards—the speaking of formulae or the carrying out of ritual acts would still bring about the same desired effects".[654] It is at this moment that the temporal distinction between mythological and contemporary time breaks down, when the practitioner undertakes the ritual instructions and recites the commands provided by or to the divine protagonist in the mythological precedent.

A final note concerns the nature of the ritual instructions and commands provided. While the exact nature of the "oil for bringing out" has been lost somewhere in the history of textual transmission—perhaps simply in copying over the turn from page 5 to 6 in the Michigan codex—, this oil, imbued with the authority and thereby efficacy of having given relief to Isis and hastened her birth, is recommended for application to the back of the squatting woman.[655] Following this, two bipartite commands are to be recited, the first of each more general, the second of each more specific. The grammar of the Coptic reveals that the commands are addressed to Isis. Thus, upon the anointing of her back

652 ⲕⲁⲉⲓ ⲙⲡⲉ[ⲕϭⲛⲧ] ⲙⲡⲉⲕϭⲓⲛⲉ ⲙⲡⲁⲣⲁⲛ: ϫⲓ ⲛⲁⲕ ⲛⲟⲩⲁⲡⲟ[ⲧ ϩⲓ] ⲟⲩϣⲏⲙ ⲙⲟⲟⲩ: ⲉⲓⲉⲓ ⲟⲩⲕⲟ[ⲩⲓ ⲛⲛⲓ]ⲃⲉ ⲉⲓⲉ ⲛⲛⲓⲃⲉ ⲛ̄ⲣⲱⲕ ⲉⲓ[ⲉ] ⲛⲛⲓϥⲉ ⲛ̄[ϣⲁⲛⲧⲕ] ⲛ̄ⲅⲙⲟⲩⲧⲉ ⲉⲡⲉⲥⲏⲧ ⲉϫⲱⲟⲩ ϫⲉ ⲡⲕⲉ̄ⲭⲏ[....] ⲡⲁⲅ-ⲅⲉⲗⲟⲥ ⲥⲛⲁⲩ ⲛⲧⲁⲩⲟⲩⲱϩ ⲉⲧⲟⲟⲧⲟⲩ ⲁⲩ[ϩⲓ]ⲛⲏϥ ⲉϫⲛ ⲁϥⲧⲓⲙⲉⲗⲉⲭ ⲛ̄ϣⲃⲉ ⲥⲛⲟⲟⲥ ⲉⲛ[ⲣⲟⲙⲡⲉ] ⲟⲩⲱϩ ⲉⲧⲟⲟⲧⲧⲏⲩⲧⲛ ⲉϩⲣⲁⲓ ⲉϫⲙ̄ ⲇⲇ (P.Schmidt 1 ll. 14–21).

653 Blumell and Dosoo 2018, 234–236.

654 Blumell and Dosoo 2018, 236.

655 Consider the oil invoked in an extract of the "song for the one in labor" in the Edfu Mammisi, demonstrating that specific oils were, in idealized cases, proscribed to ease delivery: "Sweet is the face of Isis, the great, the mother of the god … moringa-oil, anointed with myrrh, dipped in sweet salve." (*nḏm ḥr n ꜣs.t wr.t mw.t-nṯr … bꜣḳ wrḥ m ʿnt.w dḥb (i.e. ṯḥb) m skn (i.e. sgnn) nḏm*) (*Edfu Mammisi* 159.2–3). (Dagmar Budde is thanked for highlighting this passage in a personal communication.)

with oil, Isis' labor is commanded to "cease",[656] at which point her womb must be "prepared" to deliver. Here, the verb utilized is one that is found in Egyptian to refer to the preparing, establishing, and securing of body parts.[657] These bipartite commands are then followed by two single commands, the first of which is to "Serve your offspring!" Here, the full semantic range of Egyptian *šmsi̯* could be taken into consideration, deriving from its literal etymology as "to follow", which consequently comes to mean to "serve" a king or deity, and thereby in Coptic "to worship" God (ϣⲙϣⲉ). In the context of the resonances of §9 with the ritual of the *God's Birth* treated above, there is perhaps an analogy here between the role of Isis as the mother of the child-god and the fact that the child-god is both divine and royal, predestined to become the successor of his father as king of Egypt. Thus, "serve" here implies not only the crucial practical role of a mother, but also that of a subject to the divine king Horus—the mythological precedent and paradigm for the child to be delivered and suckled in the contemporary ritual. In another analogue to the role of the mother of the child-god in the ritual of the *God's Birth*, the final command of §9 is to "produce milk for Horus your son", where—as discussed above—suckling both ensured the acknowledgement of the child-god by his father, itself ensuring that he would be able to succeed him upon the throne, and bestowed the divine and royal faculties required by the child-god. In including these commands at the close of the divine drama, the desired outcomes of §9 are demonstrated to be not only that the labor cease and the safe delivery of the child be ensured, but also that the mother be able to lactate so that the child can be suckled, and thereby nourished in the crucial hours and days that follow.

While translated here as an adverbial phrase linked to the preceding imperative clause, the final line of §9 could equally be considered as referring to all the preceding imperative clauses. "Through the power of the lord god" is evidently a later addition, placed at the end of §9 at some point during its history of textual transmission. Although instantly recognizable to modern scholars as well as ancient and modern Christians as an expression ubiquitous to Christian textual culture, whether characterized as magical or otherwise, as noted above, in this

[656] As discussed in the commentary to p. 6/2, "Be healed! Be healed there!" is also a viable translation.

[657] Consider the aforementioned afterlife ritual text *P.Harkness* discussed above: "Thoth will secure your heart" (*smn ḏḥw.tỉ ỉb=t*) (*P.Harkness* 2/21) or "Thoth will come to you to establish your heart" (*ỉwi̯ n=t ḏḥw.tỉ r smnỉ ỉb=t*) (ibid. 2/30 and 3/33) and "He (i.e. Thoth) will secure your Ba-soul (to) your body daily" (*smn=f pꜣy=t by tꜣy=t ẖ.t (n-)mn*) (ibid. 4/17). A Demotic oracle question is also relevant for the semantic range of *smni̯*, which concerns "the Nubian" (*pꜣ kwr*) who is established (*smni̯*) upon his throne: "Your foot is established" (*pꜣy=k rd smnỉ*); "Your life is sound" (*pꜣy=k ʿnḫ wḏꜣ*); "Your property and your income are established for you also" (*pꜣy=k nkt nꜣ ʿḳ.w smny ẖr-ỉr=k ʿn*) (P.Vind. inv. D 12006 recto 5/14–15, ed. Stadler 2004).

particular context, both caution and a counterpoint to the assumption that such a statement is diagnostically Christian need to be expressed.[658]

As discussed more fully in the treatment of "Syncretism in the Other Direction" in **Transmitting Textual Traditions**, such elements appear in decidedly pre-Christian magical texts practiced in undoubtedly non-Christian milieux. For example, in Jewish tradition, the Greek version of the Hebrew bible sometimes terms the supreme deity κύριος "lord" (alongside Σαβαώθ in the *trishagion* of Isaiah 6:3), while in Egyptian tradition, Greek-language oracle tickets contain supplications to both κύριος and θεός "god".[659] In secular—and thus comparatively quotidian—contexts, this relates closely to secular petitioning practices in which Roman officials can be referred to as both κύριος and θεός,[660] while a letter from Tebtunis of the 1st century BCE addresses the traditional Egyptian deity Seknebtunis as ὁ κύριος θεός "the lord god".[661]

Furthermore, the 3rd and 4th centuries CE are a turning point in which Christians transition from being a persecuted fringe to the dominant superordinate cultural and religious community in Egypt. While the formulation "through the power of the lord god" comes to be used in unambiguously Christian magical texts, it is also found in texts without any other Christian or Christianized features, which might instead be considered to be direct references to Jesus and/or Christ, the Trinity, saints, and citations of scripture by non-Christians. Furthermore, there are numerous references to Jewish, Judaeo-Christian, and unambiguously Christian, motifs among the GEMP of the early and late Roman Period, including those that were certainly produced by and in circulation among non-Christian milieux.

A crucial counterpoint to stress, then, is that Jewish, Judaeo-Christian, and Christian motifs were redacted into pre- and non-Christian magical texts during the early and late Roman Period. Numerous examples of these are presented in the aforementioned discussion of "Syncretism in the Other Direction" in **Transmitting Textual Traditions**. In short, given that Christianity is not the only monotheistic tradition in Egypt during the late Roman Period, and that Judaism in Egypt predated Christianity by many centuries, caution must be expressed as to whether the closing invocation in §9 is an example of an addition that served to Christianize an otherwise unambiguously pre- and non-Christian composition, or whether instead it exhibits the appropriation of an invocation considered

[658] All prior commentators assume this to be a Christianizing addition, without considering the preceding and contemporary traditions from which it could derive or to which it could belong, see Frankfurter 2009, 242; 2018, 208; van der Vliet 2018, 159; Dosoo 2021.

[659] E.g. *SB* XVIII 13853 and 14043 (2nd century CE).

[660] E.g. *BGU* IV 1197 (7–4 BCE).

[661] *P.Tebt.* II 284.5–6.

authoritative and efficacious from elsewhere in the Graeco-Egyptian magical tradition.

On balance, this excursus has not only teased out the complexity of associations and resonances in §9 with the cosmologies and mythologies of Egyptian tradition, it has also served to contextualize this Coptic text among the milieux to which its textual content suggests it should be ascribed. That is, not the later Christian(ized) tradition of Coptic magical texts, but rather that of the Graeco-Egyptian magical tradition. Consequently, §9 is both an anchor to the plurality of traditions still circulating in Egypt of the 4th century CE and a bridge between pre-Coptic Egyptian ritual and Coptic magical texts.

§10 The Cow of Amun (pp. 6/6–7/11) (EL)

"O cow, o cow of Amun, o mother of the cattle.
They have commanded you (f.) at dawn; you should come out to pasture.
They have commanded you (f.) at evening; you should go into the fold:
Guard yourself from these seven evils against the producing of milk:
the membrane-of-the-eye,
the eyelid,
the worm of the cucumber before it has spread,
the barley before it has sprouted,
the genuine (or, precious) plants,
this one that never provides a crook for shepherds,
never makes a staff for cowherds,
never makes a goad for herdsmen."

"They have come upon me, my shepherd, my cowherd, my herdsman.
Their garments are torn, while their mouths are drooling on the front of their shoes, being fastened with black *lahmef*.
Why are you running and hastening, my shepherd, my cowherd, my herdsman, with your garments torn? Why are you drooling on the front of your shoes, being fastened with a reed-needle (or, black flax)?
Seven white sheep, seven black sheep,
seven small (or, young) calves, seven large (or, mature) cattle
—let every cow and every beast receive its offspring,
because Iaō Sabaōth has said,
Make (for) the north of Abydos, make (for) the south (of) Thinis,
until you (m.) find these two brothers as they call out and flee northwards,
so as to chase them as they flee southwards, so that you (m.) can say,
'Send forth the thoughts of your (pl.) hearts so that every beast will receive its offspring.'"

I. Narrative and Mechanics

The narrative structure of §10 is harder to discern than that of §9, partly due to a lack of any bidirectional dialogue such as features in §9, and partly due to a lack of parallels and distinct resonances in the divine drama that unfolds in the narrative. It is not immediately clear who is speaking to whom in the dialogue, nor whether this is feature of the textual structure is intentional or—seemingly more plausibly—a result of a complex history of textual transmission with losses and additions. The mythological scene setting of §10 is, however, immediately comparable to that of §9, most notably in its tripartite structure of three clauses addressing the protagonist, the Cow of Amun, before narrating her actions. There is an immediate juxtaposition—or balancing—of states, as in §9, where a cycle of *time* across a plane of *space* is described—dawn to dusk, pasture to fold. An unidentified, disembodied voice then commands the Cow of Amun to guard herself during this cycle from "these seven evils against the producing of milk", that is, the threats that may ultimately have motivated the use of the recipe, to bring about the desired outcome of successful milk production. This is in turn reminiscent of the structure of §9, in which Amun described the problem of Isis' labor and its resolution through his ritual instructions and commands.

A new address, albeit not introduced by a conjunction, unlike the preceding address that followed the mythological scene setting, appears to follow, in which the subject changes and the Cow of Amun now seems to be speaking. She describes how her shepherd, cowherd, and herdsman have come upon her, but not in their normal—or idealized—state; instead, in a dirty and disorderly state: their garments are torn, they are drooling on their shoes, and those shoes are fastened with a material evidently thought impure. As the divine drama unfolds, her herders enter into the plane of action inhabited by the Cow of Amun. She then addresses them, asking them why they are running and hastening, and why they are in such a dirty and disorderly state. Here, repetition serves to concretize the mythological precedent, framing the problem preceding its resolution. The division of speaking parts within this subsection is not entirely clear, but it could be that the answer to the Cow of Amun's question follows directly, whereby the herders cite seven white and black sheep, calves, and cattle as the cause of their coming in such a dirty and disorderly state. Although it is entirely possible that something is missing in the narrative, such as direct speech between protagonist and interlocutor, eventually it is probably the Cow of Amun, as Amun in §9, who delivers the commands to resolve the problem which caused the dirty and disorderly state of the herders. The command "let every cow and every beast receives its offspring" might otherwise relate to the delivery of offspring, but given the aforementioned reference to milk production, the absence of verbs relating to delivery here, and the presence as opposed to absence of the sheep and bovines, the suckling of offspring seems instead implicit.[662] With this command, in turn, the section appears to end. The divine drama of the dirty and disorderly herders has been resolved by the Cow of Amun herself, guarding against the threats to her own lactation and providing instructions to ensure her fellow livestock receive—suckle—their offspring.

In an apparent addition, the authority behind that command is cited as Iao Sabaoth—directly comparable to how §9 ends with "through the power of the lord god", also a later addition. The apparent resolution to the divine drama is one reason for considering this final section a later addition, and the address also changes—from a second person feminine, that is, the Cow of Amun, to a second person masculine—, which does not accord with any prior character.[663] A further mythological precedent is then introduced, which perhaps provides further elucidation as to the source of the problem, that the "two brothers" are calling out and fleeing northwards—presumably in a disorderly way and, implicitly, in an undesired direction—who themselves need to be herded southwards by being chased by a masculine protagonist so that the latter can in turn give a command reminiscent of the closing of the preceding section: "Send forth the thoughts of your (pl.) hearts so that every beast will receive its offspring". Either the plural number in the address here refers back to the "two brothers", who by sending forth the thoughts of their hearts will resolve their disorderly state and thus the problem, or this address is in the abstract and lacks a direct referent, that is, the direct referent has been lost. Nevertheless, this command apparently provides a resolution to that same problem, allowing every beast to receive—suckle—its offspring.

In what follows, a close reading of the *textual structure* and *content* will serve to elucidate—comparably to §9—the abstract divine drama that unfolds in §10, the mythological and cosmogonic resonances from Egyptian tradition that are implicit in the narrative, as well as the motifs, particularly of dirty and disorderly states, that give narrative momentum to the presentation of problem and resolution fundamental to the mechanics of this divine drama.

---

662 A Syriac parallel is found in Codex A (1802–3 CE), from Gollancz's collection of Syriac magical texts (1912, xxv–lx). A recipe titled "For the cow which dislikes, or is excited towards, her mistress (i.e., milk-maid)" seeks that "this beast may be fond of and subject herself to her mistress and to her offspring" (1912, xl–xli §24). Implicit in this invocation is the understandable anxiety among the herders that the mother's refusal to suckle the calf will cause its death. The conceivable replacement of the milk-maid with mother, or indeed wet-nurse, in the application of this recipe provides, as with §10, a practice through which human offspring could be induced to suckle.

663 Another possibility is that the second person singular masculine is used in a generic way.

II. Cow of Amun, Mother of Cattle

ⲧⲉϩⲉ ⲧⲉϩⲉ ⲛ̄ⲁⲙⲟⲩⲛ· ⲧⲙⲁⲁⲩ̈ ⲛ̄ⲛ̄ⲧ̄ⲃⲛⲟⲟⲩⲉ
tꜣ iḥ(.t) tꜣ iḥ(.t) n imn tꜣ mw.t n nꜣ tp-n-ꜥw.wt
"O cow, o cow of Amun, o mother of the cattle.
ⲁⲩϩⲱⲛ ⲉⲧⲟⲟⲧⲉ ϩⲧⲣⲟⲩ ⲉⲣⲁⲉⲓ ⲉⲃⲟⲗ ⲉⲙⲟⲟⲛⲉ·
iri̭⸗w hn r-tr.ṱ⸗t (r) twꜣ | iw⸗t r iyi̭ r-bl r mni̭
They have commanded you (f.) at dawn; you should come out to pasture.
ⲁⲩϩⲱⲛ ⲉⲧⲟⲟⲧⲉ ϩⲓ ⲣⲟⲩϩⲉ ⲉⲣⲁⲃⲱⲕ ⲉϩⲟⲩⲛ ⲉⲧⲣⲥ̣ⲱ
*iri̭⸗w hn r-tr.ṱ⸗t ḥr r(w)hi | iw⸗t r *b(ꜣ)k r-ẖn r tꜣ rsi*
They have commanded you (f.) at evening; you should go into the fold.

II.1 Textual Structure

The *textual structure* of the mythological scene setting that comprises this section is immediately reminiscent of that in §9. Pairings are again common, with two vocatives addressing the Cow of Amun, both beginning with the feminine definite article ⲧ, in turn paired with the vocative that closes the invocatory address to the Cow of Amun as "mother of the cattle", again beginning with ⲧ. The initial repetition of the simple noun ⲧ-ⲉϩⲉ is developed in the second instance with a genitive—a motif of syntactical development seen particularly clearly in §9 in the repetition of verbal objects or imperatives.[664] In this way, a pairing is nested within a bipartite structure, forming three nominal statements that in turn form the first of three clauses that comprise the mythological scene setting. The next two clauses are also pairings of two main clauses, the former beginning ⲁⲩ- and the latter ⲉⲣⲁ-. Constancy is juxtaposed with variance in so far as the action embedded in the past, "they have done something"—expressed with the same agent (subject),[665] action (verb), and patient (object)—is contrasted with the action to be undertaken in the future, "you should". The constant command is also contrasted to "coming" and "going", that is, "out" (ⲉⲃⲟⲗ) to pasture, and "into" (ⲉϩⲟⲩⲛ) the fold—pairing before and after, action and reaction. This passing of time concretized through the description of the action of the agent then resonates in the descriptions of time—from morning to evening—where the movement of the Cow of Amun through the landscape is paired with the movement of the sun through the sky; pasture to fold, east to west. The mythological scene setting thereby establishes a paradigmatic reality of command and compliance—cause and effect—through syntactical and semantic pairings of *action* that also express *place* and *time*. The *textual structure*, then, establishes something as having happened but—by framing this as a daily cycle—establishes it as something that happens over and

---

[664] Consider ⲙ̄ⲡⲉⲕϭⲛ̄ⲧ̄ | ⲙ̄ⲡⲉⲕϭⲓⲛⲉ ⲙ̄ⲡⲁⲣⲁⲛ | ⲙ̄ⲡⲉⲕϭⲓⲛⲉ ⲛ̄ⲟⲩϣⲏⲙ ⲛ̄ⲛⲉϩ ⲛ̄ⲉⲓⲛⲉ ⲉⲃⲟⲗ ϩ̄ⲙ̄ ⟨...⟩ (p. 5/18–20), and ⲁⲗⲟ ⲁⲗⲟ ⲙ̄ⲙⲁⲩ and ⲥⲙ̄ⲛⲧⲉ ⲥⲙⲛ̄-ⲧⲟⲩ-ⲟⲟⲧⲉ (p. 6/2–3).

[665] Interpreted as the three herders introduced at p. 6/15.

over, reflecting the Egyptian conceptualization of both linear (*ḏ.t*) and cyclical (*nḥḥ*) time; while the cow of Amun going out to pasture and returning into the fold is one episode that can be described linearly as beginning and ending, it also is a daily event that can be described cyclically as recurring. This provides a tension between complete and ongoing action that is about to be broken by the narrative momentum of the divine drama.

II.2 Textual Content

The protagonist of §10 appears to be the Cow of Amun. At the outset, then, the complexity of resonances in this identification needs to be considered. In Egyptian tradition, the primaeval consort of Amun (*ỉmn*) was Amunet (*ỉmn.t*),[666] the female counterpart of Amun constructed through forming a feminine of Amun's name.[667] In the Pyramid Texts, where the couple is first attested, the shadows cast by Amun and Amunet refer to their creative efficacy (*PT* 446). As a pairing, Amun and Amunet were one of four balanced pairs of male and female deities that comprised the Hermopolitan Ennead—primordial deities—, all of whom had cosmogonic aspects relating to their role in creation. In these roles, Amun is "the noble god, who came into being in the beginning, he is the wind, which is established in all things and through which one always lives"[668], while Amunet is "the north-wind, she who manifests food and sustenance through her actions, who causes trees to grow".[669] Here, the pairings of male and female counterparts are also found, with Amun being the masculine "wind" (*ṯ3w*) while Amunet is the feminine "north-wind" (*mḥ.yt*). Amunet's association with the north-wind blowing south also accounts for her common depiction wearing the crown of Lower Egypt, and her equation with Neith, a goddess from the Delta.[670] In addition, Amun and Amunet are often absent from the Ennead, being replaced with or syncretized to Nun and Nunet,[671] meaning that Amun's primeval consort

---

[666] Amunet is also found transliterated as Amaunet—compare Αμαυνι in *PGM* XIII.789 (expressing a Lower Egyptian vocalization)—, but this is erroneous as the affected stem vowel is a result of the feminine ending, and therefore the name should be transliterated as either Amunet or Amaune/Amauni.

[667] Directly comparable to the "egg" (*swḥ.t*) as the female counterpart of the "wind" (*swḥ*), discussed in the excursus to §9. Consistent with this role as the "female counterpart", Amunet was often found depicted next to an ithyphallic Amun (Sethe 1929, 85–86 §175).

[668] *ỉmn nṯr šps | ḫp(r) m-ḥ3.t | ṯ3w -pw | mn m ỉ.ḫ.t -nb.(t) | ʿnḫ=tw ỉm=f ḏ.t*, from the transcription in Sethe 1929, 78 §154.

[669] *ỉmn.t | mḥ.yt -pw | sḫpr k3.w ḏf3.w m r3-ʿ.wi=s | srd ỉ3m.w*, from transcription in Sethe 1929, 78 §154.

[670] Sethe 1929, 78 §154.

[671] As discussed in Sethe 1929, 68–70 §136–139. Consider the syncretic Amunet-Nunet at Dendera, who is "the god's wife, the god's mother, she is the goddess who was there at the beginning and who began to create the land when she came into being" (*ỉmn.t nwn.t ḥm.t-nṯr mw.t-nṯr | nṯr.t -pw š3ʿ3.t š3ỉʿ t3 m ḫp(r)=s*, from the transcription in Sethe 1929, 71 §141).

is in fact attested only rarely. Given both the temporal and spatial context of the Michigan codex, the perseverance of the cosmogony involving this Ennead and thereby Amun and Amunet into the Roman Period via the *Book of the Fayum* is particularly relevant.[672] Again partly syncretized to Nun and Nunet, respectively, the balanced pair appear as those who guard the "lake", that is the Fayum itself, and marsh, and ensure that the names "mother" and "Nunet" endure[673]—the primaeval ocean (*nwn*) of the sea (*wꜣḏ-wr*) itself being identified with the Birket el-Qarun in the Fayum.

Amid the cosmogonies and mythologies of Egyptian tradition, Amunet comes to be identified with a host of other deities, in turn appearing as the mother of Re, and thereby the mother of her own consort Amun in his form as Amun-Re, as well as even the daughter of Amun, who was with him in primaeval times.[674] Indeed, Amun's principal consort throughout Egyptian history—overshadowing Amunet – appears to be Mut, who is the wife of Amun(-Re) and mother of Khonsu in the Theban triad. Nevertheless, Amunet's principal cult site, as Amun's, is Karnak. There, a granite sanctuary constructed during, and perhaps also after, the reign of Philip Arrhidaeus (323–317 BCE) features reliefs that evidence her creative associations. In the forecourt of this sanctuary, just after the sixth pylon, two colossal statues of Amun and Amunet are found, reconstructed during the reign of Tutankhamun following the iconoclastic reign of Akhenaten, and re-erected in modern times. Directly beyond the sixth pylon, commissioned by Thutmose III and reconstructed on the same site during the reign of Alexander, lies the granite sanctuary. Interior bas-reliefs depict the purification, crowning, enthroning, and suckling of the child-king—immediately reminiscent of the ritual of the *God's Birth* discussed in the excursus to §9. As an adult, the king kneels before Amun and is crowned by him, bestowing royal office. As a child, the king is held and suckled by Amunet, bestowing royal faculties.[675] In the accompanying inscription, Amunet says to her son Philip (*plypws*) "May you suckle from my milk",[676] providing a description of the depiction—image and text serving to actualize the desired outcome that the king receive royal faculties from his divine mother. The association of both Amun and Amunet in turn with bovine manifestations is then seen in an accompanying relief, where the ithyphallic Amun-Re "Bull of his Mother" (*kꜣ mw.t⸗f*) is presented by the king with four calves—one black, one red, one white, and one spotted.[677]

[672] See Beinlich 1991.

[673] *ỉmn ỉmn.t šdỉ̭ š ḥn.t ḏḏ smn rn mw.t nw.wt* (*BF* 1192).

[674] As discussed in Sethe 1929, 34 §59.

[675] The bestowing of royal, and in the case of the child-god divine faculties through suckling is discussed in the treatment of the ritual of the *God's Birth* in the excursus to §9.

[676] *snḳ⸗k m ỉrṯ.t⸗ỉ* (*LD* IV Plates, pl. 2c).

[677] *LD* IV Plates, pl. 2b.

The association of Amunet as Amun's cow is also evidenced in the archive of the *katochoi* of the Serapeum from mid 2nd century BCE. In the narrative of a dream experienced by one of the residents of this sanctuary dating to 158 BCE, the dreamer sees, or sees himself in the form of, a pregnant cow[678] and calls Amun to come from the north;[679] the god arrives, reaches inside the cow, and delivers a bullock.[680] This in turn resonates with a mythological narrative in which the (heavenly) cow begged Amun to come to help her while she was "in need", resulting in her giving birth to the sun(-god), who later sat between her horns.[681] Although Amun's description and depiction as a bull is much more common than that of Amunet as a cow, it is in her identification with *ỉh.t*—that is, the "cow"—and, indeed, in the apparently homophonous "(heavenly) cow" (*ỉh.t*) where Amunet's relationship to §10 can instead be sought.

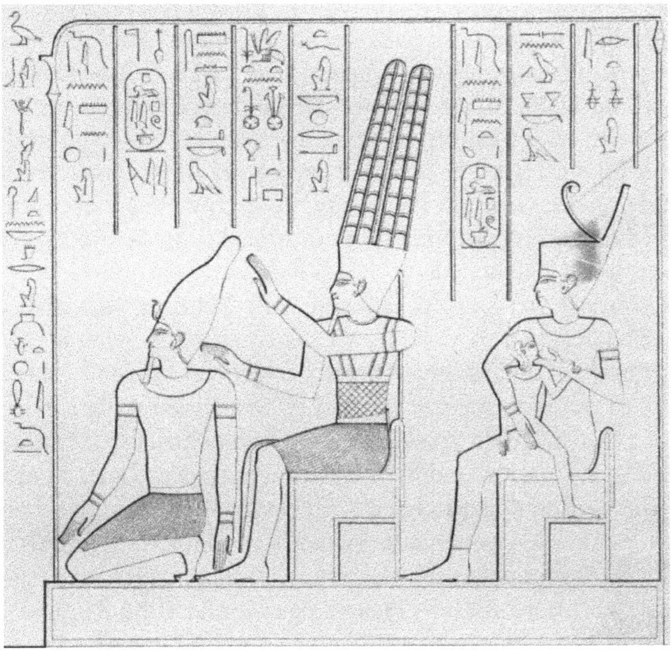

In the granite sanctuary of Philip Arrhidaeus at Karnak, the king as an adult is crowned by Amun-Re and as a child is held and suckled by Amunet. In the accompanying inscription, Amunet says to her son Philip, "May you suckle from my milk" (*LD* IV Plates, pl. 2c).

---

678 ᾤμην με βοῦν ἐν τῷ τόπῳ εἶναι κα[ὶ] οὐδείνουσα (*UPZ* I 77 recto 2/26–27).

679 ᾤμην ἐν τῷ ὕπνῳ ἐπεικαλεῖν με τὸν μέγιστον Ἄμμωνα ἔρχεσθαι ἀ[πὸ] βορρᾶ (*UPZ* I 77 recto 2/22–25).

680 ἐμβάλλει αὐτοῦ τὴν χεῖρα εἰς τὸ οἰδὴν καὶ ἐκσπᾶι ταῦρον (*UPZ* I 77 recto 2/29–30).

681 Sethe 1929, 93 §195.

The "heavenly (or, celestial) cow" is perhaps most resonant with a cosmogonic text inscribed upon the walls of the tombs of New Kingdom pharaohs in the Valley of the Kings, known variously as *The Book of the Heavenly Cow* or *The Destruction of Mankind*. The narrative itself concerns the rebellion of humanity against the sun-god, and the ensuing divine punishment. The separation of sun-god from humanity was subsequently ensured through his location upon the back of the (heavenly) cow, in that case a manifestation of Nut, the sky deity, supported by the *ḥḥ.w*-deities under the belly of the cow and in turn supported by Shu, the air deity. The protective associations of the (heavenly) cow for her son the sun-god is found in the *Book of the Dead*, where a recipe to be spoken over a figure of the cow and identifying statements in which the practitioner declares "I am the (heavenly) cow" provide a mythological precedent for "a very, very great protection that the (heavenly) cow created for her son Re". This same recipe will in turn ensure that the deceased will be able to transverse the underworld by being able to pass through all of its gates (*BD* 162). In the Esna cosmogony, preserved upon the walls of the temple of Esna constructed during the reign of Trajan, it was Neith who manifested as a cow, who bore the sun-god and carried the sun-god not on her back but between her horns. As Amunet syncretized with a host of other goddesses, so the (heavenly) cow was conceptualized as a manifestation of numerous different—but ultimately interrelated—goddesses.[682]

In the Temple of Hatshepsut at Deir el-Bahari, "Amunet in the midst of Karnak" (*ꞽmn.t ḥr.ꞽ-ꞽb ꞽp.t-s.wt*) is equated with Neith as "the mistress of life", whose creative efficacy also extends to being as one "who gives offspring", "who rescues throats", that is, gives breath and thereby life,[683] and "who causes the Two Lands to flourish through her efflux"[684]—associating the fluids coming forth from her with the Nile flood. In the aforementioned Temple of Opet at Karnak, Amunet's primaeval and creative associations are also clear in her being addressed as the "mother of mothers", "the primaeval one who came with the primaeval one" and "who conceived in the beginning".[685] Amunet is also "the mother who made the father in the beginning", and—most crucially—"the great (heavenly) cow who bore Ra".[686] This is paralleled in the Temple of Horus at Edfu, where Amunet is addressed as "the (heavenly) cow who bore Ra".[687] The (heavenly) cow is described as rearing (*rr* and *ꜣṯꞽ*) the child-king in the mam-

[682] Principally Neith, Hathor, Isis, and Tjenenet, all of whom are identified with the *ꞽh.t* or *ꞽh.t-wr.t*.

[683] For the creative associations of wind, breath, and life, see the excursus to §9.

[684] *ḥnw.t ꜥnḫ | rḏꞽ̯.t ḏꜣ(m) | nḥm(.t) ḥty.t | wꜣḏ(.t) tꜣ.wꞽ m rḏ.w⸗s* (*DEB* 55.1–3).

[685] *mw.t mw.wt | pꜣw(.tꞽ t) ꞽyꞽ̯(.t) ḫr pꜣw(.tꞽ) | ꞽ wr(.t) m-ḥꜣ.t* (*Opet* 145).

[686] *mw.t ꞽrꞽ̯(.t) ꞽt m-šꜣꜥ | ꜣh.t wr.t msꞽ̯(.t) rꜥ* (*Opet* 255).

[687] *(ꞽ)h.t msꞽ̯(.t) rꜥ* (*Edfu* II.1, 87.14).

misis of both Dendera and Edfu,[688] and thereby also conceptualized as the child-king's mother, and consequently the paradigmatic divine mother in mythological precedents.

Here, the *Book of the Fayum* is of further note because it evidences that the principal myth of the Fayum is that of the (heavenly) cow.[689] Recast in the context of a Fayumic cosmogony, the narrative begins with Re ruling over the Nile Valley—the primordial state—and ends with the sun-god enthroned upon the back of the (heavenly) cow—the contemporary state. Indeed, the enthroned sun-god is depicted suckling from the teats of his mother, manifest as the (heavenly) cow in the principal hieroglyphic manuscript of the *Book of the Fayum*.[690] This in turn relates to a passage describing how "She causes him to live through her milk", which resulted in the manifestation of the "lake", that is, the Fayum, and the sun.[691] Her role as primordial creator is explicated in the description of the Nonnad as borne by the (heavenly) cow, who is in turn the creator of the sun-god and of his mother, that is, herself.[692] In this Fayumic cosmogony, the body of the (heavenly) cow is conceptualized as the manifestation of the primaeval flood and therefore the Birket el-Qarun in the Fayum which, when raised to the sky, ensured the separation of sky and earth.[693] In turn, the Birket el-Qarun is the primordial manifestation of the Primaeval Ocean, from which the Ogdoad—the eight primordial deities—manifest.[694]

The latest attested conceptualizations of Amunet and the (heavenly) cow come from Armant (Hermonthis).[695] Dating from the reign of Nectanebo II to Diocletian, the cult of the Buchis bull (*bꜣ-ꜣẖ*), first equated with Montu and eventually also with Osiris and Re, was regenerated through a new temple during the reign of Cleopatra VI and a new mammisi during the reign of Cleopatra VII.[696] As late as the 2nd century CE, Amunet was identified with the "great (heavenly) cow" (*ꜣh.t-wr.t*), who bore Re, and therefore was the "mother of Re".[697] With the equation of the Buchis bull and Re, Amunet and the "great

[688] *Dendera Mammisi* 99.15 and *Edfu Mammisi* 34.4.

[689] Beinlich 1991, 314.

[690] See Beinlich 1991, 109 fig. 45; pl. 16.

[691] *sʿnḫ⸗s -sw m irṯ.t⸗s | ḫpr š | ḫpr rʿ* (*BF* 137–140).

[692] *psḏ.t -twy msi̯(.t) ih.t | ir.w rʿ | ir.w mw.t⸗f* (*BF* 156–158).

[693] Beinlich 1991, 315.

[694] Beinlich 1991, 316.

[695] Indeed, this is also the case for most of Egyptian textual culture in monumental contexts, given that the Buchis stelae and inscriptions are among the latest dated other than the graffiti at Philae: see Love 2016, §7.5.2–7.5.3.

[696] *LD* IV Plates, pl. 64a; *LD* IV Text, I–II.

[697] *ꜣh.t-wr.t msi̯ rʿ | imn.t mw.t rʿ ir.t rʿ nb(.t) p.t ḥn.wt nṯr.w -nb(.w)* (Stela of Commodus), see *Bucheum* II, 20 no. 21; *Bucheum* III, pl. 47.

(heavenly) cow" became identified with the "Mother of the Buchis", that is, the "mother of the sun-god",[698] whether alone or in equation with Neith.[699]

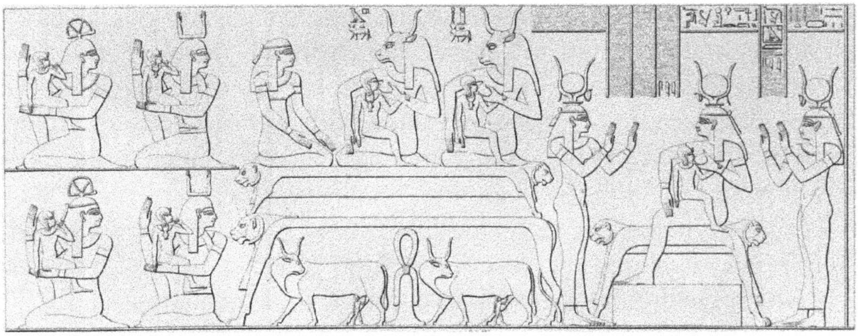

In the Temple of Armant, the "(heavenly) cow" (*ỉh.t*) is depicted as a cow-headed anthropomorph, suckling the sitting child-god on a bed, and in a bovine form suckling the standing child-god under a bed (leftmost of the pair) (*LD* IV Plates, pl. 59c).

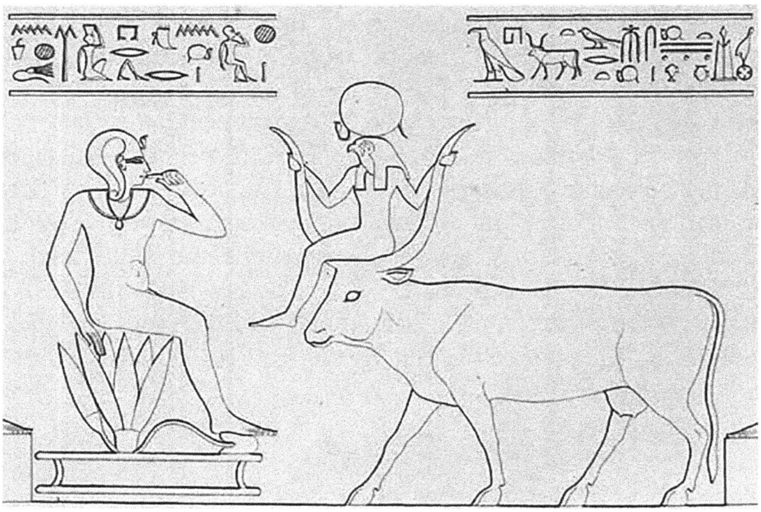

In the Temple of Armant, "the great (heavenly) cow (*ꜣh.t-wr.t*) who bore Re" is depicted carrying the sun-god, sitting between her horns, towards the seated "child of Re" (*LD* IV Plates, pl. 61g).

[698] See *Bucheum* III, pl. 51.

[699] "Words spoken by Neith the Great, Amunet, who bore the Primeval Gods, Mother of Re" (*ḏd-mdw ỉn n.t wr.t ỉmn.t pꜥpꜥ pꜣw.tyw mw.t n rꜥ*), see *LD* IV Plates, pl. 61c; *Bucheum* II, 25.

In spite of all of these associations and manifestations, the epithet "mother of the cattle"—even in a lexically younger form of Egyptian—does not appear to be clearly paralleled. The syncretic nature of the goddesses who were identified with the "(heavenly) cow", especially during the Graeco-Roman Period, meant that a host of epithets, while attested for one, can be extended with reasonable confidence to qualify others. Therefore, while Hathor is identified as "mother of the mother of the cows",[700] Neith as "mother of the gods",[701] and Tjenenet as "mother of the gods and goddesses"[702]—all these deities in turn can be equated with the "(great) (heavenly) cow". Thus, the creative associations of the "(heavenly) cow" demonstrate the appropriateness of the complementary epithet "mother of the cattle". Notwithstanding these considerations, it could be that this epithet hides further layers of meaning. In the lexicon of First Phase Egyptian, one word for "womb" was *mw.t-rmṯ,* etymologically "mother of people (i.e. humanity)". In light of the evidence of an Egyptian idiom for "humanity" as the "noble herd" (*ʿ.wt šps(.t)*),[703] here a layering of meanings could be intended. The epithet "mother of the cattle" resonates not only with the bovine manifestations and associations of the Cow of Amun, but also—or even more so—with her role as primordial creator, whose creative efficacy brought everything into being, beginning with the sun-god, ultimately meaning that she was the "mother of the herd", i.e. humanity—the "womb" of humanity. Thus, besides the deep and complex cosmogonic associations and resonances of the Cow of Amun's presence in the mythological scene setting of §10, her character also demonstrates that the bovine analogies in the divine drama itself were as applicable to humanity as they were to deities—as seen in the reliefs and texts of the aforementioned temples. Thus, it seems most parsimonious to interpret §10 as a practice applicable to a human—perhaps even principally—rather than bovine patient.[704]

At this point a digression into magical texts from Mesopotamia may demonstrate the comparable tradition of divine dramas as found in the Ancient Near East, as well as a shared tradition of motifs of herding and analogies between divine bovine mothers and mortal human mothers. *A Cow of Sîn* is the conventional title for a divine drama known in at least six versions upon five tablets from Nineveh, Boghazköy, and Ugarit of the Middle Assyrian through New-Assyrian

---

700 *mw.t-mw.wt-n.t-ỉd.wt* (*LGG* 3, 259)

701 *mw.t-nṯr.w* (*LGG* 3, 268).

702 *mw.t-n.t-nṯr.w-nṯr.wt* (*LGG* 3, 268).

703 *P.Westcar* (P.Berl. inv. 3033) 8/17, ed. Lepper 2008.

704 By contrast, Frankfurter first interpreted §10 as concerning "the fertility of cattle" (2009, 242) and subsequently as a "blessing of the expansion of the herd" (2018, 208).

Periods (1400–600 BCE).[705] Although the divine drama concerns the moon-god[706] and bull Sîn and his cow Geme-Sîn—how he impregnated her, heard her cries when in labor, and sent two lamasus or daughters of Anu to facilitate the delivery of the "Milk Calf"—the recipe itself ends with the supplication "may this woman give birth as easily as Geme-Sîn", specifying its application for the benefit of a human mother.[707] Pastoral analogies are also prominent in the divine drama, with the herdsmen following Geme-Sîn, the narrative voice describing Geme-Sîn grazing and watering, and notably that the screams of Geme-Sîn's labor were so great that: "When her days came to an end, her months were finished, the cow trembled and terrified her herdsman", so much so that "his head was bowed, all the herd boys lamented with him".[708] In turn recalling the resolution of §9 rather than §10, the lamasus who descend from heaven bring "oil from the jar" and "water of labor", the former to anoint Geme-Sîn's forehead, the latter to sprinkle over her, which—when completed three times—results in the delivery of the calf. Consequently, the "little oil for bringing out" as prescribed by Amun is §9 is directly comparable, but whether or not such liquids were utilized in the practice of *A Cow of Sîn*, or whether it was efficacious by nature of its recitation, is unclear. The closing supplications do, however, equate the lamasus from heaven directly with the human midwives: "Just as Geme-Sîn gave birth normally, may this girl in labor give birth also. Let the midwife not tarry, let the pregnant one be all right."[709] While the textual structure and content of the divine drama of Geme-Sîn are more tightly interwoven than that in §§9 and 10,[710] this comparative case study evidences not only the broader tradition of divine dramas, attested across substantial temporal and spatial frames, but also the analogous utilization of pastoral and bovine motifs in divine dramas for the benefit of human patients, as is arguably the case for §10.

---

[705] Veldhuis 1991, 4–5. For further witnesses to the broader tradition of the "cow motif" in birth incantations, which can be traced as early as Old Babylonian, see now Wasserman 2018, 18–20.

[706] As the crescent moon has horns, so the moon-god was associated with a bull. In addition, the moon was also conceptualized as a shepherd, the stars as his flock, and so the moon god often had a pastoral role, ensuring the fertility of his herds (Veldhuis 1991, 1).

[707] Veldhuis 1991, 1.

[708] Veldhuis 1991, 9.

[709] Veldhuis 1991, 9.

[710] Explicit puns appear—for example the "oil from a jar" (*šaman pūri*) prescribed for Geme-Sîn is a direct pun on "heaven" (*šamû*) and "calf" (*būru*) (Veldhuis 1991, 21–22)—, as do implicit puns, for example "cow" (*littu*) is a direct pun on a "woman in labor" (*ālittu*), where the latter does not appear in the divine drama itself (Veldhuis 1991, 22). For the textual structure of this composition, in particular the presence of parallelism, see Veldhuis 1991, 27–37.

III. Protecting Milk Production against "The Seven Evils"

ϫⲉ
ḏd
ϩⲁⲣⲉϩ ⲉⲣⲟ ⲉⲡⲓ ⲍ̅ ⲛ̅ⲃⲱⲛ ⲉⲡⲕⲁϩⲱⲣ·
ḥrḥ r-r=t r pꜣy 7 n bin r pꜣ k[711] **hꜣr*
"Guard yourself (f.) from these seven evils against the producing of milk:
ⲡⲕⲁϊϩ·
pꜣ kḥ
the membrane-of-the-eye,
ⲡⲃⲟⲩϩⲉ·
*pꜣ *bh*
the eyelid,
ⲡⲃⲛ̅ⲧ ⲛ̅ⲡϣⲱⲡⲉ ⲉⲙⲡⲁⲧⲉϥⲡⲱ̅ⲣ̅ϣ
*pꜣ *fnt n pꜣ šwb(.t)/špi | iw bw-iri̯.tw=f prš*
the worm of the cucumber before it has spread,
ⲡⲓⲱⲧ ⲉⲙⲡⲁ̅ⲧ̅ϥ̅ⲣ̅ ⲥⲏⲃⲉ·
pꜣ it̠ iw bw-iri̯.tw=f iri̯ sby.t
the barley before it has sprouted,
ⲛ̅ⲧⲏϭⲙⲉ
*(nꜣ) *ntgꜣ*[712] *mꜣꜥ.t*
the genuine (or, precious) plants,
ⲡⲁⲓ ⲉ
pꜣy iw
this one that
ⲙⲉϥⲣ̅ ⲕⲉⲗⲉⲗⲉ ⲛ̅ϣⲱⲥ·
*bw-iri̯=f iri̯ *ḳllꜣ (.t) n (nꜣ) šs*
never provides a crook for shepherds,
ⲙⲉϥⲣ̅ ϣⲃⲱⲧ ⲛ̅ⲉⲗⲟϊϩ
bw-iri̯=f iri̯ šbt(e) n (nꜣ) mr-iḥ(.w)
never makes a staff for cowherds,
ⲙⲁϥⲣ̅ ϫⲟⲟⲕⲉϥ ⲛ̅ⲉⲙⲉ·
bw-iri̯ iri̯ ḏḳꜥ=f n (nꜣ) ꜥꜣm
never makes a goad for herdsmen".

A direct quotation is introduced in the next section with the conjunction ϫⲉ. Given that the command is to a female patient addressed in the second person singular, it seems that the same unidentified, disembodied voice continues to

---

711 *kꜣ < ḥꜣꜥ*, compare the unhistorical or unetymological orthographies attested already in the 20th Dynasty (1189–1077 BCE) in Černy (*CED* 52).

712 **ntgꜣ* perhaps < *m-dgꜣ/dḳr*, cf. *dgꜣ* (*KHB* 262), cf. Vycichl (*DE* 147), see the commentary to p. 6/13.

speak to the Cow of Amun. She is commanded to "guard herself" against the "seven evils" that would prevent her from "producing milk" —that is, from lactating and thereby suckling her offspring. Consequently, the situation of *time* switches from that of a past set of commands and their ongoing fulfilment to a liminal moment immediately following delivery, during which the nourishment of the new-born is a matter of life and death, and where one threat to the survival of the child is the inability of the mother to lactate, and thereby to nourish her offspring. The implication from this opening statement is that if the Cow of Amun consumes any of the following seven types of flora and fauna during her time at pasture and before her return to the fold, she will be unable to lactate, and therefore unable to suckle her offspring.

The list of threats that follow is enigmatic. They all appear to be epithets: perhaps they are a mixture of physiological ailments—of the membrane of the eye and of the eyelid—coupled with names of flora, perhaps they are all euphemisms for particular afflictions resulting from ingesting flora and fauna, or perhaps they also carry deeper mythological associations that are—through a want of parallels—difficult to discern. Mythological names for flora are a cross-cultural phenomenon: elecampane is Latin *inula helenium*, named after Helen of Troy, and is known in English as elfdock, in German—among other names—as *Helenenkraut* "Helen's herb" and *Odinskopf* "Odin's head". In Egyptian tradition, mythological names are not uncommon,[713] while some enigmatic names are sometimes given semantic glosses. For example, in *P.London-Leiden* a plant is described as follows: "Ram's horn is its name (...), an herb which is like a wild fennel bush. Its leaves and its stem are incised like the 'love-man' plant".[714] Of note in this particular example is that the plant "ram's horn" required describing, but the reader is assumed to be familiar with the "love-man" plant.[715]

As discussed in the commentary to p. 6/13, "the genuine (or, precious) plants" recall a style of euphemism used in Greek healing and apotropaic incantations in the Byzantine tradition, in which diseases are denoted by positive epithets in place of their true names and opposite their true natures. Avoiding their true names thereby helps to protect against them.[716] Given that the predecessors of Coptic ⲃⲟⲩϩⲉ, ⲛ̄ⲧⲏϭⲙⲉ, and ⲕⲉⲗⲉⲗⲉ are not attested in pre-Coptic Egyptian,

---

[713] Consider the "great of Amun" (*ꜥꜣ ỉmn*) or "footprint of Isis" (*p(ꜣ)-tgs-ꜣs.t*) (*P.London-Leiden* recto 10/32; 27/10) plants, as well as the "plant of Anubis" (*sym n ỉnp*) (ibid. 14/21–22; 14/31) and the "heart of the fine house" (*ḥꜣ.ṱ n pr-nfr*) plant (ibid. 10/12–13).

[714] *tp n sr* ⲕⲉⲫⲁⲗⲉⲕⲏ *rn⸗f* | *wꜥ sym ỉw⸗f m-ḳty wꜥ.t bwe n šmre ẖwṱ* | *tꜣy⸗f gbe.t pꜣy⸗f ẖt ḏḳꜥ m-ḳty pꜣ mr-rmṯ* (*P.London–Leiden* verso 4/10–13).

[715] Compare also the "great of love" (*wr-mr.t*) plant (*P.London-Leiden* recto 11/23).

[716] For example, epilepsy can be called "the sweet one" (τὸ γλυκύ), while plague lesions can be called "blessing" (εὐλογία)—see further the commentary to p. 6/13.

however, it may be that these lexemes were uncommon in the higher registers of the domains of writing, that the medical texts in which they feature are not preserved, that they are regional variants brought to prominence through the emergence of regional language varieties in Coptic, or—least likely—that they are lexemes novel to the language from the 3rd century CE. This, in turn, makes it difficult to identify their meaning and resonance any further.

Nevertheless, the threat posed by consuming involuntarily a particular type of invertebrate that worms its way into immature cucumbers, those cucumbers, or unsprouted barley, seems clear. Furthermore, a type of shrub whose wood is unsuitable for being made into a crook, staff, or goad is also described through its functionality, rather than named.[717] The parallel tripartite structure in which these are introduced is reminiscent of those discussed above, as well as that which follows. This at once contextualizes the associations of the Cow of Amun within that of pastoralist practice while also prefiguring the introduction of the shepherd, cowherd, and herdsman in the next section.

IV. Shepherds, Cowherds, and Herdsmen

ⲁⲩⲉⲓ ⲉϫⲱⲓ̈
iri̯=w iyi̯ r-ḏw=i
They have come upon me,
ⲡⲁϣⲱⲥ
pꜣy=i šs
my shepherd,
ⲡⲁⲉⲗⲟⲓ̈ϩ·
pꜣy=i mr-iḥ(.w)
my cowherd,
ⲡⲁⲁⲙⲉ
pꜣy=i ꜥꜣm
my herdsman.
ⲛⲉⲩϩⲟⲓ̈ⲧⲉ ⲡⲏϩ ⲉⲣⲁⲩ ϩⲁ ϫⲓϩ ϩⲏⲧ̄ϥ̄ ⲙ̄ⲡⲉⲩⲧⲟⲟⲩⲉ ⲉϥⲧⲏϭ ⲛ̄ⲗⲁϩⲙⲉϥ ⲛ̄ⲕⲉⲙ·
nꜣy=w ẖety pẖ | iw rꜣ=w ẖr ḏꜣẖ ḥꜣ.ṯ=f n pꜣy=w twꜣ | iw=f tg n ⲗⲁϩⲙⲉϥ *n ḳm/km*
Their garments are torn, while their mouths are drooling on the front of their shoes, being fastened with black *lahmef*.
ⲁϩⲣⲟⲕ ⲉⲕⲡⲏⲧ: ⲉⲕⲓ̈ⲏⲥ ⲡⲁϣⲱⲥ ⲡⲁⲉⲗⲟⲓ̈ϩ· ⲡⲁⲁⲙ̄ⲉ ⲉ̄ⲣⲉⲛⲉⲕϩⲟⲓ̈ⲧⲉ ⲡⲏϩ·
iẖ-r=k | ıw=k pt | iw=k ys pꜣy=i šs pꜣy=i mr-iḥ(.w) pꜣy=i ꜥꜣm | iw nꜣy=k ẖety pẖ

---

[717] A letter from one Khaybekhnet to his "brother" Bennekhetef dating to the reign of Ramses II reports that "the donkey (f.) suffers (or, is ill) from the staff" (*tꜣ ꜥꜣ.t mḥr.ti m-ꜥ pꜣ šbd*) (O.Berl. inv. 12398 ll. 7–8, ed. Allam 1981, and it seems that this "illness" had already been the case for several days. However, it is not possible to tell whether this is through having eaten the wood or having been beaten by the wood—Bennekhetef is, after all, later instructed to bring the donkey back carrying his "people" as always.

Why are you running and hastening, my shepherd, my cowherd, my herdsman, with your garments torn?
ⲁϩⲣⲟⲕ ϩⲁ ϫⲓϩ· ϩⲏⲧ̅ϥ̅ ⲙ̅ⲡⲉⲕⲧⲟⲟⲩⲉ ⲧⲏⲕ ⲛ̅ⲗⲁⲁⲥ ⲕⲁⲙ·
ỉḫ-r=k ẖr ḏꜣẖ ḥꜣ.ṱ=f n pꜣy=k twꜣ tg n ls n ḳm/km
Why are you drooling on the front of your shoes, being fastened with a reed-needle (or, black flax)?

The tripartite structure describing the shrub in the preceding section prefigures the beginning of this section. Again, the narrative momentum is facilitated by an action. That the shepherd, cowherd, and herdsman have come is situated in the past tense by nature of having occurred—moving all the prior action now even further back within the mythological precedent and situating the actions that follow instead as those occurring contemporaneously. As a plural unity, the shepherd, cowherd, and herdsman of the Cow of Amun are introduced, seemingly giving identity to the plural agents who—in the mythological scene setting at the beginning of the divine drama—commanded the Cow of Amun to go out to pasture and return to the fold.[718] While at that time their commands were followed, and an idealized and thereby balanced situation of cause and effect was concretized, here something is wrong. Contravening the ideal of purity and propriety in Egyptian tradition, the herders come in a dirty and disorderly state, one that throws the divine drama into a situation of uncertainty and perhaps also reveals the underlying cause of the problem and thereby the route towards its resolution.

This motif is prominent in Egyptian divine dramas,[719] further reflecting the importance of purity and propriety over being dirty and disorderly. This is evidenced in a bilingual manuscript contemporary to the Michigan codex, *PGM* IV,[720] in the divine drama of an erotic recipe (94–113) redacted together alongside other erotic recipes containing invocations and commands in Egyptian written in Old Coptic and ritual instructions in Greek (*PGM* IV.114–153).[721] Isis, the protagonist of that divine drama, is described as "coming (down) from the desert plateau at midday in summer; <her> head covered with dust, her eyes full of

[718] Divine identities for these herders are not forthcoming. While Re is referred to as the "herdsman" (*mnỉ.w*) (11/12), "great herdsman" (*mnỉ.w-ꜥꜣ*) "who comes" to "all your (pl.) cattle" (*ỉḥ.wt r-ḏr.w=tn*) (11/13), and the "beloved herdsman" (*mnỉ.w-mry.tỉ*) (12/4) in a Hymn to Amun-Re (P.Brit.Mus. EA 10684 = P.Chester Beatty IV, ed. Gardiner 1935), this still appears to be in his role as the sun rising and setting.

[719] See now the comprehensive treatment of examples in Blumell and Dosoo 2018, 232–233.

[720] Discussed also in the excursus to §9 and **Transmitting Textual Traditions**.

[721] For the divine drama of Isis, Thoth, and Osiris' adultery, see Love 2016, §1.5 and 5.1 as well as the corrections in Love 2018/19a and new parallels in Love 2018/19b.

tears, (and) her heart full of sorrow".[722] Thus, Isis is presented as being in a dirty and disorderly state, a motif of the dutifully mourning widow who intentionally soils her hair, also attested for millennia in Egyptian textual culture.[723] After the mythological scene is set, a direct, unmediated dialogue ensues where Thoth comes before her and asks her:[724] "What is wrong with you, my daughter Isis, [since] your head is covered with dust, your eyes are full of tears, your heart is full of sorrow, (and) [the] garment of your robe is soiled (by) the tears of your eyes?".[725] Thoth's question adds a further detail to Isis' dirty and disorderly state,[726] that her very tears have soiled her clothes. This inversion of the idealized state of purity and propriety thereby has several resonances with the condition of the herders in §10.

Besides the disheveled state of the garments of the herders and of Isis—torn and soiled, respectively—both the herders and Isis are described as emitting involuntary fluids—spittle and tears, respectively. These directly comparable examples not only reflect the structured and thereby deliberate composition of such motifs, they also perhaps describe an underlying analogy. In both cases, involuntary emissions of fluid symptomatic of a problem are juxtaposed with emissions of fluid characteristic of the desired outcome. In §10, the desired outcome is the production of milk—through lactation—, a bodily fluid which the body produces involuntarily, but whose secretion can be stimulated by an infant. The undesired spittle emitted by the herders is thereby juxtaposed with the desired milk to be produced by the Cow of Amun. Given that the desired outcome of *PGM* IV.94–113 is that Isis again receives the affections and attentions of her adulterous husband Osiris—who has conceived a child with Senephthys—, a further implicit aim seems to be that *she* can conceive a child with him. Thus, as is principally the case in erotic recipes, the desired outcome is sexual intercourse, and consequently the ejaculation of a bodily fluid by Osiris produced involuntarily, but whose emission can be stimulated by a sexual partner. The undesired tears emitted by Isis are thereby juxtaposed with the desired semen produced by Osiris. As metaphors embedded within motifs, then, spittle[727] and tears are directly juxtaposed with the implicit reference to the

---

722 ⲏⲥⲉ ⲡⲉⲧⲛⲏ́ⲟⲩ ⲛ̄ⲡⲧⲟⲟⲩ ⲛ̄ⲙⲉⲣⲉ ⲛ̄ϭⲱⲙ ⲉⲧϭⲟ́ⲩ ⲁ̄ ϭ[ⲟï]ϭ ⲉⲓ̈ⲁ́ⲧⲥ· ⲭⲁ ⲉⲙⲣⲏ ⲉⲉⲧⲏ́ⲥ ⲭⲁ̀ ⲉ̀ⲟ́ⲙ (*PGM* IV.94–95).

723 Parallels discussed in Love 2016, 32 n. 70 and Love 2018/19b.

724 The comparability of this motif with that of Thoth coming before "me", i.e. Amun, in §9 is discussed in the excursus to §9.

725 ⲁⲣⲟ̑ ⲧⲁϭⲉ́ⲣⲓ̣ ⲏⲥ[ⲉ] [ⲉ]ⲧϭⲟⲩ ⲭⲁ̄ ϭⲟï̈ϭ ï̈ⲁ́ⲧⲓ· ⲁ̀ ⲉⲙⲣⲏ́ ⲭⲉ ⲉ̀ⲧⲏ ⲁ̄ ⲉⲟ̄ⲙ [ⲧ]ϭ̣ⲧⲏⲛ ⲛⲧⲉϭⲉⲛⲧⲱ ⲟⲣⲡ· ⲛⲉⲣⲙⲟⲟⲩ ⲛⲓⲉ́ⲧⲉ́ (*PGM* IV.96–98).

726 Either by intention or omission in the preceding description of Isis in the third person.

727 Potential parallels for understanding the presence of spittle are also discussed in the commentary to p. 6/17.

positive alternatives of milk and semen, both of which were conceptualized as being imbued with creative agency.

The narrative momentum is maintained by the questioner, presumably the Cow of Amun, who poses two interrogative clauses. The first interrogates the disorderly manner in which the herders have already been narrated as having come, “running and hastening”, and the dirty state in which they have come, with their garments torn. The second interrogates further that state, focusing on the spittle upon their shoes, fastened with a reed needle or black flax—an apparently impure material. This pairing results in partial repetition, also found in the divine drama of *PGM* IV.94–113, where Thoth also introduces his questions with the interrogative particle ⲁϩⲣⲟ⸗. In this section, a pairing of two bipartite structures is seen that provides repetition as well as elaboration as the divine drama unfolds. Firstly, the herders are introduced as a triplet, while three characteristics describe their dirty and disorderly state. These two statements are described in the past tense, establishing as accomplished the situation in which the herders are introduced into the divine drama. This pairing is followed by a pairing of two clauses that are interrogative, rather than descriptive, and which bring the divine drama into the present, adding to the narrative momentum. Repetition, while not exact, serves to concretize the descriptive statements. This questioning, a motif common to such divine dramas, then presupposes that a resolution to the dirty and disorderly state—itself an index of a wider problem—is both possible and forthcoming. Although a bidirectional divine dialogue is not part of the extant text of §10, as opposed to §9 and *PGM* IV.94–113, a resolution, true to the motifs and structures of such divine dramas, appears to present itself in the next section.

V. White and Black Sheep and Cows

ⲍ̄· ⲛ̄ⲉⲥⲟⲩ ϩⲏⲣ· ⲍ̄ ⲛ̄ⲉⲥⲟⲩ ⲕⲁⲙⲉ·
*7 n ỉsw *ẖrr 7 n ỉsw km*
Seven white sheep, seven black sheep,
ⲍ̄ ⲛ̄ⲃⲁϩⲥⲉ· ϣⲏⲙ· ⲍ̄ ⲛ̄ϩⲉⲱ́·
7 n bḥs(.t) ẖm 7 n ỉḥ(-)ꜣ
seven small (or, young) calves, seven large (or, mature) cattle—
ⲙⲁⲣⲉ· ⲉϩⲉ ⲛⲓⲙ· ϩⲓ ⲧ̄ⲃ̄ⲛ̄ⲏ ⲛⲓⲙ ϫⲓ ⲡⲉϥϣⲏⲣⲉ
my-ỉrỉ̯ ỉḥ -nb ḥr tp-n-ꜥw.t -nb ṯꜣỉ̯ pꜣy⸗f šrỉ
let every cow and every beast receive its offspring.

Although there is again no indication of a bidirectional dialogue, in which this section would be understood as the answer by the three herders to the questions posed by the Cow of Amun,[728] this section appears to be a purposeful unit in which a pairing of two clauses, each in turn made up of a pairing, is then complemented by a command that provides resolution. The parallelism of four groups of seven—a number of ubiquitous efficacy in the Egyptian magical tradition—can be further divided into two pairs of seven, each encompassing a particular spectrum. Each designation begins with "seven", followed by compounds in the attributive construction, completing the structure of two pairs of pairs. Comparable to the scene in §9 of Amun riding a white horse, with a black horse before him, the reference to "white" and "black" sheep may be intended to encompass the entire spectrum of color, and thereby the totality of what comes between. This is then paired with the "small"—that is, young – calves and "large"—that is, mature—cattle, perhaps also intended to encompass the entire spectrum of the lifetime of livestock. Thereby, these two pairings, idealized through there being seven of each, reflect the spectra of appearance, size, and age—prefacing a command which can by extension be seen as applying to, and thereby being efficacious for, *all* domestic animals.

As in the preceding section concerning the "seven evils", direct parallels that elucidate the resonances of the textual content in this section have not yet been found. Perhaps the motif of the spectra being encompassed in the description of those domestic animals itself serves to ground the textual referents. Just as in the preceding section, however, a further consideration is the register of language to which these lexemes belong. As discussed,[729] the pairings—ⲉⲥⲟⲩϩⲏⲣ and ⲉⲥⲟⲩⲕⲁⲙⲉ[730]—exhibit either pre-Coptic grammar or evidence construct (prenominal) forms that are not otherwise attested in written varieties of Coptic known thus far. By comparison, while ⲃⲁϩⲥⲉ ϣⲏⲙ is perfectly Coptic, ϩⲉⲱ́, from ⲉϩⲉ-ⲱ, also appears to attest a pre-Coptic lexicalized compound. These pairings seem, then, to evidence terms established in the Egyptian-Coptic language, but which are in general poorly attested in written language varieties.

The command that closes this section accords with the interpretation of the preceding pairings as encompassing spectra of appearance, size, and age, because the lexemes chosen to be the patient (object) of the command are ⲉϩⲉ and ⲧⲃ̄ⲛⲏ. These terms refer to all "cows"—that is, all bovids—and all "beasts"—that is, all domestic animals—thereby including all other livestock.

[728] Compare, for example, the bidirectional dialogue between Thoth and Isis in *PGM* IV.94–113 discussed above, as well as the common structuring of such divine dramas as studied by Blumell and Dosoo 2018, 232–236.

[729] See the commentary to p. 7/2–3; 7/3, as well as **Linguistic and Orthographic Features**.

[730] Compare with the discussion of the "white" and "black" horse in the excursus to §9 and the notes to the commentary there.

The use of ϣⲏⲣⲉ, literally "child", rather than, for example, ⲙⲁⲥ "young" or ⲙⲁⲥⲉ "young animal", which are used to refer to the offspring of animals more specifically, suggests that, although the analogies utilized in the divine drama of the Cow of Amun concern livestock, the command itself demonstrates that this recipe was more likely applied to human offspring than those of domestic animals, as in *A Cow of Sîn*. Indeed, as discussed above, given that this section closes with a command, it could be that an earlier version of this composition ended here, and that subsequently another section was added during its history of textual transmission.

The section that follows appears to be an addition whereby the subjects do not fit grammatically with the Cow of Amun, while the absence of a bidirectional dialogue means that the structure of the narrative is unclear. This section could once have been treated as the response by the three herders to the questioning by the Cow of Amun, but, if so, the narrations and/or conjunctions that would frame such a bidirectional dialogue were lost in its history of textual transmission. It is, after all, only at the end of such divine dramas that the resolution to the problem is provided, and given that the command that ends this section is almost one and the same as that which ends the next section, the case for understanding the next section as a subsequent addition is strong.

Further support for understanding this section as the conclusion to §10 at an earlier point in its history of textual transmission, then, is the recurrence in this section, for the first time in the composition, of ⲉϩⲉ, the lexeme also used to refer to the Cow of Amun. This repetition rounds off the section by bringing the points of reference back to the beginning of §10. After all, every cow and beast is commanded to "receive" its offspring, resonant in Egyptian-Coptic with the term ϫⲓ ⲉⲕⲓⲃⲉ, literally "to receive breast", the action through which offspring would be suckled by the mother[731]—specified earlier as the desired outcome of §10.

VI. A Command of Iao Sabaoth

ϫⲉ ⲡⲉϫⲉ ⲓⲁⲱ· ⲥⲁⲃⲁⲱⲑ·
ḏd pꜣy-ḏd y-ʿ-ꜣ[Go] *s-ʿ-b-ʿ-ꜣ-t-h*[Go][732]
Because Iaō Sabaōth has said,
ⲣ̄ ⲡⲉⲙϩⲓⲧ ⲛ̄ⲁⲃⲱⲧ
ỉrỉ̯ pꜣ mḥṱ n ỉbt
"Make (for) the north of Abydos,

[731] The mother then "gives breast" (ϯ ⲉⲕⲓⲃⲉ).

[732] For the transliteration of ⲓⲁⲱ ⲥⲁⲃⲁⲱⲑ into demotic with these exact orthographies, see *P.London-Leiden* recto 10/4, where they are glossed precisely as ⲓⲁⲱ ⲥⲁⲃⲁⲱⲑ. Sabaoth appears again in recto 18/2–3 and verso 22/10, compare also *s-ʿ-b-ʿ-w-t-h*[Go] glossed ⲥⲁⲃⲁⲟⲩⲑ (verso 26/6).

ⲣ̄ ⲡⲣⲏⲥ ⲧⲓⲛ·
ir̲i̲ pꜣ rs(y) (n) tny
make (for) the south (of) Thinis,
ϣⲁⲛⲧⲉⲕϭⲛ̄ ⲡⲁϊⲥⲟⲛ ⲥⲛⲁⲩ
šʿ-mtw=k gmi̲ pꜣy sn sn.wy
until you (m.) find these two brothers,
ⲉⲩⲱϣ ⲉⲩⲡⲏⲧ ϭⲁϩⲏⲧ
iw=w ʿš | iw=w pt s.t-ḫt
as they call out and flee northwards
ⲉⲡⲏⲧ ⲛ̄ⲥⲱⲟⲩ ⲉⲩⲡⲏⲧ ⲥⲁⲣⲏⲥ
r pt m-sꜣ=w | iw=w pt s.t-rs(y)
so as to chase them as they flee southwards,
ⲛ̄ⲕϫⲟⲟⲥ
mtw=k d̲d=s
so that you (m.) can say:
ϫⲉ
d̲d
ⲃⲱⲕ ⲛ̄ⲙ̄ⲙⲉⲩⲉ ⲙ̄ⲡⲉⲧⲛ̄ϩⲏⲧ ⲉⲃⲟⲗ·
**b(ꜣ)k n nꜣ mwy n pꜣy=tn ḥꜣ.t̲ r-bl*
'Send forth the thoughts of your (pl.) hearts
ϫⲉⲕⲁⲁⲥ ⲉⲣⲉ ⲧ̄ⲃⲛⲏ ⲛⲓⲙ ⲛⲁϫⲓ ⲡⲉϥϣⲏⲣⲉ:
**d̲d-kʿ=s*[733] *iw tp-n-ʿw.t -nb nʿ(y) t̲ꜣi̲ pꜣy=f šri*
so that every beast will receive its offspring.'"

VI.1 Textual Structure

This section opens by describing itself as a set of commands given by Iao Sabaoth to an anonymous male entity. The textual structure is immediately established with a pairing of imperatives, both as ⲣ̄-, a pairing of cardinal points, "north" and "south", and a pairing of toponyms, "Abydos" and "Thinis". The narrative momentum builds apace, with the imperatives followed by a construction which limits this action. That is, the addressed protagonist is only to journey north of Abydos and south of Thinis *until* they find the two brothers, who are presumably somewhere between in a mythological landscape that nonetheless has direct points of reference to the lived landscape of contemporary practitioners and patients. Such reference to *finding* prefigures the resolution of the problem, whereby the *finding* of something or someone, and thereby the *knowing* of a matter, is a fundamental mechanism in Egyptian ritual tradition, accelerating the divine drama towards completion.[734] The apparently contem-

[733] *kʿ* < *ḫꜣʿ*, compare the unhistorical or unetymological orthographies attested already in the 20th Dynasty (1189–1077 BCE) in Černy (*CED* 52).
[734] As discussed in the excursus to §9.

porary point of reference for the action of the imperatives is then seemingly set in the past through their completion, because the state of the "two brothers"—calling out and fleeing northwards—is described in the present.

Pairings are found both in the reference to the cardinal points and in the actions that relate to them: as the male and probably divine protagonist must "make north of Abydos", so the two brothers are "calling out and fleeing northwards"; as the protagonist must "make south of Thinis", so the two brothers must be "chased as they flee southwards". A pair of paired clauses, the first circumstantial clause describing the disorderly state of the two brothers—calling out and fleeing—, the second a purpose and circumstantial clause describing what must be done in response—chase them southwards—, also expresses further pairings with internally resonant structure. Of the four verbs in these two clauses, three are "to run" (ⲡⲏⲧ), drawing together all referent actions, while each of the two pairs of clauses ends with directions of movement, first northwards (ⲥⲁϩⲏⲧ), then southwards (ⲥⲁⲣⲏⲥ)—framing the pairs. The "chasing" described is itself a clear analogy to herding, whereby the two brothers must be herded in the desired direction—southwards.

The consequence of having chased them southwards is that the protagonist can then say the command that resolves the problem of the mythological precedent. This in turn suggests that, in this section, the disorderly state in which the two brothers would be found was itself part of the cause of, and thereby part of the resolution to, the problem framed in the mythological precedent. Given that they are the only plurality introduced in this section, the resolution appears to be to tell the two brothers to "send forth the thoughts" of their hearts, which will serve as the authority and thereby efficacy behind the command that ended the preceding section: "so that every beast will receive its offspring". The authority and thereby efficacy between what Iao Sabaoth "has said" and what he says "you (m.) can say" is also provided in the pairing of imperatives in this section—Iao Sabaoth commands to "make" north and south, and commands that the protagonist should command the two brothers to "send forth" the thoughts of their hearts, underlining that Iao Sabaoth is the agent who actualizes the desired outcome.

In a further way, the two closing clauses are paired with the divine drama described in the preceding clauses. That is to say, the two brothers must stop fleeing northwards, and instead be herded southwards; they must stop calling out, and instead send forth the thoughts of their hearts. The mythological precedent seems to present both the cause of the problem and its resolution as framed within the undesired and desired actions of those two brothers. As north is inverted to south and crying out is inverted to sending forth thoughts from the heart, so the problem will be inverted into a solution—the unbalanced and thereby undesired stasis is broken.

VI.2 Textual Content

The conjunction ϫⲉ that opens this section introduces a change in the discourse. If the preceding section was once understood as a response by the three herders to questions posed by the Cow of Amun, this section would then provide the authority behind the command that ended the preceding section, "Let every cow and every beast receive its offspring". As noted in the discussion of the preceding section, given that the resolution to a problem usually comes only at the end of such divine dramas, and that a command bringing about that resolution ends the previous section as well as this one, the structure of this section suggests strongly that it was a later addition. Nevertheless, it would not be unexpected for the authority and thereby efficacy behind the commands that are provided to be introduced. In the same way that §9 ended with the supplication that it was "through the power of the lord god"—a generic term for a class of superordinate deities—that the recipe was efficacious, in §10 the theonym and epithet of one specific superordinate deity—"Iao Sabaoth"[735]—is utilized in providing the authority and thereby efficacy behind that which precedes and that which follows.

Journeying is reintroduced to the divine drama, providing narrative momentum through Iao Sabaoth's imperatives to "make" for the north of Abydos and for the south of Thinis; that is, to travel downstream before traveling upstream. Such a command is paralleled in the aforementioned divine drama of *PGM* IV.94–113, whereby Isis is instructed by Thoth to "go south of Thebes and north of Abydos".[736] This is a clear reference to a significant length of the Nile Valley, a journey that the divine protagonist has to undertake in order to find a resolution to the problem posed in the mythological precedent, which itself lends authority to the resolution provided when Isis finds a character named Belf. Thus, just as in §10, *PGM* IV.94–113 requires the protagonist to find someone who will provide the resolution. By contrast, a journey that takes the divine protagonist "north of Abydos" and "south of Thinis" results in that character meeting themselves in the middle. Quite distinct from the parallels to traveling in divine dramas discussed in the excursus to §9, not only the locations of Abydos and Thinis but also what follows suggest strongly that this command is for the protagonist to journey to a particular—implicit but unnamed—place, because it is there that the two brothers will be found.

---

[735] It cannot be excluded that the compiler of §10 and thereby the Michigan codex, or earlier copyists in its history of textual transmission, meant a specific association with Yahweh here. The assumption that the invocation of this theonym and epithet are diagnostic of the Christian(ized) nature of the text has been deconstructed in the discussion of "Syncretism in the other Direction" (VI) in **Transmitting Textual Traditions**. For the meaning of Iao Sabaoth, and its associations and appearance in Coptic magical texts, see the commentary to pp. 7/5 and 8/1.

[736] [ⲧⲉ]ϭ[ⲉ]ï ⲉⲣⲏ́ⲥ ⲛ̄ⲛⲉ́ ⲉ̀ⲡⲉⲙ́ⲓ́ⲧ· ⲛ̄ⲛⲁⲃⲱⲧ (*PGM* IV.107).

A further reason for treating this section as a later addition is the change in gender of the protagonist commanded by Iao Sabaoth. Although the masculine form is sometimes used as the default in Egyptian—as in many other languages—the consistent use of the feminine in the preceding sections suggests a later addition, whose commands were addressed to a masculine protagonist. Otherwise, something substantial that preceded this section has gone missing in its history of textual transmission.

The following description of the two brothers calling out and fleeing northwards, who instead must be chased southwards, is a clear allusion to herding—presented as part of the resolution to the problem, where the disorderly noise and undesired direction of travel of the two brothers must cease. As the only plurality in this section, it must be the two brothers who, instead of "calling out", must "send out the thoughts" of their hearts, which in turn provides the efficacy behind the resolution, "so that every beast will receive its offspring".

The identity of the "two brothers" is never specified, unlike the character Belf in *PGM* IV.94–113. As an epithet, presumably of two particular deities, the "two brothers" does not yield any unambiguous parallels. P.Brook. 47.218.50 (ed. Goyon 1972), dating to c. 600–551 BCE, bearing a composition that served to confirm royal power at the new year, is divided into two rituals: the rituals of the great seat practiced during the festivals of the earth, and the ceremonies in praise of Horus who bestows inheritance. In the second composition, a goddess, perhaps Mut, is described as "the mother who bore the two brothers",[737] who then goes on to specify that she will "give the two sisters their two brothers".[738] In the first composition, reference is made to the "years of the two",[739] where Horus and Seth are meant, as appears to be the case in a damaged passage earlier in that composition which refers to Atum as "[he who judges] between Horus and Seth, causing the two …".[740] If Horus and Seth are the "two brothers", this implies deep cosmogonic resonances with the struggle between these two gods in the Egyptian tradition following Seth's murder of Osiris, and the ensuing struggle over the kingship of Egypt.

The reference to "two brothers" is also immediately reminiscent of a tale from Egyptian literature. P.D'Orbiney[741] preserves the only copy of a composition conventionally known as the *Tale of the Two Brothers*. This tale concerns an older and younger brother Anubis and Bata, the former a farmer, the latter a

[737] *ỉnk mw.t msỉ̯-sn.wỉ* (20/9), where the group is determined with two divine classifiers.

[738] *rḏỉ̯=ỉ [n sn.tỉ] {msỉ̯} sn.wỉ=sn* (20/9–10), where both groups are determined with divine classifiers—feminine and masculine, respectively.

[739] *rnp.wt sn.wỉ* (3/15), where *sn.wỉ* is determined with divine classifiers.

[740] *[ntf wpỉ̯] ⸢ḥr⸣ ḥnꜥ stš ḏd sn.wỉ* … (2/20), where *sn.wỉ* is determined with divine classifiers.

[741] P.Brit.Mus. EA 10183, ed.pr. Gardiner 1937, 9–30a; Lichtheim 1976, 203–211, dating to the 19th Dynasty, perhaps copied in the first quarter of the 13th century BCE.

herder. Anubis' wife tries to seduce Bata and, when her advances are rejected, slanders him, with the result that Anubis tries to kill him. Fortunately for Bata, the cows warn their herdsman, and Re-Horakhty produces a body of crocodile-invested water between the two. While the brothers are reconciled, Bata does not initially go home. Although the tale continues with elaborate stories within stories, more relevant here are the mythological allusions to the struggle between Osiris and Seth that are established during these first scenes, including the threats of Anubis to his brother's life, Bata cutting off his own genitals, his posthumous procreation framed within the fundamental themes of death and rebirth, and the motif of conflicting brothers as well as their reconciliation.

Understanding how the prominent motif of conflicting brothers was brought into different regionalized contexts across broad temporal frames in Egyptian history is nevertheless difficult. This is principally because isolated synchronic sources of textual evidence, known through the accident of preservation, selectiveness of excavation, or the even more pronounced selectiveness of publication, can never fully inform on the diachronic transmission of motifs, whatever the sphere of textual culture production. Consequently, while the suggestions as to the potential mythological associations of the two brothers in §10 are tentative, given that the motif of the struggle between brothers permeates much of Egyptian temple, ritual, and literary textual culture, perhaps this motif is indeed resonant in §10.

Regardless of their identity, it is these two brothers who will provide the resolution of the problem by sending forth the thoughts of their hearts, such that "every beast will receive its offspring". This command once again resonates in Egyptian-Coptic with the term ϫⲓ ⲉⲕⲓⲃⲉ, literally "to receive breast", the act of suckling. Thus, in this section, once redacted into the composition from a distinct source text, the resolution of the problem is specified as being one and the same as the preceding section, closing off the mythological precedent with reference to the authority and thereby source of efficacy in Iao Sabaoth through which the desired outcome will be brought about. Comparable to the concluding supplication of §9, which also appears to be a later addition to that composition, the significance of the appearance of Iao Sabaoth is treated further in the discussion of "Syncretism in the other Direction" (VI) in **Transmitting Textual Traditions**. Of note here is that, by the 4th century CE, Iao Sabaoth had become an essentially pan-cultural theonym for a superordinate deity ubiquitous in the Graeco-Egyptian magical tradition. It cannot be excluded that the compiler of §10 and thereby the Michigan codex, or earlier copyists in its history of textual transmission, picked up on the specific associations between Iao Sabaoth and Yahweh, while the broad utilization of Iao Sabaoth as a theonym and epithet of a superordinate deity also means that the implied association cannot be assumed to be that with the Christian God. Therefore, the section that closes §10 in its present form, but which appears to have been a later addition, is not diagnostic of an attempt to Christianize an otherwise unambiguously pre- and non-Christian composition. It is instead suggestive of the appropriation of a theonym considered authoritative and efficacious from elsewhere in the Graeco-Egyptian magical tradition.

This excursus, as the preceding, has developed the associations and resonances of settings, actions, and characters of the divine drama comprising this recipe with the cosmologies and mythologies of Egyptian tradition, alongside apparent novelties. In doing so, it has contextualized this Coptic text in the milieux to which its textual content suggests it should be ascribed: that is, not the later Christian(ized) Coptic magical tradition, but the Graeco-Egyptian magical tradition. This has further demonstrated that §§9 and 10 serve both as anchors for the plurality of traditions still circulating in Egypt of the 4th century CE, and bridges between pre-Coptic Egyptian ritual and Coptic magical texts.

§11 An Invocation to Staunch Bleeding, by the Command of Damnameneus (p. 7/11–15) (MZR)

Despite the loss of the heading, as in §3 above, there are ample grounds to regard this text as a distinct section. Besides the difference in aim from the preceding §10, the present section fits into an extensive Greek tradition, in the motif of attributing a healing command to a divinity in protective amulets.[742] As Christopher Faraone has recently argued, the motif likely arose in oral performance, which was eventually refracted in written texts, and represents two of the most common types of incantatory speech-acts; a simple imperative commands the affliction or patient or, as here, a subordinate divinity tasked with the desired healing or protection, with the command strengthened in turn by attribution to a higher divinity, with an implied threat of that divinity's anger in case of disobedience. The verb κελεύω, as used here, is the most commonly applied to this motif. In the medical collection of Marcellus Empiricus, roughly contemporary with the Michigan codex, a version of the motif is recommended for inscription on a gold ring to prevent colic, and the commander is an anonymous god (θεός); the archeological record bears out the application of similar recipes in the form of a series of rings and other amuletic objects inscribed with a similar formula.[743]

> anulus de auro texta tunica fit exusta cui insculpitur uice gemmae piscis aut delfinus sic ut olochrysus sit et habeat in ambitu rutunditatis utriusque, id est et interius et exterius, Graecis litteris scriptum: θεὸς κελεύει μὴ κύειν κόλον πόνους. obseruandum autem erit ut si in latere sinistro dolor fuerit in manu sinistra habeatur anulus aut in dextra si dextrum latus dolebit. luna autem decrescente die Iouis primum in usu habendus erit anulus.
>
> A ring is forged with gold from the burning of a tunic woven (with gold), and on it is engraved, as on a gem, a fish or dolphin, such that it is pure gold and has around each circumference, that is, both on the inside and on the outside, the writing in Greek letters: "A god commands the intestines to bear no pains." It should be observed that if the pain is on the left side, the ring be

---

742 Faraone 2009; Zellmann-Rohrer 2015a; Faraone 2018, 205, 213–217.

743 Faraone 2009, 235–243; Zellmann-Rohrer 2015a; Faraone 2018, 213–217.

> worn on the left hand, or in the right if the right side is in pain. The ring should be used for the first time when the moon is waning, on the day of Jupiter (Thursday).[744]

Relevant to bleeding specifically, some early medieval additions to Theodore Priscianus yield a command to the blood to staunch its flow, attributed to the Roman author Apuleius of Madaura, who earned a reputation for involvement in magical practices already in his own lifetime:

> in chartas ad aurem ipsius: sanguis, imperat tibi Apuleius Madaurensis ut cursus tuus stet.
> (Write) on pieces of papyrus (and place) at his ear: "Blood, Apuleius of Madaura commands you that your flow stop."[745]

In the papyri the motif circulated elsewhere in the context of bilingual Greek-Egyptian collections. A command in some phylacteries in the Paris magical codex of the late third or early fourth century CE (*PGM* IV) is attributed to an Egyptian-sounding *Entho phenen thropioth*;[746] in the same manuscript, a variant with the synonymous verb ἐπιτάσσει appears, subject "the great living god", whose names suggests Judaeo-Christian influence.[747] The latter verb is also applied, subject Helios, in a bilingual (Demotic and Greek) papyrus of the third century CE (*PGM* LXI), addressing a beetle used in the accompanying ritual.[748]

---

[744] Marcellus Empiricus, *De medicamentis* 29.23 (cf. Heim 1893, 479 no. 53). Two metal amulets of the Roman period found at Avignon and Mondragon feature similar inscriptions, commanding a subordinate divinity to ward off hail from a field, on the order of the "god Oamoutha" (*GMA* 11: κελεύẹι θεὸς Ωαμουθ̣α).

[745] Additions to the *Euporiston* (1.14), ed. Rose 1894, 276, with Önnerfors 1993, 207 no. 10.

[746] *PGM* IV.710–711, μή με καταλείψῃς ὅτι κελεύει σοι Ενθο φενεν θροπιωθ, "Do not abandon me, for *Entho phenen thropiōth* commands you." The element Ενθο is likely derived from *nṯr-ꜥꜣ* "Great God", cf. ⲡⲛⲉⲧⲟ (*pꜣ nṯr-ꜥꜣ*) in *PGM* III.421 (*PGM* III.B verso 3/15 in the new reconstruction of Love 2017), and θρο from *Ḥw.t-Ḥr ꜥꜣ.t*, cf. αθροϊ in *PGM* XII.471 (glossing Demotic *ꜣthr ꜥꜣ-y*, according to the new reading in *GEMF* 15 19/26), while πιωθ renders exactly *pꜣ iṭ* "the father", cf. ⲡ-ⲓⲱⲧ.

[747] *PGM* IV.1038, ἐπιτάσσει σοι ὁ μέγας ζῶν θεός, "the great, living God commands you." The "living God", a Hebraism introduced via the Greek bible translations, is more commonly θεὸς (ὁ) ζῶν, but cf. Esther 8:12q, of the Jews as "children of the greatest, living God" (υἱοὺς τοῦ μεγίστου ζῶντος θεοῦ).

[748] The bilingual *PGM* LXI.35–36, for the releasing of erotic magic, addressed to a "sun-beetle" (κάνθαρος ἡλιακός), "Consume my love-charm, image of the Sun: he himself commands you to do so" (ῥύφησον τὸ ὀμὸν φίλτρον, ἴδωλον Ἡλίου· αὐτός σοι ἐπιτάσσει ποιῆ[σ]αι).

More common in the later Coptic tradition is a related motif in which the commanding utterance is placed in the mouth of the divinity, but without the direct specification of command. This is reflected already in the phrase ⲡⲉϫⲉ ⲓⲁⲱ at p. 7/5 above, and can be found e.g. in a prayer against reptiles:

> ⲧⲁⲓ ⲧⲁⲡⲣⲟ ⲙⲡⲟ̅ⲥ̅ ⲥ̅ⲁ̅ⲃ̅ⲁ̅ⲱⲑ ⲧⲉⲛⲧⲁⲥϫⲉ ⲡⲁⲓ· ϫⲉ ⲛⲡⲉⲣⲧⲣⲉⲗⲁⲁⲩ ⲛϫⲁⲧⲃⲉ ⲗⲟⲕⲥⲧ ⲁⲛⲟⲕ ⲁⲗⲗⲁ ⲙⲁⲣⲉⲛϫⲁⲧⲃⲉ ⲧⲏⲣⲟⲩ ⲙⲡⲕⲁϩ ϣⲱⲡⲉ ⲛⲱⲛⲉ ⲛⲡⲁⲉⲙⲧⲟ ⲉⲃⲟⲗ ⲛⲧⲉⲛⲉⲧϩⲓϫⲛ ⲡⲕⲁϩ ⲧⲏⲣⲟⲩ ϣⲱⲡⲉ ⲛⲑⲉ ⲛⲟⲩⲱⲛⲉ ⲙⲛ ⲟⲩⲡⲉⲛⲓⲡⲉ ⲙⲡⲁⲉⲙⲧⲟⲩ ⲉⲃⲟⲗ ϫⲉ ⲧⲁⲡⲣⲟ ⲡⲟ̅ⲥ̅ ⲥ̅ⲁ̅ⲃ̅ⲁ̅ⲱ̅ⲑ̅ ⲧⲉⲛⲧⲁⲥϫⲉ ⲛⲁⲓ ⲁⲩⲱ ⲛϣⲁϫⲉ ⲙⲡϫⲟⲉⲓⲥ ϩⲛⲙⲉ ⲛⲉ.
> It is (the) mouth of the lord Sabaoth that has said this, that no reptile bite me, I (so-and-so), but let all reptiles of the earth turn to stone before me, and all those upon the earth be like stone and iron before me, for (the) mouth of the lord Sabaoth is the one that has said these (words), and the words of the lord are true.[749]

A further variation, found in the spell from Saqqara cited above and treated in the appendix, proceeds directly to making the divinity the subject of a verb denoting the healing or protecting itself. As it is claimed there, " It is Eiao who loosens you. It is Adone who releases you. It is Eloe who gives (a) path for you to save (or, preserve) yourself immediately" (ⲉ̣̅ⲓ̣̅ⲁ̅ⲱ̣̅ ⲡⲉⲧⲃⲟⲗ ⲙⲙⲱⲕ `ⲁ̣´ⲁ̣ⲱⲛⲉ ⲡⲉⲧⲕⲱ ⲙⲙⲱⲕ ⲉⲃⲟⲗ ⲉⲗⲱⲉ ⲡⲉⲧ†ϩⲓⲏ ⲛⲁⲕ ⲉⲛⲁϩⲙⲉⲕ ⲛⲧⲉⲓⲟⲩⲛⲟⲩ).[750]

The shadowy figure of Damnameneus (Δαμναμενεύς), the issuer of the command in the present text, is said to be one of the Idaean Dactyls as early as Hesiod (fr. 282 M-W). He was associated with magic in Greek mythology from at least the fourth century BCE,[751] and his name, glossed as "the Sun, which masters", was thought to figure among the so-called *Ephesia grammata*.[752] He is invoked in an apotropaic capacity in some early Greek metrical incantations preserved on lead,[753] and in a healing capacity on a Greek fever amulet on papyrus.[754] In Coptic, a spell for gathering in customers to a workshop

---

[749] *P.Ryl.Copt*. 104 §4, 12–18; similarly the formulary P.Heid. inv. K 686 (ed. Kropp 1966), p. 14/ 239, "It is the mouth of the lord Jesus Christ that has said these (words)" (ⲧⲁⲡⲣⲁ ⲡⲟ̅ⲥ̅ ⲓ̅ⲥ̅ ⲡⲭ̅ⲥ̅: ⲥ̅ⲁ̅ⲃ̅ⲁ̅ⲱ̅ⲑ̅ = ⲧⲉ ⲛⲧⲁⲥϫⲉ ⲛⲁⲓ =).

[750] P.Saqqara inv. F.17.10 (ed. van der Vliet 2018; see now the appendix), 11–15.

[751] See Faraone and Kotansky 1988, commentary to line 25 (for the text see now *SEG* XXXVIII 1926); *Suppl.Mag*. I 19.2–4 with commentary; Martín Hernández 2010, 149; add *CIIP* II 1679.4; Andreeva 2020.

[752] Clement of Alexandria, *Stromata* 5.8.45, Δαμναμενεὺς δὲ ὁ ἥλιος ὁ δαμάζων, with Bernabé 2013, 88–89.

[753] The reconstructed archetype of the Getty Hexameters and Phalasarna tablet (and others), 2/42: see Janko 2013 with *SEG* LXIV 680.

[754] *Suppl.Mag*. I 19.2–4.

performatively arrays four divinities around the person of the practitioner, one of whom, Damdamenneos (sic), is said to have his back.[755]

§12 A *Charitesion* with Solar and Angelic Salutations (pp. 7/16–8/4) (MZR)

The χαριτήσιον, a procedure to gain favor, is well attested among the Greek ritual formularies on papyrus.[756] An external witness is the mention by Irenaeus, writing in the second century CE, of χαριτήσια in a list of "magic arts" (τέχναι μαγικαί), without details on the means, but situated in the context of the cult of angels,[757] who also figure in the Michigan text. The text opens with a salutation of the Sun, closely paralleled in two other ritual recipes from the Graeco-Roman period: the first another *charitesion* with a longer invocation, from a third-century papyrus (P.Mich. inv. 3404);[758] the second an invocation of the Sun to torment an unfaithful lover, in a papyrus formulary of the early first century (P.Berl. inv. 21243).[759] The three texts are presented here in parallel:

[755] P.Moen III (ed. Satzinger and Sijpesteijn 1988), hair side, 76–81, "Ablanathanabla on my right, Akramachamari on my left, Damdamenneos behind me, Sēnsēnkēbarphagēs in front of me" (ⲁⲃⲗⲁⲛⲁⲑⲁⲛⲁⲃⲗⲁ ϩⲓ ⲟⲩⲛⲁⲙ ⲙⲟⲓ̈ ⲁⲕⲣⲁⲙⲁⲭⲁⲙⲁⲣⲓ ϩⲓ ϩϥⲃⲟⲩⲣ ⲙⲙⲟⲓ̈ ⲇⲁⲙⲇⲁⲙⲉⲛⲛⲉⲟⲥ ϩⲓ ⲡⲁϩⲟⲩ ⲙⲙⲟⲓ̈ ⲥⲏⲛⲥⲏⲛⲕⲏⲃⲁⲣⲫⲁⲅⲏⲥ ϩⲓ ⲑⲏ ⲙⲙⲟ[ⲓ̈]).

[756] χαριτί(σιον) (l. χαριτήσιον) as a rubric in e.g. *PGM* XXXVI.274; in invocations e.g. *P.Oxy*. LXV 4468 verso 1/16, "grant me (the results of) *charitesia*" (δωρήσατέ μοι χαριτήσια). On the genre, see Brashear 1991, 71–73; Quack 2011.

[757] *Adversus haereses* 1.20.2, including also love-charms (φίλτρα), the summoning of supernatural assistants (πάρεδροι), and the sending of dreams (ὀνειροπομποί); the practices are imputed to the sect of Carpocrates, noted for their belief in the creation of the cosmos by angels (ἄγγελοι κοσμοποιοί), who granted such powers.

[758] 1/2–9, ed. Cohn 2012.

[759] 2/9–10, ed. *Suppl.Mag*. II 72, here following the new readings of Zellmann-Rohrer 2020a, 27–34: the last limb of the salutation is perhaps to be read τ̣ὸ̣ π̣λ̣ο̣ῖ̣ο̣ν̣ "the boat" in reference to the solar bark, but another possibility is the more general ὁ̣ κ̣ό̣σ̣μ̣ο̣ς̣ "the universe". The Sun dominates the rest of the central motif, despite the invocation of Aphrodite in the hexametrical coda (24–25), and so it seems unnecessary to insert her or Isis here following Daniel and Maltomini.

P.Mich. inv. 3404

[χαιρέτω ὁ θ]εὸς
[ἀνα]τέλλων,
χερέτω ὁ τὸ φῶς
[φέρων,]
[χαι]ρέτω[σα]ν καὶ οἱ
συνανατέ[λλ]οντε[ς
θεοί,]
[χαιρέτ]ω καὶ ὁ [ἀ]γαθ̣ός
σου ὀχευτής.
χα[ι]ρέτ[ω τὸ c. 6–8]ον
τό σε βαστάζ̣[ο]ν,
χαιρέτωσαν δὲ [οἱ c.
6–8]ν̣τες σε
χαιρέτω̣ καὶ τ̣ὸ ἀγαθόν
σου [c. 6–8]
χαιρέτωσαν [δ]ὲ καὶ αἱ
ἀκτεῖ[ν]ές σου.
[χαιρέτω] ὁ τ̣όπος ἐν ᾧ̣
ἀνα̣τ[έλ]λ̣ις.
χαιρέτωσαν αἱ πύλαι [c.
6–8]π̣[ο]ρεύη̣.
χαιρέτω [ὁ τ]όπ̣ο̣ς ἐν ᾧ̣
κατ̣αδύνις

Michigan 136

ⲭⲁⲓⲣⲉ ⲡⲣⲏ
ⲭⲁⲓⲣⲉ ⲛⲉⲧⲛ̄ⲙ̄ⲙⲁⲕ
ⲭⲁⲓⲣⲉ ⲡⲉⲧⲉⲡⲱϥ ⲡⲉ
ⲡⲉⲭⲁⲓⲣⲉ
ⲭⲁⲓⲣⲉ ⲙⲓⲭⲁⲏⲗ
ⲭⲁⲓⲣⲉ ⲅⲁⲃⲣⲓⲏⲗ
ⲭⲁⲓⲣⲉ ⲥⲉⲙⲉⲥⲓⲗⲁⲙⲯ

P.Berl. inv. 21243

χαῖρε Ἥλιε,
χαῖρε ἀνατέλλων,
χαιρέτωσαν δὲ οἱ σὺν
σοὶ ἀνατέλλοντες
θεοί,
χαιρέτω δὲ κ̣α̣ὶ . . . .

Hail the god at his rising.
Hail the one who brings
the light,
and hail the gods who
rise with (him),
and hail your noble
vehicle.
Hail the [boat (?)] that
carries you,
and hail those who [...]
you,
and hail your noble [...],
and hail too your rays.
Hail the place in which
you rise.
Hail the gates [through
which (?)] you pass.
Hail the place in which
you set.

Hail, Sun.
Hail, those who are with
you.
Hail, the one to whom
"hail" belongs.
Hail, Michaēl.
Hail, Gabriēl.
Hail, Semesilamps.

Hail, Sun.
Hail at your rising,
and hail, the gods who
rise with you,
and hail too [your boat
(?)]

Michigan 136 shortens what appears to be a traditional Egyptian invocation of the sun-god Re and his companions on the solar bark (see further the discussion on **Transmitting Textual Traditions** in the introduction), the essential core shared by all three invocations ([χαιρέτω ὁ θ]εὸς [ἀνα]τέλλων, ... [χαι]ρέτω[σα]ν καὶ οἱ συνανατέ[λλ]οντε[ς θεοί; χαῖρε Ἥλιε, χαῖρε ἀνατέλλων, χαιρέτωσαν δὲ οἱ σὺν σοὶ ἀνατέλλοντες θεοί; ⲭⲁⲓⲣⲉ ⲡⲣⲏ ⲭⲁⲓⲣⲉ ⲛⲉⲧⲛ̄ⲙ̄ⲙⲁⲕ). Equivalent expressions in Demotic to ⲛⲉⲧⲛ̄ⲙ̄ⲙⲁⲕ, for "the ones who are with you", are common in invocations for deities cohabiting in a particular place with the main addressee.[760] This phraseology subsequently made its way into the Greek-language examples of "Letters to Gods" from Ptolemaic and Roman Egypt. The opening invocation in the so-called "Curse of Artemisia" from Saqqara, more accurately an early Ptolemaic petition to Oserapis, addresses the latter and "the

[760] E.g., the petitioners of the late Ptolemaic P.Brit.Mus. EA 10845 (ed. Migahid 1987, 115–121 no. 9) refer to themselves as "the ones who speak before the Ibis, the Falcon, the Baboon, and the gods who rest with them" (*nꜣ nty ḏd m-bꜣḥ pꜣ hb pꜣ bk pꜣ ꜥꜥny ỉrm nꜣ ntr.w ntỉ ḥtp ỉrm=w*, 2–3); the petitioner of P.Cair. inv. 31255 (ed. Migahid 1987, 54–73 no. 4), in 155 BCE, invokes Isis (*ꜣs.t-nꜣ-nfr.t-ỉrị-šy*) and Harpsenesis (*ḥr-pꜣ-šrỉ-(n-)ꜣs.t*) and likely "[the gods and] the goddesses who rest with her" (*[nꜣ ntr.w ỉrm] nꜣ ntr.wt ntỉ ḥtp ỉrm=s*) (lines 4–6). The gods and goddess who rest with a particular deity comprise their entourage, but this formulation was employed particularly in cults of sacred animals, to refer to the mummified animals lying in the catacombs of that deity, and is therefore also found in numerous votive inscriptions, see Love fc. e, §6.3.2.1.

gods who sit with", or "about Oserapis."[761] A petition from Esna-Latopolis of the first or second century CE addresses "images of Athena, greatest gods", seeking protection from them and from "all the gods who are with you".[762]

To this core the Michigan text adds salutations of three angels, belonging at least originally to the Jewish tradition. In a neat doubled tricolon, the three hailings of the Sun are matched by one for each of the angels, Michael, Gabriel, and Semesilamps, unified by anaphora of ⲭⲁⲓⲣⲉ. The latter device, attested already in an Old Coptic portion of the Paris magical codex (*PGM* IV) in an address to the "God of Abraham, God of Isaac, God of Jacob" to cast out demons, proved popular in the later Coptic tradition: one invocation on an ostracon repeats ⲭⲁⲓⲣⲉ 17 times, and similar lengthy anaphoric strings are not uncommon.[763] A fragmentary formulary on a papyrus codex leaf of the second or third century CE offers a procedure for a "petition" (ἐντυχία) before the Sun, useful for every necessity and particularly court cases and angry confrontations with those in power: the luminary is saluted with the same verb χαῖρε and a series of traditional Egyptian epithets combined with others associated with Judaism ("the one who (presides) over the Cheroubim", [ὁ ἐπάνω] Χερουβι) and Gnosticism ("Abrasax, the one called the ethereal sire, Elōeu", Αβρασα̣[ξ ὁ] καλούμενος αἰθ̣έ̣[ριος γενν]ήτωρ Ελωευ).[764]

A parallel of particular note from the fourth century is a papyrus sheet from Oxyrhynchus, recycled from an original use for a documentary text to receive a formula for an invocation with salutations, an anaphora of χαῖραι (for χαῖρε) eight times, addressing divinities some of whom bear epithets in syntactical Old Coptic.[765] As at p. 7/18 of the Michigan text, ⲭⲁⲓⲣⲉ may also refer metonymic-

[761] *PGM* XL.1, 7–10, οἱ θεοὶ οἱ μετὰ τοῦ Ὀσεράπιος, or ἀμπ' Ὀσερᾶπι, καθήμενοι. The latter has also been read ἐμ Ποσερᾶπι "in Poserapis", most notably by Wilcken (*UPZ* I, p. 104), as a transliteration of Egyptian *pr-wsỉr-ḥp*, the designation of the temple of Osiris-Apis at Saqqara, also known as the Memphite Serapeum.

[762] *P.Worp* 7.1–2, εἰδώλοις Ἀθηνᾶς θεοῖς μεγίστοις, and 10, τῶν σὺν ὑμῖν ἁπάντων θεῶν.

[763] Old Coptic invocation: *PGM* IV.1231–1232 (Love 2016, §1.10), ⲭⲁⲓⲣⲉ ⲫⲛⲟⲩⲑⲓ ⲛ̄ⲁⲃⲣⲁⲁⲙ· ⲭⲁⲓⲣⲉ ⲡⲛⲟⲩⲧⲉ ⲛ̄ⲓ̈ⲥⲁⲕ ⲭⲁⲓⲣⲉ ⲡⲛⲟⲩⲧⲉ ⲛ̄ⲓ̈ⲁⲕⲱⲃ (see further the commentary in Love 2016, §6.2.2). Ostracon: O.Cair. inv. 49547 (ed. Girard 1927); cf. Frankfurter 2018, 202–204. For other lengthy instances of this anaphora see *P.HermitageCopt*. 56 and 71; P.CtYBR 1791, first text (ed. Emmel 1994, 346–351 no. 2), 31–46; P.Heid. inv. K 686 (ed. Kropp 1966), p. 1/6–18; P.Fribourg AeT inv. 2006.5 (ed. Müller 2009), 58–65; most recently *P.Köln* XV 640. In Greek: *PGM* IV.1115–1169; VII.1017–1026; LXXXI (see below); P.Mich. inv. 3404 (see above); P.Berl. inv. 9873 (ed. *P.Philammon*) p. 23.17–26 (see below); for a partial collection and discussion of Greek instances see recently Blanco 2015.

[764] P.Duk. inv. 729 (ed. Jordan 2006), 28–54.

[765] *P.Oxy*. XII 1566 (*PGM* LXXXI), e.g. πετ'κη ερχε νενκαμ τηρου (5–6: read from a facsimile, possibly to be normalized ⲡⲉⲧⲕⲏ ⲉϩⲣⲏⲓ ⲛⲛϭⲁⲙ ⲧⲏⲣⲟⲩ, "the one who is set [i.e., presides] over all powers"; πετ'κηιερχενειγκαμτηρου eds.).

ally to such invocations and salutations.[766] In a Christian context, the salutation of Gabriel to Mary, Luke 1:28, "Hail, you who have received grace" (ⲭⲁⲓⲣⲉ ⲧⲉⲛⲧⲁⲥϭⲛ̄ ϩⲙⲟⲧ, rendering χαῖρε κεχαριτωμένη), provides one obvious motivation for the continued use of the motif in invocations of angelic powers.[767] The Michigan text then proceeds to the substance of the request itself. The desired power, strength, and favor are specified as belonging to three further divinities, Iao, Abrasax, and Sabaoth, respectively. This motif, enhancing the promised benefits by their attribution to higher powers, is neatly paralleled by yet another invocation of the Sun in a collection of ritual recipes belonging to the municipal official Aurelius Philammon from mid-fourth century Hermopolis, as well as an invocation via salutations of angels in the contemporary ritual handbook *PGM* VII.[768] Opening in a similar anaphoric salutation with tricolon of χαῖρε,[769] the request is likewise couched in comparisons to a cast of divinities, in this case for the beneficiary to be made "good like Iao, wealthy like Sabaoth, beloved like Lailam, great like Barbaras, honored like Michael, glorious like Gabriel."

[766] P.CtYBR inv. 1791, first text (ed. Emmel 1994, 346–351 no. 2), 1/23, an introductory section describing ritual preparations before the bulk of the invocation is given (1/29 and following), i.e. ⲭⲁⲓⲣⲉ ⲕⲁ, "'Hail-'(invocation) 21 (times)"; the invocation itself contains the salutation ⲭⲉⲣⲉ (χαῖρε) at least 16 times (see further the commentary of Emmel 1994, 349); compare among Greek formularies e.g. the instruction in *PGM* XIII.117–118 "make salutations to the Sun each day for seven days" (τὸν ἥλιον χαιρέτισον ἐπὶ ἑπτὰ ἡμέρας καθ' ἡμέραν), introducing an invocation.

[767] This event is cited in the amuletic prayer of Mary, the so-called *Oratio Mariae ad Bartos*, in P.Lond.Copt. inv. Or 4714 (1) (ed. Crum 1897; cf. *P.Lond.Copt.* I 368, and further Kropp 1965), p. 5; and in the invocation for erotic magic in P.Vind. inv. K 192 (ed. Stegemann 1934, 12–14 text I; with Till 1935, 196–200 and Polotsky 1937, 120–127), 14–15.

[768] P.Berl. inv. 9873 (ed. *P.Philammon*), p. 23/17–26; *PGM* VII.1018–1021. For the salutations of the Sun and the angels Γαβριήλ, Ῥαφαήλ, and Μιχαήλ at 1017–1018 see above; the restorations of Preisendanz are based on parallels in the Berlin papyrus codex and a similar motif within a longer invocation in *PGM* XXXV for favor (χάρις) and victory (νίκη), in which the invoked divinities are adjured "by the power of Iaō and the strength of Sabaōth and the garment of Elōe and the might of Adōnai and the crown of Adōnai" (διὰ τὴν δύναμιν τοῦ Ιαω καὶ τὴ⟨ν⟩ ἰσχὺν τοῦ Σαβαωθ καὶ τὸ ἔνδυμα τ⟨ο⟩ῦ Ελωε καὶ τὸ κράτος τοῦ Αδωναι καὶ τὸν στέφανον τοῦ Αδωναι, 19–22).

[769] P.Berl. inv. 9873 (ed. *P.Philammon*), ibid., χαῖρε Ἥλιε· χαῖρ[ε Ἥ]λ̣ιε· χαῖρε ὑ̣π' [ο]ὐρανὸν θεέ.

P.Philammon	Michigan 136	*PGM* VII
ποίησ̣[όν] με	ⲙⲁϯ ⲛⲁⲓ̈	[δός μοι]
καλὸν παρ᾽ αὐτῇ	ⲛ̄ⲧϭⲟⲙ ⲛ̄ⲓⲁ̄ⲱ̄	τὴ[ν ἐξουσίαν] καὶ τὴν
γενέσθαι ὡς Ιαω,	ⲡⲧⲁϫⲣⲟ ⲛ̄ⲁⲃⲣⲁⲥⲁⲝ	δύναμιν τοῦ
πλούσιον ὡς Σαβαωθ,	ⲧⲉⲭⲁⲣⲓⲥ ⲛ̄ⲥⲁⲃⲁⲱⲑ	Σαβ[α]ω[θ,]
φιληθῆναι ὡς Λαιλαμ,		[τὸ] κρ[άτος τοῦ Ιαω]
μέγαν ὡς Βαρβαραν,		[κ]αὶ τὴν ἐπιτυχίαν τοῦ
ἔντιμος ὡ̣ς Μιχαηλ,		Αβλαναθα[ναλβα]
ἔν̣δοξας [ὡς] Γαβριηλ		κα[ὶ τὴν ἰσχὺν τοῦ
		Α]κρα[μ]μαχα[μ]αρει
Make me	Give to me	Give to me
good in her eyes like Iaō,	the power of Iaō,	the power and force of
wealthy like Sabaōth,	the strength of Abrasax,	Sabaoth,
beloved like Lailam,	the favor of Sabaōth	the strength of Iao
great like Barbaras,		and the success of
honored like Michael,		Ablanathanalba
glorious like Gabriel.		and the might of
		Akrammachamarei

This motif resembles another found in contemporary ritual texts, in which each member of a list of angels or angelic powers is asked for a specific benefit. Such "angelic rosters" appear in a few Coptic invocations with comparably structured clauses around the verb ϯ "give"[770] and may derive in turn from a much older motif of claiming or requesting to be surrounded by divinities. There are ancient Mesopotamian parallels for the latter, which entered Egypt by the Graeco-Roman period and later became widespread in the Jewish tradition.[771]

The invocation in the Michigan text closes with a further specification, that the favor be given before all people, but especially before one person in particular, whose name is left to be filled in with the placeholder ⲇⲇ.[772] The Hermopolite formulary in fact offers a similar specification, at an intermediate stage between the solar salutation and the main body of the request, "Give me stead-

770 P.Brit.Mus. inv. EA 10434a (ed. Crum 1934, 199 text C), 23–32; P.Lond.Copt. Or. 5525 (ed. Kropp, *AKZ* I, text C), 116–119; P.Lond.Copt. Or. 6796 (2–3) recto (ed. Kropp, *AKZ* I, text G), 89–100, and verso (ed. Kropp, *AKZ* I, text H), 43–56.

771 Ancient Mesopotamia: e.g. the text ed. Geller 2007, tablet 3, lines 108–110. Egypt: *P.London-Leiden* recto 9/19, "Horus is before me, Isis behind me, Nephthys as my diadem" (see now also *P.Kramer* 2.3–5). Jewish tradition: Levene, Marx, and Bharyo 2014; for medieval Hebrew, e.g. the text edited by Bohak 2014, 217 (cod. p. 176/14–16).

772 That is, an abbreviation of a metronymic identification, τὸν δ(εῖνα) (τῆς) δ(εῖνος) or (ὃν ἔτεκεν ἡ) δ(εῖνα). On the metronym see the commentary to p. 3/9 above.

fast favor before all the race of men and all women, especially before so-and-so (ϕϕ)."[773] Another contemporary formulary, with the same Fayum provenance as the Michigan text, closes an invocation requesting victory, favor, repute, and success with the specification, "before all men and all women, especially before him, N, whom she, N, bore."[774]

§13 A Textual Amulet for Pain with Analogic Deletion (p. 8/5–13) (MZR)

The recipe prescribes an amulet (φυλακτήριον) against stomach- and headache. The amulet consists of ritual text and designs to be inscribed on tin. Two sequences of the seven Greek vowels are written out on either side of the central design in normal, then inverse order, respectively, hence forming a palindrome, then repeated in following lines with the progressive deletion of the last letter. The motif belongs to a tradition of manipulation of text as an analogy for the desired removal of sickness and malevolent supernatural powers. Christopher Faraone has traced this tradition from its origins in oral performance, in ancient Greece, through its cooption in the production of textual amulets in the Graeco-Roman period.[775] Taken up particularly for healing amulets, the motif, attested across formulary recipes and surviving amulets on papyrus, metal sheets, and gemstones, features most often the name of a disease or demon slated for deletion. The seven vowels, as found here, and Αβλαναθαναλβα and similar palindromes are significant exceptions to this general rule.[776] The same palindrome αεηιουω ωυοιηεα is used in a fever amulet on papyrus, where it has been suggested that a solar association carried by the seven vowels may have been felt particularly appropriate for banishing a demonic influence believed to be causing fever.[777]

The amuletic application of the seven vowels to stomach-ache, as in the Michigan text, can also be paralleled in contemporary practice. The historian Ammianus Marcellinus records a death sentence meted out by Festus of Raetian Tridentum while proconsular governor of Asia in the fourth century, against a young man who "counted out the seven vowel letters" as a remedy for this same ailment.[778] Marcellus Empiricus also prescribes for intestinal pain the inscription

---

[773] P.Berl. inv. 9873 (ed. *P.Philammon*), ibid., δọ́[ς] μοι χάριν στ[άσι]μον πρὸς πᾶσαν ἀνθρωπίνην γε[ν]ẹὴṿ καὶ πάσας γυναῖκας, μάλιστα πρὸς τὸν ϕϕ.

[774] *PGM* XXXVI.45–47, πρὸς πάντας ἀνθρώπους καὶ πρὸς πάσας γυνε̂κας, μάλιστα πρὸς τὸν δεῖνα ὃν ἔτοκεν ἡ δεῖνα.

[775] Faraone 2012; the present recipe is no. 36 in the catalogue.

[776] For the latter, see also the bilingual fever amulet *P.Köln* X 425.

[777] *Suppl.Mag*. I 3; Faraone 2012, 22–23 and 31–33 with catalogue no. 2.

[778] Ammianus Marcellinus 29.2.28, "a young man who was seen in the baths to apply the fingers of both hands to the marble and to his chest by turns, and to count out the seven vowel

of some "signs" (*charactēres*), which appear to be a sequence of seven Greek letters ending in A, and may well represent a distorted form of an original (αεηιουω) ωυοιηεα.[779] It is difficult in this case to establish any direct connection between the vowels and stomach-ache (or headache),[780] and one might therefore suppose that they represent a more abstract manipulation of text as analogy for the healing power claimed by the amulet.

§14 Pharmacologic and Ritual Treatment for Dysuria (pp. 9/1–17, 10/7–16) (MZR)

The recipe was apparently added to the codex at a tertiary phase of its composition, on two pages left blank after Phase 1 (pp. 9–10), and after Phase 2 had added a separate recipe (§15) at the top of the second page, around which §14 had to be fitted. The writer marks the interruption and resumption by a reference-sign (~) in the bottom margin of p. 9 and the left margin of p. 10. The treatment requires first the preparation of a drug, mixed from plant and liquid ingredients, which is administered in an elaborate therapeutic regimen over the course of three days, accompanied by visits to the bath, a technique ubiquitous in the Greek medical tradition.[781]

The chief interest lies in the combination in that regimen of ritual means, namely bringing the patient to a horse-wallow (ϩⲛ̄ ⲧⲕⲉⲗⲓⲥⲧⲣⲁ, Greek κυλίστρα) and causing him to roll about therein in a manner recalling that of a horse (i.e., with legs bent backwards). As so far seems to have gone unnoticed, this prescription appears to exploit analogous features of equine behavior: spatial and temporal concentration of the urination of a herd, and more generally, the most

letters, thinking that this was useful as a remedy for stomach-ache" (*uisus adulescens in balneis admovere marmori manus utriusque digitos alternatim et pectori, septemque uocales litteras numerasse, ad stomachi remedium prodesse id arbitratus*). The accompanying action of the fingers might have functioned as an analogy, applying the cool solidity of the marble to the disturbed contents of the chest. On Festus, see Jones, Martindale, and Morris 1971, 334–335 s.v. 3.

779 *De medicamentis* 29.26 (cf. Heim 1893, 533 no. 197). The signs are to be written on a gold sheet with a gold pen, to be worn in a gold tube; as transmitted they run L Ψ M Θ K I A, thrice repeated.

780 The common element might be instead the solar associations: compare another prescription of Marcellus Empiricus for stomach pain (20.98), with a figural amulet of a serpent emanating seven rays carved on a jasper gem (*in lapide iaspide exculpe draconem radiatum, ut habeat septem radios*) and worn about the neck in a gold setting.

781 Note particularly their reflection in the late ancient Latin compilation of Marcellus Empiricus, *De medicamentis* for dysuria and related complaints, combining the administration of a drug with bathing: 26.21, 32, 96, 132; for the division of a potion into a number of drinks, administered in the bath, as a remedy for sciatica, see also 25.14; and §31 in the Michigan codex, with the excursus below.

copious animal urination that a patient would be likely to encounter.[782] In modern times, some distant reflex of such traditions might be discerned in the recommendation to encourage a horse to wallow in a sheep-fold and sniff the sheep dung as a cure for dysuria.[783]

More broadly, this conjunction of ritual medicine fits within contemporary healing practice that embraced animal analogies. For bladder- and related complaints alone, there is for example a procedure mentioned by Pliny the Elder and picked up by Marcellus Empiricus, to treat incontinence: the patient should urinate in a place where a dog sleeps and announce that he is doing so in order that like a dog he himself not urinate where he sleeps.[784] Marcellus also gives two versions of a remedy for kidney-stones, in which the blood of a kid fed laurel and denied water for seven days, collected in a state of ritual purity, is given to the patient with wine, ideally in the bath,[785] which also figures in the Michigan text. The ashes of burnt horse hooves, and goat urine, are recommended against kidney-stones, as is powdered horse tooth for disorders of the male genitals.[786] The analogical use of human urine itself may also be noted: for dysuria in a Coptic handbook, and for incontinence in Marcellus.[787]

§15 A Stray Invocation (p. 10/1–6) (MZR)

The circumstances by which this text likely came to be surrounded by the unrelated matter of §14 have been treated in the previous excursus. The text itself proves to be a general-purpose request, with no specific aim expressed. The absence of a main verb, where e.g. an imperative denoting giving or granting might be expected in construction with ϩⲛ̄ ϩⲱⲃ ⲛⲓⲙ ⲉⲉⲓⲟⲩⲁϣϥ, suggests

[782] Compare the English idiom "piss like a (race)horse".

[783] Pye 1807, 516. Further lore on ritual healing for equine dysuria is recorded by Aelian: a maiden should untie her girdle and strike a horse with it (*De natura animalium* 11.18; the same is attributed to Julius Africanus in *Corpus Hippiatricorum Graecorum, Hippiatrica Cantabrigiensia* 24.6, ed. Hoppe and Oder 1927, whence it has been included in Viellefond's edition of the *Cesti,* 3.11).

[784] Pliny, *Naturalis historia* 28.215; Marcellus Empiricus, *De medicamentis* 26.129; cf. also [Pliny], *De medicina* 2.19.1, with Önnerfors 1993, 185–186.

[785] *De medicamentis* 26.30 and 94–95; note also at 26.47, a woman who has given birth to twins should step on the back over the kidneys, the dual number perhaps analogous to the two kidneys, and the birthing to the evacuation of stones.

[786] Horse hooves: Marcellus Empiricus, *De medicamentis* 26.92; horse tooth: ibid. 33.38; mountain-goat urine: the medieval Latin antidotary ed. Rose 1894, 396 (*Antodotarium Bruxellense* §199).

[787] P.Cair. inv. 42573 (ed. Chassinat 1955), f. 1v/6–9; Marcellus Empiricus, *De medicamentis* 26.130.

that the beginning of the original might have been omitted in this copy or its exemplar.

As it stands, the text begins with, or in the midst of, the name of a deity, who is qualified with the epithet "the one who has a hold over the four corners of the universe," before the insertion of the name of the user himself. The clause ϩⲛ̄ ϩⲱⲃ ⲛⲓⲙ ⲉⲉⲓⲟⲩⲁϣ̄ϥ suggests that the request is for something similar to the favor-procedure (*charitesion*) in §12.

The epithet of the divinity invoked, whose name contains a form of the well-known Ia(ō) Sabaōth, has affinities with the extensive and originally Jewish tradition of angelic catalogues, best attested in Greek formularies and amulets. In these, angelic powers are listed and invoked, each of which is said to preside, in various phrasings, over physical or more abstract spheres of competence.[788] The Michigan text stands at a transitional point between the Greek and Coptic traditions, as does a bilingual Greek-Coptic invocation copied in a private letter from a Manichaean milieu in fourth-century Kellis.[789] That text, which aims at setting two parties at odds, opens with a Greek invocation, "I invoke you, the one who presides over rule, the one seated over the Cheroubim and Seraphim," and continues in Coptic, "who stands [i.e., presides] over hatreds and quarrels,"[790] before progressing to the substance of the request.

There is obvious Greek influence in the loanword ⲕⲟⲥⲙⲟⲥ (κόσμος) and the closing exhortation ⲏⲇⲏ ⲏⲇⲏ ⲧⲁⲭⲩ ⲧⲁⲭⲩ (ἤδη ἤδη, ταχὺ ταχύ), and in the presence of the Hebrew divine names ⲓ̈ⲁⲥⲁⲃⲁⲱ̄ⲑ̄ ⲁⲇⲱⲛⲁⲓ, likely due to a Greek intermediary. The formula of metronymic identification, however, ⲁⲛⲟⲕ ⲛⲓⲙ ⲡϣⲉ ⲛⲓⲙ, remains, or has been fully converted to, a purely Egyptian phrasing, in contrast to the Greek-derived ⲇⲇ used in the *charitesion* in §12 (for the abbreviation see the commentary there)[791], from the original phase of the copying.

[788] For Coptic reflexes of this tradition see the commentary to P.MMA acc. 34.1.226 in the edition of Zellmann-Rohrer 2017a; for Greek, the commentary to *P.Oxy*. LXXXII 5312.

[789] *P.Kell.Copt*. I 35, with Mirecki, Gardner, and Alcock 1997.

[790] Greek: ἐπικαλοῦμαί σε τὸ̣ν ἐπὶ ἀρχῆς ὄντα, τὸν καθήμενον· ἐπάνω Χερουβιν καὶ Σαρουφιν (the first epithet is rendered "who has been from the beginning" in *P.Kell.Copt*., and "the one who rules" in the discussion of Mirecki, Gardner, and Alcock 1997); Coptic: ⲡⲉⲧⲁϩⲁⲣⲉⲧϥ ⲁⲭ̣ⲛ̄ ⲙ̄ⲙⲓϣⲉ ⲙⲛ̄ ⲛ̄ϯ ⲧⲕⲱⲛ.

[791] As with modern abbreviations such as "&" that are read in accordance with their frame language, ⲇⲇ might have been read ⲛⲓⲙ ⲡϣⲉ ⲛⲓⲙ or similar by a Coptophone, or simply parsed as a non-phonetic marker to be replaced with the proper names.

§18 A Stele-amulet for Demoniacs (p. 11/1–8) (MZR)

This recipe promises relief for affliction, broadly defined as sickness of the heart or mind (ϩⲏⲧ), attributed to demonic possession. The prescription calls for an amulet in the form of an Egyptian apotropaic stele, within which some signs (*charaktēres*), a divine name (ⲭⲟⲩⲃⲁⲣⲟⲩⲭ), and a short prayer (ⲡⲉⲧϫⲱⲛⲉ ⲙⲁ ⲧⲟⲩϫⲉ) are to be inscribed. The signs accompanying the stele are noteworthy for including a symbol possibly derived from Christian cult, the rho-headed staurogram (⳨), which would be the only certain mark of Christian influence in the codex. That this recipe was added in a later stage of the manuscript's composition should be borne in mind in this connection. Given the background of the stele in pre-Christian Egyptian traditions, discussed below, the meaning of that same sign as the *ꜥnḫ*-sign, the hieroglyph for "life" (*ꜥnḫ*), may in fact be preferred, as it is indeed found on some Egyptian apotropaic stelae, and common in general on lunettes of hieroglyphic stelae of the Pharaonic and Graeco-Roman Period.

Demonic possession, not prominent in ancient Egyptian medical diagnostics, began to be targeted in earnest in the Graeco-Roman period. A bilingual Greek-Coptic spell (λόγος) in *PGM* IV invokes in its Coptic portion the Judaeo-Christian "God of Abraham, God of Isaac, God of Jacob," along with Jesus Christ and the holy spirit, to cause Iao Sabaoth to cast out "this unclean demon" (ⲡⲁⲓ ⲡⲁⲕⲁⲑⲁⲣⲧⲟⲥ ⲛ̄ⲇⲁⲓⲙⲱⲛ); the Greek portion adjures the demon itself.[792] As in the Michigan text, the procedure includes two recipes for amulets, in this case to be inscribed on tin leaves and given to the patient to wear after the demon has been cast out, the first a series of magical words followed by a short prayer ("protect so-and-so", φύλαξον τὸν δεῖνα), the second giving only a single "sign" (σημεῖον). Exorcistic formulae also become increasingly popular in contemporary finished products, amulets on gold and silver sheets as well as papyrus.[793]

The attribution of mental illness in particular to demonic possession is already a feature of the religious landscape of the Christian gospels, continuing a Jewish tradition exemplified by the evil spirit inflicted upon Saul, calmed by David's harp-playing.[794] The disturbed and sometimes violent demoniac is a stock character in the accounts of miraculous healings by saints in later Christian hagiography; in one text the devil himself boasts of having driven a man out of his mind and reduced him to madness (ἔκφρονα γενάμενον εἰς μανίαν ἀπήγαγον).[795] Better-educated churchmen, more conversant in the learned Graeco-

[792] *PGM* IV.1227–1264, see the excursus to §12 and Love 2016, §1.10; §6.

[793] Kotansky 1995; the commentary to *P.Oxy*. LXXXII 5306.4; de Bruyn 2017, 204–212.

[794] For the background, see Sorensen 2002, Bohak 2008, 88–114, Nicolotti 2011.

[795] *Historia monarchorum in Aegypto* 13.5–6, ed. Festugière 1961, with Wortley 2010, 124 no. 164.

Roman medical tradition, might also react against the overly broad diagnosis of mental disorder as demonic possession, as in the case of a much-commented letter of John Chrysostom to a monk suffering from depression (ἀθυμία) who believed himself to be so possessed (δαιμονιάω).[796] Modern medical research has suggested a correlation between belief in demons and worsened mental health, even as those suffering from the latter are more likely to turn to religious experts than to any other potential source of help.[797]

The term στήλη, as borne out by the accompanying drawing, denotes a figure approximating the shape of an Egyptian amuletic monument (e.g. stelae such as the common Horus *cippi*). Amuletic stelae with inscribed texts are attested since the New Kingdom.[798] One, from Ptolemaic Boubastis,[799] bears symbols of the decans, a feature that might already suggest the path by which ritual signs (*charaktēres*) came to be included in the present design. A close parallel is found in the Greek fever-amulet *Suppl.Mag.* I 23, where the drawing itself is invoked in turn as "holy stele" (ἁγία στήλη), in conjunction with "mighty signs (*charaktēres*)" (εἰσχυροὶ χαρακτῆρες), also drawn, to heal the bearer. The Michigan text is the only attestation so far in Coptic texts of this use of the stele in the original sense. In Greek handbooks, already the term can be applied more generally to drawings, employed for a wider range of purposes,[800] or to the text of invocations alone (so too the ⲥⲧⲏⲗⲏ in the curse of *P.KölnÄgypt.* I 11, discussed in the excursus to §3 above), without specification of inscription.[801] In this way the Michigan example may once again be seen to preserve a vestige of traditional Egyptian practice that did not survive the transitional, fourth-century period of bilingual compilation and translation.

The substrate for the amulet, a "uterine stone" (ⲱⲛⲉ ⲛ̄ⲟⲟⲧⲉ), apparently a lithic growth expelled from a human womb, is unparalleled as such. There is no obvious connection between such a stone and demonic possession generally considered. One avenue of interpretation might be pursued, in light of some beliefs about a specific kind of demon active in the human body. Already present in ancient Greece, and reflected in Greek texts throughout Late Antiquity and Byzantium, was the conception of the human womb as a quasi-demonic

796 *Ad Stagirum ascetam a daemonio vexatum*, PG 47:423–494, with Wright 2015.

797 Correlation: Nie and Olson 2016; treatment preferences: Stanford 2007, Mercer 2013 (exorcism).

798 Kákosy 1980, 1162–1164. For the tradition of amulets in both Pharaonic and Graeco-Roman Egypt, see now Quack 2020.

799 Cairo Museum, JdÉ 39505: ed. Bey Kamal 1908 with Daressy 1910.

800 *PGM* VII.215 (drawing with magical words inside, recipe for favor [χαριτήσιον], on a tin leaf), 940 (magical words beside drawing, a recipe to restrain anger [θυμοκάτοχος] on papyrus), and V.423 (similarly, alongside an invocation for divination); text alone to be inscribed, *PGM* XIII.54, 61, 127, 132 (for an invocation); oral invocation that may also be inscribed, *PGM* V.96.

801 *PGM* IV.1115, 1167, 2573, 3249, 3252.

entity, liable to wander from its natural seat about a woman's body and produce a range of ill effects conceptualized under the heading of hysteria.[802] Medical writers prescribed fumigations in the first instance to encourage the womb to return to its proper place, but incantations and textual amulets are also attested in formularies and the archaeological record, most extensively documented in a series of Byzantine metal pendants, whose textual formulae have roots in the Egyptian or Egyptianizing ritual texts of Late Antiquity, as shown by characteristic elements in a version recorded by the physician Aetius of Amida.[803] A feature of the Byzantine tradition is a confusion over the scope of the original prescriptions, which nevertheless continued to circulate in manuscript collections under more general indications that came to include men as well as women, for internal disorders very broadly conceived. It is just possible that the present protection against demons was meant originally for the demonic womb in particular, suggested by an analogic connection between a uterine stone and an immobilized womb turned to stone or weighed down in place, then extended over time to more general use. In this connection a previously obscure recipe in a late Coptic iatromagical formulary on paper may be mentioned (*P.Ryl.Copt.* 104 §7): a rubric ⲟⲩⲙⲁⲁⲩ ⲉϣⲁⲥⲁϩⲉⲣⲁⲧⲥ ϩⲓⲟⲩⲥϩⲓⲙⲉ rendered by the first editor "When a mother stands by a woman" more likely calques a Greek phrase with μήτρα "womb", i.e. "A womb that stands (aside from its natural place) in a woman". The procedure centers on an incantation, whose text is poorly preserved but surely begins with a narrative motif involving Jesus going somewhere (ⲛⲉⲣ̣ⲉ̅ⲓ̅ⲥ̅ ⲉⲓ), in which he probably encounters and heals a patient suffering from an analogous affliction.[804] From the Greek tradition an incantation in a post-Byzantine manuscript may be compared:

> ἑτέρη εὐχή· ''στέρα μελανή, μελανωμένη, αἷμαν τρώεις, αἷμαν πίνεις, εἰς ποταμὸν διαβαίνεις. 'στέρα στεροφαγοῦσα, ἀπὸ τῶν ιβʹ φλεβῶν κρατεῖς καὶ τοὺς οβʹ ὁρμοὺς καὶ πλοκάμους ποτίζεις καὶ τὴν δούλην τοῦ θεοῦ τὴν δεῖνα κολάζεις. θέλεις ἄνθρωπον νά σου δώσω; θέλεις παῖδα νὰ ποίσῃς; — ἐγὼ ἄνδραν θέλω, καὶ νὰ φάγω καὶ νὰ πίω καὶ παῖδα νὰ ποίσω. καὶ εἶπον αὐτῆς· μὴν κλαίῃς, μὴν θλίβεσαι καὶ νὰ φάγῃς καὶ νὰ πίῃς καὶ τὴν δούλην τοῦ θεοῦ τὴν δεῖνα μὴν κολάζῃς· μὴ ὡς κάβουρος πιάνῃς καὶ ὡς θηρίον ἔχῃς εἰς

[802] Faraone 2011.

[803] Metal pendants: Spier 1993; Björklund 2016. Late Antiquity: Aetius of Amida, *Iatrica* 16.67 bis, ed. Romano 1994, 598–599, with use of the characteristic Egyptian metronym formula alongside adjurations in the name of the Judaeo-Christian god and reference to the demonological precedent of Solomon.

[804] Ibid., note in particular ⲁϥϩⲉ ⲟⲩϩ̣ⲣ̣ⲟⲩ "he encountered a sound", sc. of a woman in pain, followed after a lacuna by ⲟ̣ⲩ̣ⲥϩⲓⲙⲉ ⲡⲉ "it is a woman", presumably a shift to dialogue form with the answer to a question about what the source of the noise is.

αὐτὴν καὶ ὡς δράκαινα φαρμακόννης τὴν βρῶσιν καὶ τὴν πόσιν αὐτῆς, ἀλλὰ ἄπελθε καὶ ἔπαρον τοὺς πόνους σου καὶ τὴν φλόγαν σου ἀπὸ τὴν δούλην τοῦ θεοῦ τὴν δεῖνα καὶ ῥῖψον εἰς ἄγρια ὄρη ὅπου σημάνδρου φωνὴ οὐκ ἀκούεται· ἐπὶ ὀνόματος τοῦ πατρὸς καὶ τοῦ υἱοῦ καὶ τοῦ ἁγίου πνεύματος, ἀμήν.'
Another prayer: "Womb, black, blackened, you eat blood, you drink blood, you cross a river. Womb, devouring womb, you take hold of the twelve veins and moisten the 72 joints and tresses, and you chastise her, the servant of God so-and-so. Do you want me to give you a man? Do you want to make a child? 'I want a man, to eat and drink and make a child.' I said to it, 'Do not cry, do not be distressed, and eat and drink, and do not chastise her, the servant of God so-and-so. Do not clutch like a crab and behave like a wild animal in her and like a serpent poison her food and drink, but go and take your pains and your fire from her, the servant of God so-and-so, and cast them into the wild mountains, where the sound of the bell is not heard, in the name of the father and the son and the holy spirit, amen.'"[805]

The identity of the first-person speaker, the interlocutor of the demonic womb, is left unspecified, but the obvious authority reposed in the personage, who can command it to depart, suggests a holy figure, one of the saints who often figure in such motifs in the medieval tradition or perhaps Christ himself.

In view of the parallels in Late Antiquity for the attribution of mental illness to demonic possession, finally, the Coptic term ϩⲏⲧ in the rubric of the Michigan text is taken as "mind" in the first instance, but the broader sense "heart" to denote internal malady more generally may also have been felt, with a potential conflation between ϩⲏⲧ and ϩⲏ "womb, belly".

§31 A Ritual Treatment for Sciatica (p. 14/1–20) (MZR)

The final recipe in the codex is an elaborate prescription for the treatment of sciatica. The primary component is the mixing of a compound ointment, applied to the affected leg, but the preparation and administration contain some interesting ritual and other features that show the influence of Graeco-Roman popular medicine. First is the gathering of a frond from a palm-tree never before harvested, which has not been touched by iron (sc. of a cutting implement). The stricture on keeping iron away from medicinal substances, especially plants, is found already in Pliny the Elder, and becomes widespread in herbal lore

[805] St. Petersburg, National Library of Russia cod. gr. 575, ff. 32v–33r (unpublished).

throughout Late Antiquity, the Middle Ages, and modern Europe.[806] It has been observed that the reference by the Sibyl of Cumae to the impossibility of using iron to cut the golden bough (*Aeneid* 6.148) might relate to this same complex of beliefs. Herb-gathering lore is already found in the Graeco-Egyptian papyri, notably *PGM* IV, which gives a spell to accompany this activity (βοτανήαρσις), addressing the plant directly.[807]

Once prepared, the ointment is to be applied to the affected leg with the hand of the corresponding side of the body. A parallel prescription for a sciatica-like condition in an early medieval Latin recipe, which combines a potion made with an herb gathered under ritual strictures, here the offering of Christian prayers, prescribes that the patient lie on the afflicted side after its administration.[808] Examples of side-strictures may be multiplied from the collection of Marcellus Empiricus: in a prescription for sciatica, a potion is administered with the patient facing east, with him receiving the cup from his right side and returning it to his left, without looking at the person furnishing it, an arrangement also recalled by a further element in the Michigan text (see below).[809] In some Greek medical recipes later attributed to Galen, a procedure for sciatica recommends catching a swallow, plucking its feathers with the right hand and stepping on its wings with the right foot if that is the one that is affected, and vice versa for the left.[810] An unpublished Greek recipe in a Byzantine codex prescribes an inscription on the afflicted area and a spoken incantation, preceded by the placement of the healer's hand from the same side of the body as that on which the pain is felt.[811]

---

[806] Pliny, *Naturalis historia* 15.124, 23.263 (examples could be multiplied); for medicinal substance gathered without iron for similar conditions see also Marcellus Empiricus, *De medicamentis* 25.13 (for *nescia*, an herb incanted and gathered with the fingers and not iron); 25.14 (another herb for the same affliction, to be gathered without iron); additions to Theodore Priscianus, *Euporiston* (post 1.31, ed. Rose 1894, 289: for *ischiadici*, an herb to be applied without having been touched by iron); on the stricture in general, Delatte 1961, 168–170.

[807] *PGM* IV.286–295. Note also the incantation accompanying the gathering of an herb for sciatica, in Leiden, cod. VLQ 9, ed. Piechotta 1887, vii §57. On herb-gathering incantations in Latin texts, see Önnerfors 1993, 203–205.

[808] Glasgow, University Library Ms. Hunter 96 (T.4.13), f. 167r, ed. Sigerist 1923, 146.

[809] Marcellus Empiricus, *De medicamentis* 25.11; cf. also the directions for the amulet prescribed ibid. 29.26, discussed in the excursus to §11 above, for intestinal pain, written on a gold sheet, placed in a tube, and affixed to the right foot if the right side of the body is in pain, or vice versa for the left.

[810] [Galen], *De remed. parab.* 14:386–387 Kühn.

[811] Paris, Bibliothèque nationale de France cod. suppl. gr. 764, f. 68r, "Another, for sciatica: you should measure from the outer ankle of the foot that is in pain with the big finger of the hand (of that side), one inch; then you should place the first segment of the big finger of the hand, where the nail is, on the tip of the ankle of the foot at the part near the leg" (ἕτερον εἰς ἰσχιάδα· ἵνα μετρήσῃ ἀπὸ τοῦ ἔξωθεν ἀστραγάλου τοῦ ποδὸς τοῦ ἀλγοῦντος μετὰ τοῦ μεγάλου δακτύλου τῆς χειρὸς οὐγγίαν· εἶτα ἵνα θήσῃς τὸν πρῶτον ἁρμὸν τοῦ μεγάλου δακτύλου τῆς χειρὸς ἔνθα ὁ ὄνυξ ἀπὸ τοῦ ἄκρου τοῦ ἀστραγάλου τοῦ ποδὸς ὡς τὸ πρὸς τὸ σκέλος). The inscription consists of the

The administration also includes strictures against speaking to anyone. In Pliny, the juice of an herb is to be applied in the morning before the patient speaks, as part of what is said to be an Egyptian remedy for bleary eyes.[812] For cough, Marcellus Empiricus gives two remedies applied before bed, after which the patient should avoid speech.[813]

The procedure ends with the patient lying on a brick in the bath. The prevalence of bath-therapy in the Graeco-Roman popular healing tradition has already been noted (see the excursus to §14 above). It is once again the collection of Marcellus Empiricus that provides the closest parallel to the present case: for sciatica, an ointment is applied to the patient on the affected side while he is lying down, and he is then brought to the bath and left for as long as possible in the heated section.[814]

The specification of the palm-tree may be noted, finally, as a sign of the integration of native Egyptian flora into a procedure that to all appearances arrived from elsewhere. The palm is, perhaps not surprisingly, uncommon in the sort of popular medical collections exemplified by Marcellus.

names of the saints Cosmas, Damian, and Panteleemon, performers of healing miracles, while the incantation addresses the disorder itself and commands it to flee.

[812] *Naturalis historia* 27.105.

[813] Marcellus Empiricus, *De medicamentis* 16.18, 16.33.

[814] Marcellus Empiricus, *De medicamentis* 25.22; note also two potions for sciatica administered in the bath, ibid. 25.32, 46.

Bibliography

Abbreviations

For papyrological publications the abbreviations from the papyri.info *Checklist* are used <http://papyri.info/docs/checklist>.

BD = Naville, E., 1886, *Das aegyptische Todtenbuch der XVIII. bis XX. Dynastie*. Berlin.

BE = Various eds., 1888– , *Bulletin épigraphique* (in *Revue des études grecques* 1–). Paris.

BF = Beinlich, H., 1991, *Das Buch vom Fayum: Zum religiösen Eigenverständnis einer ägyptischen Landschaft*. Ägyptologische Abhandlungen 51. Wiesbaden.

Bucheum II–III = Mond, R., and O. H. Myers, 1934, *The Bucheum* 2: *The Inscriptions*; *The Bucheum* 3: *The Plates*. Memoirs of the Egypt Exploration Society 41. London.

Cavallo-Maehler, *GB* = Cavallo, G., and H. Maehler, 1987, *Greek Bookhands of the Early Byzantine Period, A.D. 300–800*. University of London, Institute of Classical Studies Bulletin Supplement 47. London.

CC = Kasser, R., 1964, *Compléments au dictionnaire copte de Crum*. Bibliothèque d'études coptes 7. Cairo.

CD = Crum, W. E., 1939, *A Coptic Dictionary*. Oxford.

CDD = Oriental Institute, University of Chicago, 2001, *The Demotic Dictionary of the Oriental Institute of the University of Chicago*. Chicago.

CED = Černý, J., 1976, *Coptic Etymological Dictionary*. Cambridge.

CIIP II = H. M. Cotton et al., eds., 2012, *Corpus inscriptionum Iudaeae/Palaestinae* 2: *Caesarea and the Middle Coast*. Berlin.

CT = Buck, A. de, 1935–1961, *The Egyptian Coffin Texts*. University of Chicago Oriental Institute Publications. Chicago.

DE = Vycichl, W., 1983, *Dictionnaire étymologique de la langue copte*. Leuven.

DEB = Laskowska-Kusztal, E., 1984, *Le sanctuaire ptolémaïque de Deir el-Bahari*. Deir el-Bahari 3. Warsaw.

Dendera II = Chassinat, É., 1934, *Le temple de Dendara* II. Publications de l'IFAO. Cairo.

Dendera Mammisi = Daumas, F., 1959, *Les mammisis de Dendara*. Publications de l'IFAO. Cairo.

DG = Erichsen, W. 1954. *Demotisches Glossar*. Copenhagen.

Edfu II.1 = Chassinat, É., 1987, *Le temple d'Edfou* II.1. Mémoires publiés par les membres de la Mission archéologique française au Caire 11. Cairo.

Edfu Mammisi = Chassinat, É., 1939, *Le mammisi d'Edfou*. Mémoires publiés par les membres de l'Institut français d'archéologie orientale 16. Cairo.

GDG = Gauthier, H., 1925–1931, *Dictionnaire des noms géographiques contenus dans les textes hiéroglyphiques*. Cairo.

GMA = Kotansky, R., 1994, *Greek Magical Amulets: The Inscribed Gold, Silver, Copper, and Bronze Lamellae*. Part I: *Published Texts of Known Provenance*. Papyrologica Coloniensia 22. Opladen.

GMP = Andorlini, I. (ed.), 2001– , *Greek Medical Papyri*. Florence.

KHB = Westendorf, W., 1965–1977, *Koptisches Handwörterbuch*. Heidelberg.

Kropp, *AKZ* = Kropp, A. M., 1930–1931, *Augewählte koptische Zaubertexte*. Brussels.

LBG = Trapp, E., 1994–2017, *Lexikon zur byzantinischen Gräzität, besonders des 9.–12. Jahrhunderts*. Österreichische Akademie der Wissenschaften. Philosophisch-Historische Klasse. Denkschriften 238, 250, 276, 293, 326, 352, 417, 494. Vienna.

LD IV Plates = Lepsius, C. R., 1849–1858, *Denkmäler aus Ägypten und Äthiopien: Nach den Zeichnungen der von Seiner Majestät dem König von Preussen Friedrich Wilhelm IV. nach diesen Ländern gesendeten und in den Jahren 1842–1845 ausgeführten wissenschaftlichen Expedition* 2,9/10: Tafeln; 9/10, Abtheilung IV/V, *Denkmäler aus der Zeit der griechischen und römischen Herrschaft, äthiopische Denkmäler*. Osnabrück.

LD IV Text = Lepsius, C. R., 1901, *Denkmäler aus Ägypten und Äthiopien: Nach den Zeichnungen der von Seiner Majestät dem König von Preussen Friedrich Wilhelm IV. nach diesen Ländern gesendeten und in den Jahren 1842–1845 ausgeführten wissenschaftlichen Expedition* 1,4: Text; 4, *Oberaegypten*. Osnabrück.

LGG = Leitz, C., D. Budde, F. Förster, D. von Recklinghausen, and B. Ventker, 2002–2003, *Lexikon der ägyptischen Götter und Götterbezeichnungen*. Orientalia Lovaniensia analecta 110–116, 129. Leuven.

Opet = de Wit, C., 1958–1968, *Les inscriptions du temple d'Opet à Karnak*. Bibliotheca Aegyptiaca 11–13. Brussels.

Monuments = Champollion, J. F., 1835–1845, *Monuments de l'Égypte et de la Nubie*. Paris.

P.Borg.Copt. = Zoëga, G., 1810, *Catalogus codicum Copticorum manuscriptorum qui in museo Borgiano Velitris adservantur*. Leipzig.

P.Harkness = Smith, M. J. 2005. *Papyrus Harkness (MMA 31.9.7)*. Oxford.

P.London-Leiden = Griffith, F. L., and H. Thompson, 1904, *The Demotic Magical Papyrus of London and Leiden*. Vol. 1: *Transliteration and Translation*. London.

P.Med.Bouriant = Bouriant, U., 1887, "Fragment d'un livre de médecine en copte thébain", *Comptes rendus des séances de l'Académie des Inscriptions et Belles-Lettres* ser. 4, 15, 374–379.

P.Med.Chassinat = Chassinat, É., 1921, *Un papyrus médical copte*. Mémoires publiés par les membres de l'Institut français d'archéologie orientale 32. Cairo.

Philä II = Junker, H., and E. Winter, 1965, *Das Geburtshaus des Tempels der Isis in Philä*. Österreichische Akademie der Wissenschaften. Philosophisch-Historische Klasse. Philä-Publikation 2. Vienna.

PT = Allen, J. P., 2013, *A New Concordance of the Pyramid Texts*. Providence, RI.

SEG = J. J. E. Hondius et al., eds. 1923– , *Supplementum Epigraphicum Graecum*. Leiden.

Suppl.Mag. I–II = Daniel, R. W., and F. Maltomini, 1990, *Supplementum magicum*. Papyrologica Coloniensia 16. Opladen.

TEAD = *The Excavations at Dura-Europos: Preliminary Reports*. New Haven, 1929–1952.

TM = *Trismegistos: An Interdisciplinary Portal of the Ancient World* <www.trismegistos.org>.

Works Cited

Aitken, J. K., 2015, *The T&T Clark Companion to the Septuagint*. Bloomsbury Companions. London and New York.

Allam, S., 1981, "Ostracon Berlin P. 12398", *Mitteilungen des Deutschen Archäologischen Instituts, Abteilung Kairo* 37, 9–13.

Almazov, A. I., 1901, "Apokrifičeskija molitvy, zaklinanija i zagovory", *Lětopis' istoriko-filologičeskago obščestva pri Imperatorskom Novorossijskom Universitetě* 9, 221–340.

Altenmüller, H., 1979, "Ein Zauberspruch zum Schutz des Leibes", *Göttinger Miszellen* 33, 7–12.

Amundsen, D. W., and G. B. Ferngren, 1978, "The Forensic Role of Physicians in Ptolemaic and Roman Egypt", *Bulletin of the History of Medicine* 52, 336–353.

Andrade, N., 2015, "The Jewish Tetragrammaton: Secrecy, Community, and Prestige among Greek-writing Jews of the Early Roman Empire", *Journal for the Study of Judaism* 46, 198–223.

Andreeva, E. N., 2020, "A New Spherical Amulet from Taman", *Zeitschrift für Papyrologie und Epigraphik* 216, 169–172.

Assmann, J., 1998, "Mono-, Pan-, and Cosmotheism: Thinking the 'One' in Egyptian Theology", *Orient* 33, 130–149.

Assmann, J., 2005, *Death and Salvation in Ancient Egypt*, Ithaca, NY.

Aune, D., 1996, "Iao", in *Reallexikon für Antike und Christentum* 17, 1–12. Stuttgart.

Bagnall, R. S., 1982, "Religious Conversion and Onomastic Change", *Bulletin of the American Society of Papyrologists* 19, 105–124.

Bagnall, R. S., 1987, "Conversion and Onomastics: A Reply", *Zeitschrift für Papyrologie und Epigraphik* 69, 243–250.

Bagnall, R. S., 1993, *Egypt in Late Antiquity*, Princeton.

Bagnall, R. S., 2017, "Zones of Interaction between Greek and Egyptian in Roman Egypt", in E. Grossman, P. Dils, T. S. Richter, and W. Schenkel (eds.), *Greek Influence on Egyptian-Coptic: Contact-Induced Change in an Ancient African Language (DDGLC Working Papers 1)*, 19–26. Lingua aegyptia. Studia monographica 17. Hamburg.

Bagnall, R. S., and K. A. Worp, 2004, *Chronological Systems of Byzantine Egypt*, 2nd ed., Leiden.

Bain, D. M., 2006. "Koiraniden", in *Reallexikon für Antike und Christentum* 21, 224–232. Stuttgart.

Barb, A. A., 1948, "St. Zacharias the Prophet and Martyr: A Study in Charms and Incantations", *Journal of the Warburg and Courtauld Institutes* 11, 35–67.

Batibo, H. M., 2005, *Language Decline and Death in Africa: Causes, Consequences, and Challenges*. Multilingual Matters 132. Buffalo, NY.

Beltz, W., 1983, "Die koptischen Zauberpapyri der Papyrus-Sammlung der Staatlichen Museen zu Berlin", *Archiv für Papyrusforschung* 29, 59–86.

Beltz, W., 1984, "Die koptischen Zauberpergamente der Papyrus-Sammlung der Staatlichen Museen zu Berlin", *Archiv für Papyrusforschung* 30, 83–104.

Bernabé, A., 2013, "The Ephesia Grammata: Genesis of a Magical Formula", in C. A. Faraone and D. Obbink (eds.), *The Getty Hexameters: Poetry, Magic, and Mystery in Ancient Selinous*, 71–95. Oxford.

Betz, H. D. (ed.), 1986, *The Greek Magical Papyri in Translation: Including the Demotic Spells*, Chicago.

Bey Kamal, A., 1908, "Notes prises au cours des inspections. IX", *Annales du Service des antiquités de l'Égypte* 9, 192–193.

Björklund, H., 2016, "Classical Traces of Metamorphosis in the Byzantine Hystera Formula", *Dumbarton Oaks Papers* 70, 151–166.

Blanco, M., 2015, "¡Salve, Helio! Estudio estilístico-funcional de la fórmula χαῖρε en los textos mágicos", in E. Suárez, M. Blanco, and E. Chronopoulou (eds.), *Los papiros mágicos griegos: Entre lo sublime y lo cotidiano*, 111–131. Colección Clásicos Dykinson. Madrid.

Bleeker, C. J. 1958. "Isis and Nephthys as Wailing Women", *Numen* 5, 1–17.

Blid, J., Fr. Maximous el-Antony, H. Lundhaug, J. Zaborowski, M. Polliack, M. Gobezieworku, and S. Rubenson, 2016, "Excavations at the Monastery of St Antony at the Red Sea", *Opuscula: Annual of the Swedish Institutes at Athens and Rome* 9, 133–215.

Blumell, L. H., and K. Dosoo, 2018, "Horus, Isis, and the Dark-Eyed Beauty: A Series of Magical Ostraca in the Brigham Young University Collection", *Archiv für Papyrusforschung* 64, 199–259.

Boak, A. E. R., 1959–1960, "The Building of the University of Michigan Papyrus Collection", *Michigan Alumnus Quarterly Review: A Journal of University Perspectives* 66, 35–42.

Bohak, G., 2008, *Ancient Jewish Magic: A History*. Cambridge.

Bohak, G., 2014, *A Fifteenth-Century Manuscript of Jewish Magic: MS New York Public Library, Heb. 190 (formerly Sassoon 56)*. Meḳorot u-meḥḳarim be-sifrut ha-ḳabalah 44. Los Angeles.

Bohak, G., 2016, "The Diffusion of the Greco-Egyptian Magical Tradition in Late Antiquity", in I. Rutherford (ed.), *Greco-Egyptian Interactions: Literature, Translation, and Culture, 500 BCE–300 CE*, 357–381. Oxford.

Bohak, G., Y. Harari, and S. Shaked (eds.), 2011, *Continuity and Innovation in the Magical Tradition*. Jerusalem Studies in Religion and Culture 15. Leiden and Boston.

Boles, A., 2015, *Coptic Colour Terminology*. Unpublished MPhil thesis. Oxford.

Bonner, C., 1950, *Studies in Magical Amulets, Chiefly Graeco-Egyptian*. University of Michigan Studies, Humanistic Series 49. Ann Arbor.

Bonner, G., 1964, "The Crum Papers", *The British Museum Quarterly* 28, 59–67.

Borghouts, J. F., 1971, *The Magical Texts of Papyrus Leiden I 348*. Oudheidkundige mededelingen uit het Rijksmuseum van Oudheden te Leiden 51. Leiden.

Brashear, W. M., 1991, *Magica Varia*. Papyrologica Bruxellensia 25. Brussels.

Brashear, W. M., 1995, "The Greek Magical Papyri: An Introduction and Survey; Annotated Bibliography (1928–1994)", in *Aufstieg und Niedergang der römischen Welt* II.18.5, 3380–3684. Berlin.

Brugsch, H., 1878, *Reise nach der großen Oase El Khargeh in der Libyschen Wüste: Beschreibung ihrer Denkmäler und wissenschaftliche Untersuchungen über das Vorkommen der Oasen in den altägyptischen Inschriften auf Stein und Papyrus*. Leipzig.

Brunner, H., 1977, "Götter, Kinder", in W. Helck et al. (eds.), *Lexikon der Ägyptologie* 2, 648–651. Wiesbaden.

Buck, A. de, and B. H. Stricker, 1940, "Teksten tegen schorpioenen naar Pap. I 349", *Oudheidkundige mededelingen uit het Rijksmuseum van Oudheden* 21, 53–62.

Budde, D., 2010a, "Child Deities", in *UCLA Encyclopedia of Egyptology* 1(1). <https://escholarship.org/uc/item/9cf2v6q3>.

Budde, D., 2010b, "Das Kind, das mit allem beginnt: Zu einer Bezeichnung der Hathor von Dendera, von Kindgöttern und vom König in griechisch-römischen Tempeltexten", in D. Kurth and W. Waitkus (eds.), *Edfu: Materialien und Studien*, 1–23. Inschriften des Tempels von Edfu. Begleithefte 6. Gladbeck.

Budde, D., 2011, *Das Götterkind im Tempel, in der Stadt und im Weltgebäude: Eine Studie zu drei Kultobjekten der Hathor von Dendera und zur Theologie der Kindgötter im griechisch-römischen Ägypten*. Münchner ägyptologische Studien 55. Mainz.

Budde, D., 2021, "Hymnische Texte im Mammisi von Edfu", in L. Bricault and M. A. Stadler (eds.), *Hymnen und Aretalogien im antiken Mittelmeerraum: Von Inana bis Isis*, 83–116. Philippika 154. Wiesbaden.

Caminos, R. A., 1954, *Late-Egyptian Miscellanies*. Brown Egyptological Studies 1. London.

Capone Ciollaro, M., 2003, *Demetrio Pepagomeno, Prontuario medico*. Hellenica et Byzantina Neapolitana. Collana di Studi e Testi 21. Naples.

Cavallo, G., 1975, "Γράμματα Ἀλεξανδρῖνα", *Jahrbuch der österreichischen Byzantinistik* 24, 23–54.

Chassinat, É., 1921, *Un papyrus médical copte*. Mémoires publiés par les membres de l'Institut français d'archéologie orientale du Caire 32. Cairo.

Chassinat, É., 1955, *Le manuscrit magique copte nº 42573 du Musée Égyptien du Caire*. Bibliothèque d'études coptes 4. Cairo.

Choat, M., 2013, "Was Coptic a Part of Papyrology? Crum, Bell, and 'Worrell's Complaint' in 1936", *Chronique d'Égypte* 88, 161–181.
Clarysse, W., and M. Depauw, 2013, "How Christian Was Fourth Century Egypt? Onomastic Perspectives on Conversion", *Vigiliae Christianae* 67, 407–435.
Clarysse, W., and M. Depauw, 2015, "Christian Onomastics: A Response to Frankfurter", *Vigiliae Christianae* 69, 327–329.
Cohn, M., 2012, "P.Mich. 3404 recto: An Unpublished Magical Papyrus", *Zeitschrift für Papyrologie und Epigraphik* 182, 243–257.
Collins, D., 2008, "The Magic of Homeric Verses", *Classical Philology* 103, 211–236.
Cribiore, R., 1996, *Writing, Teachers, and Students in Graeco-Roman Egypt*. American Studies in Papyrology 36. Atlanta.
Crislip, A. T., 2005, *From Monastery to Hospital: Christian Monasticism & the Transformation of Health Care in Late Antiquity*. Ann Arbor.
Crislip, A. T., 2006, "A Coptic Request for Materia Medica", *Zeitschrift für Papyrologie und Epigraphik* 157, 165–167.
Crum, W. E., 1897, "A Coptic Palimpsest", *Proceedings of the Society of Biblical Archaeology* 19, 210–222.
Crum, W. E., 1902, "A Bilingual Charm", *Proceedings of the Society of Biblical Archaeology* 34, 329–331.
Crum, W. E., 1934, "Magical texts in Coptic: II", *Journal of Egyptian Archaeology* 20, 195–200.
Curbera, J. B., 1999, "Maternal Lineage in Greek Magical Texts", in D. R. Jordan, H. Montgomery, and E. Thomassen (eds.), *The World of Ancient Magic: Papers from the First International Samson Eitrem Seminar at the Norwegian Institute at Athens 4–8 May 1997*, 195–213. Skrifter utgitt av det Norske institutt i Athen 4. Bergen.
Daressy, G., 1910, "La semaine des égyptiens", *Annales du Service des antiquités de l'Égypte* 10, 21–23.
Daumas, F., 1958, *Les mammisis des temples égyptiens*. Annales de l'Université de Lyon. Troisième série, Lettres 32. Paris.
Daumas, F., 1977, "Geburtshaus", in W. Helck et al. (eds.) *Lexikon der Ägyptologie* 2, 462–475. Wiesbaden.
Davies, N. de Garis, 1908, *The Rock Tombs of El-ʿAmarna*, Part 6: *Tombs of Parennefer, Tutu and Ay*. Archaeological Survey of Egypt Memoir 18. London.
De Bruyn, T., 2017, *Making Amulets Christian: Artefacts, Scribes, and Contexts*. Oxford Early Christian Studies. Oxford.
De Haro Sanchez, M., 2004, "Catalogue des papyrus iatromagiques grecs", *Papyrologica Lupiensia* 13, 37–60.
De Haro Sanchez, M., 2010, "Le vocabulaire de la pathologie et de la thérapeutique dans les papyrus iatromagiques grecs: Fièvres, traumatismes et 'épilepsie'", *Bulletin of the American Society of Papyrologists* 47, 132–141.
De Haro Sanchez, M., 2012, "Mise en texte et contexte des papyrus iatromagiques grecs: recherches sur les conditions matérielles de réalisation des formulaires et des amulettes", in P. Schubert (ed.), *Actes du 26e Congrès international de papyrologie, Genève 16–21 août 2010*, 159–169. Recherches et rencontres 30. Geneva.
Delatte, A., 1961, *Herbarius: Recherches sur le cérémonial usité chez les anciens pour la cueillette des simples et des plantes magiques*, 3rd ed. Mémoires de la Classe des lettres 54.4. Brussels.
Delattre, A., 2014, "Un phylactère copte contre une inflammation de la luette", *Analecta Papyrologica* 26, 383–389.

Dieleman, J., 2004, "Ein spätägyptisches magisches Handbuch: Eine neue PDM oder PGM?", in F. Hoffmann and H. J. Thissen, (eds.), Res severa verum gaudium: *Festschrift für Karl-Theodor Zauzich zum 65. Geburtstag am 8. Juni 2004*, 121–128. Studia demotica 6. Leuven.

Dieleman, J., 2005, *Priests, Tongues, and Rites: The London-Leiden Magical Manuscripts and Translation in Egyptian Ritual (100–300 CE)*. Religions in the Graeco-Roman World 153. Leiden.

Dieleman, J., 2006, "Abundance in the Margins: Multiplicity of Script in the Demotic Magical Papyri", in S. L. Sanders (ed.), *Margins of Writings, Origins of Cultures*, 67–81. University of Chicago Oriental Institute Seminars 2. Chicago.

Dieleman, J., 2010, "What's in a Sign? Translating Filiation in the Demotic Magical Papyri", in A. Papaconstantinou (ed.), *The Multilingual Experience in Egypt, from the Ptolemies to the Abbasids*, 127–152. Farnham.

Dieleman, J., 2019, "The Greco-Egyptian Magical Papyri", in D. Frankfurter (ed.), *Guide to the Study of Ancient Magic*, 293–321. Religions in the Graeco-Roman World 189. Leiden and Boston.

Dieleman, J., and I. S. Moyer, 2010, "Egyptian Literature", in J. J. Clauss and M. Cuypers (eds.), *A Companion to Hellenistic Literature*, 429–447. Blackwell Companions to the Ancient World. Chichester.

Donadoni, S., 1965–1966, "Un incantesimo amatorio copto", *Atti della Reale Accademia delle Scienze di Torino, scienze morali, storiche e filologiche* 100, 285–292.

Dosoo, K., 2016a, "A History of the Theban Magical Library", *Bulletin of the American Society of Papyrologists* 53, 251–274.

Dosoo, K., 2016b, "Magical Discourses, Ritual Collections: Cultural Trends and Private Interests in Egyptian Handbooks and Archives", in T. Derda, A. Łajtar and J. Urbanik (eds.), *Proceedings of the 27th International Congress of Papyrology Warsaw, 29 July–3 August 2013*, 2, 699–716. Journal of Juristic Papyrology Supplements 28. Warsaw.

Dosoo, K., 2018, "Zōdion and Praxis: An Illustrated Coptic Magical Papyrus in the Macquarie University Collection", *Journal of Coptic Studies* 20, 11–22.

Dosoo, K., 2021, "Isis in Christian Egypt: The Cultural Context of Michigan Ms. Copt. 136 ll.17–34", in L. Bricault and M. A. Stadler (eds.), *Hymnen und Aretalogien im antiken Mittelmeerraum: Von Inana bis Isis*, 195–234. Philippika 154. Wiesbaden.

Drexler, W., 1899, "Alte Beschwörungsformeln", *Philologus* 58, 594–616.

Drioton, E., 1946, "Parchemin magique copte", *Le Muséon* 59, 479–489.

Drower, E. S., 1943, "A Mandaean Book of Black Magic", *Journal of the Royal Asiatic Society* 75, 149–181.

Dzwiza, K., 2019, "Magical Signs: An Extraordinary Phenomenon or Just Business as Usual? Analysing Decoration Patterns on Magical Gems", in K. Endreffy, A. M. Nagy and J. Spier (eds.), *Magical Gems and Magical Gems in Their Contexts: Proceedings of the International Workshop Held at the Museum of Fine Arts, Budapest, 16–18 February 2012, Rome, 2019*, 59–84. Studia Archaeologica 229. Rome.

Edmonds, R., 2019, *Drawing Down the Moon: Magic in the Ancient Greco-Roman World*, Princeton.

Emmel, S., 1994, "Appendix: Previously Unpublished Coptic Texts of Ritual Power in the Beinecke Library, Yale University", in M. Meyer and R. Smith (eds.), *Ancient Christian Magic: Coptic Texts of Ritual Power*, 343–356. San Francisco.

Engsheden, Å., and A. Winkler, 2017, "Three Coptic Letters in the Museum Gustavianum", *Journal of Juristic Papyrology* 47, 101–115.

Erman, A., 1901, *Zaubersprüche für Mutter und Kind aus dem Papyrus 3027 des Berliner Museums*. Abhandlungen der Königlichen Akademie der Wissenschaften zu Berlin. Berlin.

Ewers, M., 2009, *Marcellus Empiricus, De medicamentis: Christliche Abhandlung über Barmherzigkeit oder abergläubische Rezeptsammlung?* Bochumer altertumswissenschaftliches Colloquium 83. Trier.

Fairman, H. W., 1974, *The Triumph of Horus: An Ancient Egyptian Sacred Drama*. London.

Faraone, C. A., 1999, *Ancient Greek Love Magic*. Cambridge, MA, and London.

Faraone, C. A., 2000, "Handbooks and Anthologies: The Collection of Greek and Egyptian Incantations in Late Hellenistic Egypt", *Archiv für Religionsgeschichte* 2, 195–214.

Faraone, C. A., 2009, "Stopping Evil, Pain, Anger, and Blood: The Ancient Greek Tradition of Protective Iambic Incantations", *Greek, Roman, and Byzantine Studies* 49, 227–255.

Faraone, C. A., 2011, "Magical and Medical Approaches to the Wandering Womb in the Ancient Greek World", *Classical Antiquity* 30, 1–32.

Faraone, C. A., 2012, *Vanishing Acts on Ancient Greek Amulets: From Oral Performance to Visual Design*. Bulletin of the Institute of Classical Studies Supplement 115. London.

Faraone, C. A., 2013, "The Amuletic Design of the Mithraic Bull-Wounding Scene", *Journal of Roman Studies* 103, 96–116.

Faraone, C. A., 2018, *The Transformation of Greek Amulets in Roman Imperial Times*. Empire and After. Philadelphia.

Faraone, C. A., 2020, "The Late-Antique Transfer of Circular Gem-Designs to Papyri and Foil: The *Ouroborus* and Solomon's Seal", in R. Hernandez Martín (ed.), *Drawing Magic: Images of Power and the Power of Images in Ancient and Late-Antique Magic*, 69–84. Studies in the History and Anthropology of Religion. Leuven.

Faraone, C. A., and R. Kotansky, 1988, "An Inscribed Gold Phlactery in Stamford, Connecticut", *Zeitschrift für Papyrologie und Epigraphik* 75, 257–266.

Faraone, C. A., and D. Obbink (eds.), 1991, *Magika Hiera: Ancient Greek Magic and Religion*, New York and Oxford.

Fernández Marcos, N., 1975, *Los thaumata de Sofronio: Contribución al estudio de la "Incubatio" cristiana*. Manuales y anejos de Emérita 31. Madrid.

Festugière, A.-J., 1961, *Historia monachorum in Aegypto*. Subsidia hagiographica 34. Brussels.

Festugière, A.-J., and A. D. Nock, 1945–1954, *Corpus Hermeticum*. Collection des universités de France. Paris.

Fewster, P., 2002, "Bilingualism in Roman Egypt", in J. N. Adams, M. Janse, and S. Swain, (eds.), *Bilingualism in Ancient Society: Language Contact and the Written Text*, 220–245. Oxford.

Förster, H., 2002, *Wörterbuch der griechischen Wörter in den koptischen dokumentarischen Texten*. Texte und Untersuchungen zur Geschichte der altchristlichen Literatur 148. Berlin.

Fournet, J.-L., 2009, "The Multilingual Environment of Late Antique Egypt: Greek, Latin, Coptic, and Persian Documentation", in R. S. Bagnall (ed.), *The Oxford Handbook of Papyrology*, 418–451. Oxford.

Fournet, J.-L., 2020, *The Rise of Coptic: Egyptian versus Greek in Late Antiquity*. The Rostovtzeff Lectures 5. Princeton.

Frankfurter, D., 1995, "Narrating Power: The Theory and Practice of the Magical Historiola in Ritual Spells", in M. Meyer and P. Mirecki (eds.), *Ancient Magic and Ritual Power*, 457–476. Religions in the Graeco-Roman World 129. Leiden.

Frankfurter, D., 1998, *Religion in Roman Egypt: Assimilation and Resistance*. Princeton.

Frankfurter, D., 2007, "Illuminating the Cult of Kothos: The Panegryic on Macarius and Local Religion in Fifth-Century Egypt", in J. E. Goehring and J. A. Timbie (eds.), *The World of Early Egyptian Christianity: Language, Literature, and Social Context. Essays in Honor of David W. Johnson*, 176–188. Washington, DC.

Frankfurter, D., 2009, "The Laments of Horus in Coptic: Myth, Folklore, and Syncretism in Late Ancient Egypt", in U. Dill and C. Walde (eds.), *Antike Mythen: Medien, Transformationen und Konstruktionen*, 229–247. Berlin.

Frankfurter, D., 2018, *Christianizing Egypt: Syncretism and Local Worlds in Late Antiquity*. Martin Classical Lectures. Princeton.

Frankfurter, D. (ed.), 2019, *Guide to the Study of Ancient Magic*. Religions in the Graeco-Roman World 189. Leiden and Boston.

Franz, A. 1909. *Die kirchlichen Benediktionen im Mittelalter*. Freiburg im Breisgau.

Funk, W.-P., 1988, "Dialects Wanting Homes: A Numerical Approach to the Early Varieties of Coptic", in J. Fisiak (ed.), *Historical Dialectology: Regional and Social*, 149–192. Trends in Linguistics Studies and Monographs 37. Berlin.

Gardiner, A. H., 1905, "Hymns to Amon from a Leiden Papyrus", *Zeitschrift für Ägyptische Sprache und Altertumskunde* 42, 12–42.

Gardiner, A. H., 1935, *Hieratic Papyri in the British Museum*. London.

Gardiner, A. H., 1937, *Late-Egyptian Miscellanies*. Bibliotheca Aegyptiaca 7. Brussels.

Garel, E., 2016, "Lettre concernant l'envoi d'un papyrus iatro-magique et une réquisition de laine de mouton (P.Vindob. inv. K 55)", *Journal of Coptic Studies* 18, 44–55.

Geller, M. J., 2007, *Evil Demons: Canonical Utukku Lemnutu Incantations*. State Archives of Assyria Cuneiform Texts 5. Helsinki.

Gillam, R. A., 2005, *Performance and Drama in Ancient Egypt*. Duckworth Egyptology. London.

Gillam, R. A., 2009, "Drama", *UCLA Encyclopedia of Egyptology* 1(1). <https://escholarship.org/uc/item/6tv88003>.

Girard, L. S.-P., 1927, "Un fragment de liturgie magique copte sur ostrakon", *Annales du Service des antiquités de l'Égypte* 27, 62–65.

Gollancz, H., 1912, *The Book of Protection: Being a Collection of Charms*. London.

Gordon, R. L., 2014, "Charaktêres Between Antiquity and the Renaissance: Transmission and Re-Invention", in V. Dasen and J.-M. Spieser (eds.), *Les savoirs magiques et leurs transmission de l'Antiquité à la Renaissance*, 253–300. Micrologus' Library 60. Florence.

Goyon, J.-C., 1972, *Confirmation du pouvoir royal au nouvel an: Brooklyn Museum Papyrus 47.218.50*. Cairo.

Goyon, J.-C., 1984, "Räucherung", in W. Helck et al. (eds.), *Lexikon der Ägyptologie* 5, 83–85. Wiesbaden.

Green, M., 1987, "A Late Coptic Magical Text from the Collection of the Rijksmuseum van Oudheden, Leiden", *Oudheidkundige Mededelingen uit het Rijksmuseum van Oudheden te Leiden* 67, 29–43.

Griffith, F. L., 1900, *Stories of the High Priests of Memphis: The Sethon of Herodotus and The Demotic Tales of Khamuas*, Oxford.

Grinevald, C., and M. Bert, 2011, "Speakers and Communities", in P. K. Austin and J. Sallabank (eds.), *The Cambridge Handbook of Endangered Languages*, 45–65. Cambridge Handbooks in Language and Linguistics. Cambridge.

Grob, E. M., 2010, *Documentary Arabic Private and Business Letters on Papyrus: Form and Function, Content and Context*. Archiv für Papyrusforschung, Beiheft 29. Berlin and New York.

Guignard, C., 2009, "Sources et constitution des Géoponiques à la lumière des versions orientales d'Anatolius de Béryte et de Cassianus Bassus", in M. Wallraff and L. Mecella (eds.), *Die Kestoi des Julius Africanus und ihre Überlieferung*, 243–344. Texte und Untersuchungen zur Geschichte der altchristlichen Literatur 165. Berlin.

Guignard, C., 2014, "L'agriculture en syriaque: L'Anatolius Syriacus ('*Géoponiques syriaques*')", in E. Villey (ed.), *Les sciences en syriaque*, 215–252. Études syriaques 11. Paris.

Gundacker, R., 2019, "Ist ḥśjw-mw 'Wasserzauber' ein 'Älteres Kompositum'? Untersuchungen zu einem terminus technicus der ägyptischen lingua magica", *Lingua Aegyptia* 27, 77–129.

Guy, J.-C., 1993–2005, *Les apophtegmes des pères, Collection systématique*. Sources chrétiennes 387, 474, 498. Paris.

Harari, Y., 2017, *Jewish Magic: Before the Rise of Kabbalah*, translated by B. Stein. Raphael Patai Series in Jewish Folklore and Anthropology. Detroit.

Heim, R. M., 1893, "Incantamenta magica graeca latina", *Jahrbücher für classische Philologie* suppl. 19, 463–576.

Herbin, F. R., 1994, *Le livre de parcourir l'éternité*. Orientalia Lovaniensia analecta 58. Leuven.

Hevesi, K., 2018, "P. Stras. K 204 and K 205: An Unpublished Coptic Magical Collection from the Bibliothèque nationale et universitaire de Strasbourg", in S. Kiyanrad, C. Theis, and L. Willer (eds.), *Bild und Schrift auf 'magischen' Artefakten*, 49–118. Materiale Textkulturen 19. Berlin and Boston.

Hevesi, K., 2019, "A Few Remarks on the Persistence of Native Egyptian historiolae in Coptic Magical Texts", in M. Peterková Hlouchová, D. Belohoubková, J. Honzl, and V. Nováková (eds.), *Current Research in Egyptology 2018: Proceedings of the Nineteenth Annual Symposium, Czech Institute of Egyptology, Faculty of Arts, Charles University, Prague, 25–28 June 2018*, 42–54. Access Archaeology. Oxford.

Hickey, T. M., 2009, "Tebtunis on the Arno and Beyond: Two 'Archives'", in G. Bastianini and A. Casanova (eds.), *100 anni di istituzioni fiorentine per la papirologia*, 67–81. Studia e Testi di Papirologia n.s. 11. Florence.

Hickey, T. M., A. Maravela, and M. Zellmann-Rohrer, 2015, "Historical and Textual Notes on Magical Texts in the Papyrus Collection of the University of Oslo", *Symbolae Osloenses* 89, 156–182.

Hoch, J. E., 1994, *Semitic Words in Egyptian Texts of the New Kingdom and Third Intermediate Period*. Princeton.

Hoffmann, F., 1995, "Neue Fragmente zu den drei großen Inaros-Petubastis Texten", *Enchoria* 22, 27–39.

Hoppe, K., and E. Oder, 1927, *Corpus Hippiatricorum Graecorum* 2, Leipzig.

Houston, S. D., 2008, "The Small Deaths of Maya Writing", in J. Baines, J. Bennet, and S. D. Houston (eds.), *The Disappearance of Writing Systems: Perspectives on Literacy and Communication*, 231–252. Oakville, CT.

Hunt, T., 1990, *Popular Medicine in Thirteenth-Century England: Introduction and Texts*. Cambridge.

Janko, R., 2013, "The Hexametric Incantations against Witchcraft in the Getty Museum: From Archetype to Exemplar", in C. A. Faraone and D. Obbink (eds.), *The Getty Hexameters: Poetry, Magic, and Mystery in Ancient Selinous*, 31–56. Oxford.

Janssen, J. M. A., 1954, "Over farao Bocchoris", in Anonymous (ed.), *Varia historica: Aangeboden aan Professor Doctor A. W. Byvanck ter gelegenheid van zijn zeventigste verjaardag*, 17–29. Assen.

Jastrow, M., 1903, *A Dictionary of the Targumim, the Talmud Babli and Yerushalmi, and the Midrashic Literature*. London.

Johnson, J. H., 1975, "The Demotic Magical Spells of Leiden I 384", *Oudheidkundige mededelingen uit het Rijksmuseum van Oudheden* 56, 29–64.

Johnson, J. H., 1977, "Louvre E3229: A Demotic Magical Text", *Enchoria* 7, 55–102.

Johnston, S. I., 2008, *Ancient Greek Divination*. Blackwell Ancient Religions. Malden, MA and Oxford.

Jones, A. H. M., J. R. Martindale, and J. Morris, 1971, *The Prosopography of the Later Roman Empire* 1: *A.D. 260–395*. Cambridge.

Jones, P. M., 2007, "Amulets: Prescriptions and Surviving Objects from Late Medieval England", in S. Blick (ed.), *Beyond Pilgrim Souvenirs and Secular Badges: Essays in Honour of Brian Spencer*, 92–107. Oxford.

Jordan, D. R., 2006, "P.Duk.inv. 729: Magical Formulae", *Greek, Roman, and Byzantine Studies* 46, 159–173.

Jordan, D. R., H. Montgomery, and E. Thomassen, 1999, *The World of Ancient Magic: Papers from the First International Samson Eitrem Seminar at the Norwegian Institute at Athens, 4–8 May 1997*. Skrifter utgitt av det Norske institutt i Athen 4. Bergen.

Kaimakis, D. V., 1976, *Die Kyraniden*. Beiträge zur klassischen Philologie 76. Meisenheim am Glan.

Kákosy, L., 1971, "Ein magischer Papyrus des Kunsthistorischen Museums in Budapest", *Acta Antiqua Academiae Scientiarum Hungaricae* 19, 159–177. [Repr. in id., *Selected Papers (1956–73)*, 239–258 Studia Aegyptiaca 7. Études publiées par les chaires d'histoire ancienne de l'Universtié Loránd Eötvös de Budapest. Budapest, 1981.]

Kákosy, L., 1980, "Magische Stelen", W. Helck et al. (eds.), *Lexikon der Ägyptologie* 3, 1162–1164. Wiesbaden.

Kanavou, N., 2020, "Legal Narratives from a Late Antique Codex and the Ancient Novel Tradition", *Zeitschrift für Papyrologie und Epigraphik* 214, 80–86.

Kotansky, R., 1991, "Incantations and Prayers for Salvation on Inscribed Greek Amulets", in C. A. Faraone and D. Obbink (eds.), *Magika Hiera: Ancient Greek Magic and Religion*, 107–137. New York and Oxford.

Kotansky, R., 1995, "Greek Exorcistic Amulets", in M. Meyer and P. Mirecki (eds.), *Ancient Magic and Ritual Power*, 243–277. Religions in the Graeco-Roman World 129. Leiden.

Kotansky, R., P. Kovács, and P. Prohászka, 2015, "A Gold Lamella for Migraine from Aquincum", *Journal of Ancient Judaism* 6, 127–142.

Kropp, A., 1965, *Oratio Mariae ad Bartos: Ein koptischer Gebetstext aus den Giessener Papyrus-Sammlungen*. Berichte und Arbeiten aus der Universitätsbibliothek Giessen 7. Giessen.

Kropp, A., 1966, *Der Lobpreis des Erzengels Michael (vormals P. Heidelberg Inv. Nr. 1686)*. Brussels.

Kurth, D., 1986, "Wind", in W. Helck et al. (eds.), *Lexikon der Ägyptologie* 6, 1266–1272. Wiesbaden.

Lagarde, P., 1860, *Geoponicon in sermonem Syriacum versorum quae supersunt*. Leipzig.

Lagarde, P., 1867, *Der Pentateuch koptisch*. Leipzig.

Lalanne, B., and G. Métra, 2017. *Le texte médical du Papyrus Ebers*. Langues et cultures anciennes 28. Brussels.

Lange, H. O., 1927, *Der magische Papyrus Harris*. Historisk-filologiske meddelelser 14.2. Copenhagen.

Layton, B., 2000, *A Coptic Grammar with Chrestomathy and Glossary: Sahidic Dialect*. Porta linguarum orientalium n.S. 20. Wiesbaden.

Legendre, M., 2015, "Perméabilité linguistique et anthroponymique entre copte et arabe: L'exemple de comptes en caractères coptes du Fayoum fatimide", in C. Louis and T. S. Richter (eds.), *Coptica Argentoratensia: Textes et documents de la troisième université d'été de papyrologie copte (Strasbourg, 18–25 juillet 2010) (P. Stras. Copt.)*, 325–461. Cahiers de la Bibliothèque copte 19. Paris.

Leitz, C., 1999, *Magical and Medical Papyri of the New Kingdom*. Hieratic Papyri in the British Museum 7. London.

Lepper, V. M., 2008, *Untersuchungen zu pWestcar: Eine philologische und literaturwissenschaftliche (Neu-)Analyse*. Ägyptologische Abhandlungen 70. Wiesbaden.

Levene, D., D. Marx, and S. Bharyo, 2014, "Gabriel is on Their Right", *Studia Mesopotamica* 1, 185–198.

Lichtheim, M., 1976, *Ancient Egyptian Literature: A Book of Readings*. Volume 2: *The New Kingdom*. Berkeley.

Litinas, N., 2014, "Reading Aristophanes Amid the Sands of Egypt", *Chronique d'Égypte* 89, 325–348.

Love, E. O. D., 2016, *Code-switching with the Gods: The Bilingual (Old Coptic-Greek) Spells of PGM IV (P. Bibliothèque Nationale Supplément Grec. 574) and their Linguistic, Religious, and Socio-Cultural Context in Late Roman Egypt*. Zeitschrift für ägyptische Sprache und Altertumskunde, Beiheft 4. Berlin.

Love, E. O. D., 2017, "The "*PGM* III" Archive – Two Papyri, Two Scribes, Two Scripts, and Two Languages", *Zeitschrift für Papyrologie und Epigraphik* 202, 1–14.

Love, E. O. D., 2018/19a, "The Old Coptic of *PGM* IV: (Re)considerations on Readings, Scripts, and Transmission", *Enchoria* 36, 95–108.

Love, E. O. D., 2018/19b, "The Old Coptic of *PGM* IV: Fresh Parallels for Interscript and Intralingual Transmission", *Enchoria* 36, 109–115.

Love, E. O. D., 2020, "The Literary vs The Literal: The Narration of Magical Practices, Texts, and their Practitioners in Setne I and II Compared with the Co-called Demotic and Greek Magical Papyri", in F. Naether (ed.). *Cult Practices in Ancient Literatures: Egyptian, Near Eastern and Graeco-Roman Narratives in a Cross-cultural Perspective. Proceedings of a Workshop at the Institute for the Study of the Ancient World, New York, May 16–17, 2016*. ISAW Papers 18. <http://dlib.nyu.edu/awdl/isaw/isaw-papers/18/>.

Love, E. O. D., 2021a, *Script Switching in Roman Egypt: Case Studies in Script Conventions, Domains, Shift, and Obsolescence from Hieroglyphic, Hieratic, Demotic, and Old Coptic Manuscripts*. Archiv für Papyrusforschung, Beiheft 46. Berlin/Boston.

Love, E. O. D., 2021b, "The Nature of Old Coptic 1: Approaching & Contextualising Old Coptic (§§1–4); Old Coptic at Oxyrhynchus (§5)", *The Journal of Coptic Studies* 23, 91–143.

Love, E. O. D., fc. a, "GEMF 14 (BM EA 10808)", in C. A. Faraone and S. Torallas-Tovar (eds.), *Greek and Egyptian Magical Formularies: Text and Translation* Volume 1. Berkeley.

Love, E. O. D., fc. b, "A Coptic Curse on Lead (Köln T. 10)", in C. Armoni (ed.), *Kölner ägyptische Papyri (P. Köln ägypt.)*. Cologne.

Love, E. O. D., fc. c, "Bilingualism and 'Digraphia' at the Nexus of Magical Traditions: The Case Studies of Egyptian-Greek and Coptic-Arabic Bilingual Magical Texts from Roman, Coptic, and Islamic Egypt", in L. Berkes (ed.), *Christians and Muslims in Early Islamic Egypt*. American Studies in Papyrology. Ann Arbor.

Love, E. O. D., fc. d, "'Crum's Chicken': Alpak, Demonised Donkeys, and Avianised Demons among the Figures of Demotic, Greek, and Coptic Magical Texts", in K. Dosoo and J.-C. Coulon (eds.), *Magikon Zōon: Animal and Magic*.

Love, E. O. D., fc. e, *Petitioning Osiris: The Old Coptic Schmidt Papyrus and Curse of Artemisia in Context among the Letters to Gods from Egypt*. Zeitschrift für ägyptische Sprache und Altertumskunde, Beiheft. Berlin.

Love, E. O. D., and M. Zellmann-Rohrer, fc., "Releasing Everything Bound in the Knot: P.Saqqara inv. F.17.10", *Archiv für Papyrusforschung* 68 [2022].

Mariette, A., 1871, *Les papyrus égyptiens du Musée de Boulaq*. Paris.

Marshall, A., 2015, *Maternité et petite enfance en Égypte ancienne*. Monaco.

Martín Hernández, R., 2010, *Orfeo y los magos: La literatura órfica, la magia y los misterios*. Lecturas de historia. Madrid.

Martín Hernández, R., and S. Torallas Tovar, 2012, "'You Who Impose Sleep upon Abimelech for Seventy Two Years': An Egyptian Spell against Insomnia", in M. Piranomonte and F. M. Simón (eds.), *Contesti magici = Contextos mágicos: Convegno internazionale Contesti magici, contextos magicos (2009, Rome, Italy)*, 309–312. Rome.

Matthews, J., 2010. *Roman Perspectives: Studies in the Social, Political and Cultural History of the First to Fifth Centuries*. Swansea.

Matthews, P. H., 2007, *The Concise Oxford Dictionary of Linguistics*. Oxford.

Mercer, J., 2013, "Deliverance, Demonic Possession, and Mental Illness: Some Considerations for Mental Health Professionals", *Mental Health, Religion and Culture* 16, 595–611.

Meyer, M. W., 1996, *The Magical Book of Mary and the Angels (P. Heid. Inv. Kopt. 685)*. Veröffentlichungen aus der Heidelberger Papyrus-Sammlung n.F. 9. Heidelberg.

Meyer, M. W., and P. A. Mirecki, 1995, *Ancient Magic and Ritual Power*. Religions in the Graeco-Roman World 129. Leiden.

Meyer, M. W., and R. Smith, 1994, *Ancient Christian Magic: Coptic Texts of Ritual Power*. Princeton.

Meyerhoff, M., 2002. "Communities of Practice", in J. K. Chambers, P. Trudgill, and N. Schilling-Estes (eds.), *The Handbook of Language Variation and Change*, 526–548. Blackwell Handbooks in Linguistics. Chichester.

Meyrat, P., 2014, "The First Column of the Apis Embalming Ritual, Papyrus Zagreb 597–2", in J. F. Quack (ed.), *Ägyptische Rituale der griechisch-römischen Zeit*, 263–337. Orientalische Religionen in der Antike 6. Tübingen.

Michl, J., 1962, "Engel I–IX", in *Reallexikon für Antike und Christentum* 5, 53–258. Stuttgart.

Migahid, A., 1987, *Demotische Briefe an Götter von der Spät- bis zur Römerzeit: Ein Beitrag zur Kenntnis des religiösen Brauchtums im alten Ägypten*. Würzburg.

Mirecki, P. A., I. Gardner, and A. Alcock, 1997, "Magical Spell, Manichaean Letter", in P. Mirecki and J. BeDuhn (eds.), *Emerging from Darkness: Studies in the Recovery of Manichaean Sources*, 1–32. Nag Hammadi and Manichaean Studies 43. Leiden.

Mirecki, P. A., and M. W. Meyer, 2002, *Magic and Ritual in the Ancient World*. Religions in the Graeco-Roman World 141. Leiden.

Morenz, S., 1950, "Ägypten und die altorphische Kosmogonie", in S. Morenz (ed.), *Aus Antike und Orient: Festschrift Wilhelm Schubart zum 75. Geburtstag*, 64–111. Leipzig.

Mullany, L., 2006, "Speech Communities", in C. Llamas, L. Mullany, and P. Stockwell (eds.), *The Routledge Companion to Sociolinguistics*, 84–91. London.

Munier, H., 1930, *La scala copte 44 de la Bibliotheque nationale de Paris: Transcription et vocabulaire*. Bibliothèque d'études coptes 2. Cairo.

Möller, G., 1913, *Die beiden Totenpapyrus Rhind des Museums zu Edinburg*. Leipzig.

Müller, M., 2009, "Koptische magische Texte in Fribourg", in A. Giewekemeyer, G. Moers, and K. Widmaier (eds.), *Liber amicorum Jürgen Horn zum Dank*, 57–68. Göttinger Miszellen Beihefte 5. Göttingen.

Müller, M., 2017, Review of C. Ziegler, ed., *Les tombes hypogées* (etc.), *Journal of Egyptian Archaeology* 103, 129–131.

Nagel, S., 2019, *Isis im Römischen Reich*. Philippika 109. Wiesbaden.

Nicolotti, A., 2011, *Esorcismo cristiano e possessione diabolica tra II e III secolo*. Instrumenta patristica et mediaevalia 54. Turnhout.

Nie, F., and D. V. A. Olson, 2016, "Demonic Influence: The Negative Mental Health Effects of Belief in Demons", *Journal for the Scientific Study of Religion* 55, 498–515.

Niedermann, M., 1916, *Marcelli De medicamentis liber*. Corpus medicorum Latinorum 5. Leipzig.

Nongbri, B., 2014, "The Acquisition of the University of Michigan's Portion of the Chester Beatty Biblical Papyri and a New Suggested Provenance", *Archiv für Papyrusforschung* 60, 93–116.

Nongbri, B., 2018, *God's Library: The Archaeology of the Earliest Christian Manuscripts*. New Haven.

Nutton, V., 1977, "Archiatri and the Medical Profession in Antiquity", *Papers of the British School at Rome* 45, 191–226.

Oder, E., 1901, *Claudii Hermeri Mulomedicina Chironis*. Bibliotheca scriptorum Graecorum et Romanorum Teubneriana. Leipzig.

Oikonomu-Agorastu, I., 1982, *Kritische Erstausgabe des Rezeptsbuch des Cod. Par. gr. 2316, f. 348v–374v*. Thessaloniki.

Önnerfors, A., 1964, *Plinii Secundi Iunioris qui feruntur de medicina libri tres*. Corpus medicorum Latinorum 3. Berlin.

Önnerfors, A., 1993, "Magische Formeln im Dienste römischer Medizin", in *Aufstieg und Niedergang der römischen Welt* II.37.1, 157–224. Berlin.

Önnerfors, A., 2006, Physica *Plinii quae fertur Sangallensis (cod. Sang. 751 pp. 183 – 280)*. Lund.

Orsini, P., 2008, "La maiuscola biblica copta", *Segno e Testo* 6, 121–150.

Osing, J., 1976a, *Die Nominalbildung des Ägyptischen*. Mainz am Rhein.

Osing, J., 1976b, *Der spätägyptische Papyrus BM 10808*. Ägyptologische Abhandlungen 33. Wiesbaden.

Pache, C. O., 2004, *Baby and Child Heroes in Ancient Greece*. Traditions. Urbana, IL.

Pachoumi, E., 2017, *The Concepts of the Divine in the Greek Magical Papyri*. Studien und Texte zu Antike und Christentum 102. Tübingen.

Papaconstantinou, A. (ed.), 2009, *The Multilingual Experience in Egypt from the Ptolemies to the 'Abbāsids*. Farnham.

Papadopoulos-Kerameus, A., 1909, *Varia Graeca sacra: Sbornik grecheskich neizdannykh bogoslovskikh tekstov IV–XV vi͡ekov*. Zapiski ist.-filol. fak. Imp. S.-Peterburg. univ. 95. St. Petersburg.

Papathomas, A., 2000, "Das erste antike Zeugnis für die veterinärmedizinische Exzerptensammlung des Anatolios von Berytos", *Wiener Studien* 113, 138–146.

Parássoglou, G. M., 1974, "A Christian Amulet against Snakebite", *Studia Papyrologica* 13, 107–110.

Patrick, P. L., 2002, "The Speech Community", in J. K. Chambers, P. Trudgill, and N. Schilling-Estes (eds.), *The Handbook of Language Variation and Change*, 573–597. Blackwell Handbooks in Linguistics. Chichester.

Pedley, J. G., 2012, *The Life and Work of Francis Willey Kelsey: Archaeology, Antiquity, and the Arts*. Ann Arbor.

Pernigotti. S., 1979, "Nuovi papiri magici in copto, greco e aramaico", *Studi classici e orientali* 29, 19–53.

Pernigotti, S., 1993, "Una rilettura del P.Mil. Vogl. Copto 16", *Aegyptus* 73, 93–125.

Pernigotti, S., 1995, "La magia copta: I testi", in *Aufstieg und Niedergang der römischen Welt* II 18.5, 3386–3730. Berlin.

Peust, C., 1999, *Egyptian Phonology: An Introduction to the Phonology of a Dead Language*. Monographien zur ägyptischen Sprache 2. Göttingen.

Piechotta, J., 1887, *Ein anecdotum Latinum*. Programme Jahres-Bericht des Königlichen katholischen Gymnasiums zu Leobschütz über das Schuljahr 1886/87. Leobschütz.

Pierret, P., 1873, *Études Égyptologiques*. Paris.

Pietrogrande, A. L., and V. De Marco, 1938, "Construzioni d'epoca imperiale scoperte in Via di S. Basilio", *Atti della Accademia Nazionale dei Lincei, Notizie degli scavi di antichità*, ser. 16, 14, 351–425.

Podemann Sørensen, J., 1986, "Three Varieties of Ritual Drama", *Temenos* 22, 79–92.

Polotsky, H. J., 1937, "Zwei koptische Liebeszauber", *Orientalia* n.s. 6, 119–131.

Posener, G., 1980, *Catalogue des ostraca hiératiques littéraires de Deir el Médineh*. Tome III.3: *Nos. 1607–1675*. Documents de fouilles 20. Cairo.

Pye, H. J., 1807, *The Sportsman's Dictionary, Containing Instructions for Various Methods to Be Observed in Riding, Hunting, Fowling, Setting, Fishing, Racing, Farriery, Breeding and Feeding Horses for the Road and Turf; the Management of Dogs, Game and Dunghill-cocks, Turkeys, Geese, Ducks, Doves, Singing-birds, etc.; and the Manner of Curing Their Various Diseases and Accidents*, 5th ed. London.

Quack, J. F., 1998, "Kontinuität und Wandel in der spätägyptischen Magie", *Studi Epigrafici e Linguistici* 15, 77–94.

Quack, J. F., 2001, "Ein Standardhymnus zum Sistrumspiel auf einem demotischen Ostrakon (Ostrakon Corteggiani D 1)", *Enchoria* 27, 101–119.

Quack, J. F., 2003, "'Ich bin Isis, die Herrin der beiden Länder' – Versuch zum demotischen Hintergrund der memphitischen Isisaretalogie", in S. Meyer (ed.), *Egypt – Temple of the Whole World – Ägypten – Tempel der gesamten Welt: Studies in Honour of Jan Assmann*, 319–366. Studies in the History of Religions 97. Leiden.

Quack, J. F., 2004, "Griechische und andere Dämonen in den spätdemotischen magischen Texten", in S. Thomas (ed.), *Das Ägyptische und die Sprachen Vorderasiens, Nordafrikas und der Ägäis: Akten des Basler Kolloquiums zum ägytisch-nichtsemitischen Sprachkontakt, Basel 9.–11. Juli 2003*, 427–507. Alter Orient und Altes Testament 310. Münster.

Quack, J. F., 2008, "Demotische magische und divinatorische Texte", in B. Janowski and G. Wilhelm (eds.), *Omina, Orakel, Rituale und Beschwörungen*, 331–385. Texte aus der Umwelt des Alten Testaments n.F. 4. Gütersloh.

Quack, J. F., 2009, *Einführung in die altägyptische Literaturgeschichte* III: *Die demotische und gräko-ägyptische Literatur*, 2nd ed. Einführungen und Quellentexte zur Ägyptologie 6. Münster.

Quack, J. F., 2010, "Inhomogenität von ägyptischer Sprache und Schrift in Texten aus dem späten Ägypten", in K. Lembke, M. Minas-Nerpel, and S. Pfeiffer (eds.), *Tradition and Transformation: Egypt under Roman Rule. Proceedings of the International Conference, Hildesheim, Roemer- and Pelizaeus-Museum, 3–6 July 2008*, 313–341. Culture and History of the Ancient Near East 41. Leiden.

Quack, J. F., 2011. "From Ritual to Magic. Ancient Egyptian Forerunners of the Charitesion and their Social Setting", in G. Bohak, Y. Harari, and S. Shaked (eds.), *Continuity and Innovation in the Magical Tradition*, 43–84. Jerusalem Studies in Religion and Culture 15. Leiden.

Quack, J. F., 2013, "Zauber ohne Grenzen: Zur Transkulturalität der spätantiken Magie", in A. H. Pries, L. Martzolff, R. Langer, and C. Ambos, (eds.), *Rituale als Ausdruck von Kulturkontakt, "Synkretismus" zwischen Negation und Neudefinition*, 177–199. Studies in Oriental Religions 67. Wiesbaden.

Quack, J. F., 2016a, "Translating the Realities of Cult", in I. Rutherford (ed.), *Greco-Egyptian Interactions: Literature, Translation, and Culture, 500 BCE–300 CE*, 267–286. Oxford and New York.

Quack, J. F., 2016b, "The Last Stand? What Remains Egyptian in Oxyrhynchus", in K. S. B. Ryholt and G. Barjamovic (eds.), *Problems of Canonicity and Identity Formation in Ancient Egypt and Mesopotamia*, 105–126. CNI Publications 43. Copenhagen.

Quack, J. F., 2017, "How the Coptic Script Came About", in E. Grossman, P. Dils, T. S. Richter, and W. Schenkel, (eds.), *Greek Influence on Egyptian-Coptic: Contact-Induced Change in an Ancient African Language (DDGLC Working Papers 1)*, 27–96. Lingua Aegyptia Studia Monographica 17. Hamburg.

Quack, J. F., 2019a, "From Egyptian Traditions to Magical Gems: Possibilities and Pitfalls in Scholarly Analysis", in K. Endreffy, Á. Nagy, and J. Spier (eds.), *Magical Gems and Their Contexts*, 233–249. Studia archaeologica 229. Rome.

Quack, J. F., 2019b, "Ein demotisch und altkoptisch überliefertes Losorakel", in J. F. Quack and K. Ryholt (eds.), *Demotic Literary Texts from Tebtunis and Beyond*, 285–353. CNI Publications 36. The Carlsberg Papyri 11. Copenhagen.

Quack, J. F., 2020, *Altägyptische Amulette und ihre Handhabung*. Orientalische Religionen in der Antike 31. Wiesbaden.

Quack, J. F., and K. Ryholt, 2000, "Notes on the Setne Story P. Carlsberg 207", in P. J. Frandsen and K. Ryholt (eds.), *A Miscellany of Demotic Texts and Studies*, 141–163. CNI Publications 22. The Carlsberg Papyri 3. Copenhagen.

Quaegebeur, J., 1975, *Le dieu égyptien Shaï dans la religion et l'onomastique*. Orientalia Lovaniensia analecta 2. Leuven.

Ray, J. D., 1978, "The Non-Literary Material from North Saqqâra: A Short Progress Report", *Enchoria* 8 Sonderband, 29–30.

Ray, J. D., 2011, *Texts from the Baboon and Falcon Galleries: Demotic, Hieroglyphic and Greek Inscriptions from the Sacred Animal Necropolis, North Saqqara*, ed. C. J. Martin. Texts from Excavations 15. London.

Ray, J. D., 2013, *Demotic Ostraca and Other Inscriptions from the Sacred Animal Necropolis, North Saqqara*. Texts from Excavations 16. London.

Reggiani, N., 2018, "I papiri greci di medicina come fonti storiche: Il caso dei rapporti dei medici pubblici nell'Egitto romano e bizantino", *Aegyptus* 98, 107–130.

Reggiani, N. (ed.), 2019, *Greek Medical Papyri: Text, Context, Hypertext*. Archiv für Papyrusforschung, Beiheft 40. Berlin.

Reitzenstein, R., 1904, *Poimandres: Studien zur griechisch-ägyptischen und frühchristlichen Literatur*. Leipzig.

Richter, T. S., 2002, "Miscellanea Magica", *Journal of Egyptian Archaeology* 88, 247–252.

Richter, T. S., 2003, "Spätkoptische Rechtsurkunden neu bearbeitet (III): P.Lond.Copt. I 487: Arabische Pacht in Koptischem Gewand", *Journal of Juristic Papyrology* 33, 213–230.

Richter, T. S., 2007, "Miscellanea magica, III: Ein vertauschter Kopf? Konjekturvorschlag für P. Berlin P 8313 ro, col. II, 19–20", *Journal of Egyptian Archaeology* 93, 259–263.

Richter, T. S., 2009, "Greek, Coptic and the 'Language of the Hijra': The Rise and Decline of the Coptic Language in Late Antique and Medieval Egypt", in H. M. Cotton, R. G. Hoyland, J. J. Price, and D. J. Wasserstein (eds.), *From Hellenism to Islam: Cultural and Linguistic Change in the Roman Near East*, 401–446. Cambridge.

Richter, T. S., 2014, "Neue koptische medizinische Rezepte", *Zeitschrift für ägyptische Sprache und Altertumskunde* 141, 154–194.

Richter, T. S., 2017, "Medical Care on the Theban Westbank in Late Antiquity", *Journal of Coptic Studies* 19, 151–163.

Richter, T. S., 2020, "P.Berlin P.8316 (= BKU I, 21), ein koptisches Rezept zur Purpur-Imitation durch Krapp-Färbung auf gebeizter Wolle", *Journal of Coptic Studies* 22, 151–186.

Ritner, R. K., 1993, *The Mechanics of Ancient Egyptian Magical Practice*. Studies in Ancient Oriental Civilization 54. Chicago.

Ritner, R. K., 1995, "Egyptian Magical Practice under the Roman Empire: The Demotic Spells and their Religious Context", in *Aufstieg und Niedergang der römischen Welt* II.18, 3333–3379. Berlin.

Ritner, R. K., 1998, "The Wives of Horus and the Philinna Papyrus (PGM XX)", in W. Clarysse, A. Schoors, and H. Willems, (eds.), *Egyptian Religion: The Last Thousand Years. Studies Dedicated to the Memory of Jan Quaegebeur*, 1027–1041. Leuven.

Romano, R., 1994, "Ricette superstiziose ed esorcismi ginecologici nella tradizione di Aezio Amideno", in C. Curti and C. Crimi (eds.), *Scritti classici e cristiani offerti a Francesco Corsaro*, 595–600. Catania.

Rose, V., 1894, *Theodori Prisciani Euporiston libri III cum physicorum fragmento et additamentis pseudo-Theodoreis*. Bibliotheca scriptorum Graecorum et Romanorum Teubneriana. Leipzig.

Ross, M. C., 1965, *Catalogue of the Byzantine and Early Mediaeval Antiquities in the Dumbarton Oaks Collection* 2. Washington, DC.

Roth, A. M., 1992, "The psš-kf and the 'Opening of the Mouth' Ceremony: A Ritual of Birth and Rebirth", *Journal of Egyptian Archaeology* 78, 113–147.

Roth, A. M., and C. H. Roehrig, 2002, "Magical Bricks and the Bricks of Birth", *Journal of Egyptian Archaeology* 88, 121–139.

Rumpf, H., 1866, "Ein Amulet des Museums zu Wiesbaden", *Neue Jahrbücher für Philologie und Paedagogik* 93, 716–720.

Sarrazin, R. B., 2017a, "Catalogue des textes magiques coptes", *Archiv für Papyrusforschung* 63, 367–408.

Sarrazin, R. B., 2017b, "Une malédiction copte sur un ostracon d'Antinoupolis", *Analecta Papyrologica* 29, 119–22.

Satzinger, H., 1975, "The Old Coptic Schmidt Papyrus", *Journal of Egyptian Archaeology* 12, 37–50.

Satzinger, H., 1994, "An Old Coptic Text Reconsidered: PGM 94 ff.", in S. Giversen, M. Krause, P. Nagel, and R. Kasser (eds.), *Coptology: Past, Present, and Future. Studies in Honour of Rodolphe Kasser*, 213–224. Orientalia Lovaniensia analecta 61. Leuven.

Satzinger, H., and P. J. Sijpesteijn, 1988, "Koptisches Zauberpergament Moen III", *Le Muséon* 101, 51–63.

Schäfer, P., and H. G. Kippenberg, 1997, *Envisioning Magic: A Princeton Seminar and Symposium*. Studies in the History of Religions 75. Leiden.

Schönbach, A., 1893, "Eine Auslese altdeutscher Segensformeln", in *Analecta Graeciensia. Festschrift zur 42. Versammlung deutscher Philologen und Schulmänner in Wien 1893*, 25–50. Graz.

Sethe, K., 1929, *Amun und die acht Urgötter von Hermopolis: Eine Untersuchung über Ursprung und Wesen des ägyptischen Götterkönigs*. Abhandlungen der Preussischen Akademie der Wissenschaften. Philosophisch-historische Klasse. Berlin.

Shaked, S., 2005, *Officina Magica: Essays on the Practice of Magic in Antiquity*. IJS Studies in Judaica 4. Leiden.

Sigerist, H., 1923, *Studien und Texte zur frühmittelalterlichen Rezeptliteratur*. Studien zur Geschichte der Medizin 13. Leipzig.

Smith, M., 1993, *The Liturgy of Opening the Mouth for Breathing*. Oxford.

Smith, M., 2002, *On the Primaeval Ocean*. Carlsberg Papyri 5. CNI Publications 26. Copenhagen.

Smith, M., 2005, *P. Harkness (MMA 31.9.7)*. Oxford.

Smith, M., 2009, *Traversing Eternity: Texts for the Afterlife from Ptolemaic and Roman Egypt*. Oxford.

Smith, M., 2017, *Following Osiris: Perspectives on the Osirian Afterlife from Four Millenia*. Oxford.

Sorensen, E., 2002, *Possession and Exorcism in the New Testament and Early Christianity*. Wissenschaftliche Untersuchungen zum Neuen Testament. 2. Reihe 157. Tübingen.

Spiegelberg, W., 1911, "Aus der Strassburger Sammlung demotischer Ostraka", *Zeitschrift für ägyptische Sprache und Altertumskunde* 49, 33–41.

Spiegelberg, W., 1917a, *Der ägyptische Mythus vom Sonnenauge (der Papyrus der Tierfabeln-"Kufi") nach dem Leidener demotischen Papyrus I 384*. Strasbourg.

Spiegelberg, W., 1917b, "Varia", *Zeitschrift für ägyptische Sprache und Altertumskunde* 53, 91–115.

Spier, J., 1993, "Medieval Byzantine Magical Amulets and Their Tradition", *Journal of the Warburg and Courtauld Institutes* 56, 25–62.

Stadler, M. A., 2004, *Isis, das göttliche Kind und die Weltordnung: Neue religiöse Texte aus dem Fayum nach dem Papyrus Wien D. 12006 Recto*. MPER n.S. 28.2. Wien.

Stadler, M. A., 2017a, *Théologie et culte au temple de Soknopaios: études sur la religion d'un village égyptien pendant l'époque romaine*. Paris.

Stadler, M. A., 2017b, "New Light on the Universality of Isis (pVienna D. 6297+6329+10101)", in S. Nagel, J. F. Quack, and C. Witschel (eds.), *Entangled Worlds: Religious Confluences between East and West in the Roman Empire*, 232–243. Orientalische Religionen in der Antike 22. Tübingen.

Stanford, M. S., 2007, "Demon or Disorder: A Survey of Attitudes toward Mental Illness in the Christian Church", *Mental Health, Religion and Culture* 10, 445–449.

Stegemann, V., 1934, *Die koptischen Zaubertexte der Sammlung Papyrus Erzherzog Rainer in Wien*. Sitzungsberichte der Heidelberger Akademie der Wissenschaften, Philosophisch-historisch Klasse. Heidelberg.

Sudhoff, K., 1917, "Codex medicus Hertensis (Nr. 192)", *Archiv für Geschichte der Medizin* 10, 265–313.

Tait, W. J., 1991, "P. Carlsberg 207: Two Columns of a Setna-text", in P. J. Frandsen (ed.), *Demotic Texts from the Collection*, 19–46. The Carlsberg Papyri 1. CNI Publications 15. Copenhagen.

Teeter, E., 2011, *Religion and Ritual in Ancient Egypt*. Cambridge.

Thissen, H. J. 1991. "Nubien in demotischen magischen Texten", in D. Mendel and C. Ulrike (eds.), *Ägypten im Afro-Orientalischen Kontext: Aufsätze zur Archäologie, Geschichte und Sprache eines unbegrenzten Raumes: Gedenkschrift Peter Behrens*, 369–376. Afrikanistische Arbeitspapiere. Cologne.

Thompson, D. J., 2009, "The Multilingual Environment of Persian and Ptolemaic Egypt: Egyptian, Aramaic, and Greek Documentation", in R. S. Bagnall (ed.), *The Oxford Handbook of Papyrology*, 395–417. Oxford.

Thompson, H., 1931, "Magical Texts from a Bilingual Papyrus in the British Museum", *Proceedings of the British Academy* 17, 235–287.

Till, W. C., 1935, "Zu den Wiener koptischen Zaubertexten", *Orientalia* n.s. 4, 195–221.

Till, W. C., 1943, "Bemerkungen zu koptischen Textausgaben 7–8", *Orientalia* n.s. 12, 327–337.

Till, W. C., 1951a, *Die Arzneikunde der Kopten*. Berlin.

Till, W. C., 1951b, "Eine koptische Rezeptsammlung", *Le Muséon* 64, 69–81.

Till, W. C., 1955, "Zum Sprachtabu im Ägyptischen", in O. Firchow (ed.), *Ägyptologische Studien*, 322–337. Deutsche Akademie der Wissenschaften zu Berlin, Institut für Orientforschung, Veröffentlichung 29. Berlin.

Till, W. C., 1961, *Koptische Grammatik (Saïdischer Dialekt)*, 2nd ed. Lehrbücher für das Studium der orientalischen und afrikanischen Sprachen 1. Leipzig.

Töpfer, S., 2014, "The Physical Activity of Parturition in Ancient Egypt: Textual and Epigraphical Sources", *Dynamis* 34, 317–335.

Töpfer, S., 2015, *Das Balsamierungsritual: Eine (Neu-)Edition der Textkomposition Balsamierungsritual (pBoulaq 3, pLouvre 5158, pDurham 1983.11 + pSt. Petersburg 18128)*. Studien zur spätägyptischen Religion 13. Wiesbaden.

Torallas Tovar, S., R. Martín Hernández, and E. O. D. Love, fc., "GEMF 55 = *PGM* III.1 & III.2", in C. Faraone and S. Torallas-Tovar (eds.), *Greek and Egyptian Magical Formularies: Text and Translation* Volume 2. Berkeley.

Tremel, J., 2004, *Magica agonistica: Fluchtafeln im antiken Sport*. Nikephoros Beiheft 10. Hildesheim.

Turner, E. G., 1977, *The Typology of the Early Codex*. Haney Foundation Series 18. Philadelphia.

van den Broek, R., 2017, "A Greek Iatromagical Papyrus", *Zeitschrift für Papyrologie und Epigraphik* 202, 208–213.

van der Vliet, J., 1991, "Varia Magica Coptica", *Aegyptus* 71, 217–242.

van der Vliet, J., 2000, "Les anges du soleil: A propos d'un texte magique copte récemment découvert à Deir-en-Naqloun (N. 45/95)", in N. Bosson (ed.), *Études coptes* VII: *Neuvième journeé d'études, Montpellier 3–4 juin 1999*, 319–337. Cahiers de la bibliothèque copte 12. Paris and Leuven.

van der Vliet, J., 2018, "Charming a Clogged Nose: A Late Coptic Magical Spell", *Journal of Ancient Near Eastern Religions* 18, 145–166.

van Minnen, P., 1995, "Medical Care in Late Antiquity", in P. J. van der Eijk, H. F. J. Horstmanshoff, and P. H. Schrijvers (eds.), *Ancient Medicine in its Socio-Cultural Context: Papers Read at the Congress Held at Leiden University, 13–15 April 1992* I, 153–169. Clio Medica 27. Amsterdam and Atlanta.

Veldhuis, N., 1991, *A Cow of Sîn*. Library of Oriental Texts, first series, 2. Groningen.

Vittmann, G. 1996. "Semitisches Sprachgut im Demotischen", *Wiener Zeitschrift für die Kunde des Morgenlandes* 86, 435–447.

Vleeming, S. P., 1990, "Transliterating Old Egyptian in Demotic", *Göttinger Miszellen* 117/118, 219–223.

Vleeming, S. P., 2004, "A Hieroglyphic-Demotic Stela from Akhmin", in F. Hoffmann and H. J. Thissen (eds.), Res severa verum gaudium: *Festschrift für Karl-Theodor Zauzich zum 65. Geburtstag am 8. Juni 2004*, 623–637. Studia demotica 6. Leuven.

Walters, C. C., 1989, "Christian Paintings from Tebtunis", *Journal of Egyptian Archaeology* 75, 191–208.

Wasserman, N., 2018, "Labor Pains, Difficult Birth, Sick Child: Three Old Babylonian Incantations from a Private Collection", *Bibliotheca Orientalis* 75, 14–25.

Weber, M., 1972, "Ein koptischer Zaubertext aus der Kölner Papyrussammlung", *Enchoria* 2, 55–61.

Wespi, F., 2017, "Das Bücherhaus (Pr-mḏꜣ.t) des späten ägyptischen Tempels", in S. Baumann and H. Kockelmann (eds.), *Der ägyptische Tempel als ritueller Raum: Theologie und Kult in ihrer architektonischen und ideellen Dimension. Akten der internationalen Tagung, Haus der Heidelberger Akademie der Wissenschaften, 9.–12. Juni 2015*, 271–287. Wiesbaden.

Westendorf, W., 1965–1977, *Koptisches Handwörterbuch*. Heidelberg.

Whitehorne, J., 1995, "The Pagan Cults of Roman Oxyrhynchus", in *Aufstieg und Niedergang der römischen* Welt II.18.5, 3050–3091. Berlin.

Wilfong, T. G., 1999, "Agriculture among the Christian Population of Early Islamic Egypt: Practice and Theory", *Proceedings of the British Academy* 96, 217–235.

Wilkinson, R. J., 2015, *Tetragrammaton: Western Christians and the Hebrew Name of God, from the Beginnings to the Seventeenth Century*. Studies in the History of Christian Traditions 179. Leiden.

Wilson, P., 1997, *A Ptolemaic Lexikon: A Lexicographical Study of the Texts in the Temple of Edfu*. Orientalia Lovaniensia analecta 78. Leuven.

Worrell, W. H., 1930, "A Coptic Wizard's Hoard", *American Journal of Semitic Languages and Literatures* 46, 239–262.

Worrell, W. H., 1935a, "Coptic Magical and Medical Texts", *Orientalia* n.s. 4, 1–37.

Worrell, W. H., 1935b, "Coptic Magical and Medical Texts (Continued)", *Orientalia* n.s. 4, 184–194.

Worrell, W. H., 1941, "Notice of a Second-Century Text in Coptic Letters", *American Journal of Semitic Languages and Literatures* 58, 84–90.

Wortley, J., 2010, "The Repertoire of Byzantine 'Spiritually Beneficial Tales'", *Scripta & e-Scripta* 8–9, 93–306.

Wright, J., 2015, "Between Despondency and the Demon: Diagnosing and Treating Spiritual Disorders in John Chrysostom's Letter to Stageirios", *Journal of Late Antiquity* 8, 352–367.

Wünsch, R., 1898, *Sethianische Verfluchungstafeln aus Rom*. Leipzig.

Zakrzewska, E. D., 2015, "L* as a Secret Language: Social Functions of Early Coptic", in G. Gabra and H. N. Takla (eds.), *Christianity and Monasticism in Middle Egypt: Al-Minya and Asyut*, 185–198. Cairo and New York.

Zandee, J., 1947, *De hymnen aan Amon van Papyrus Leiden I 350*. Oudheidkundige mededelingen uit het Rijksmuseum van Oudheden te Leiden, nieuwe reeks, 28. Leiden.

Zauzich, K.-T., 1983, "Das Lamm des Bokchoris", in *Festschrift zum 100-jährigen Bestehen der Papyrussammlung der Österreichischen Nationalbibliothek, Papyrus Erzherzog Rainer*, 165–174. Vienna.

Zellmann-Rohrer, M., 2015a, "Protective Iambic Incantations on Two Inscribed Octagonal Rings", *Greek, Roman, and Byzantine Studies* 55, 250–255.

Zellmann-Rohrer, M., 2015b, "Three Magical Papyri from the Michigan Collection", *Zeitschrift für Papyrologie und Epigraphik* 194, 176–192.

Zellmann-Rohrer, M., 2016, "Homeric and Pharmacologic Medical Recipes in a Greek Papyrus Formulary", *Bulletin of the American Society of Papyrologists* 53, 5–16.

Zellmann-Rohrer, M., 2017a, "Seth on Mount Sinai: A Coptic Magical Formulary with a Prayer and Theophany of the Biblical Seth", *Zeitschrift für ägyptische Sprache und Altertumskunde* 144, 240–254.

Zellmann-Rohrer, M., 2017b, "Five Private Letters on Papyrus in the British Library", *Archiv für Papyrusforschung* 63, 135–170.

Zellmann-Rohrer, M., 2018, "'Psalms Useful for Everything': Byzantine and Post-Byzantine Manuals for the Amuletic Use of the Psalter", *Dumbarton Oaks Papers* 72, 113–168.

Zellmann-Rohrer, M., 2019a, "Incantations in Byzantine and Post-Byzantine Greek: Change and Continuity", in L. M. Bortolani, W. Furley, S. Nagel, and J. F. Quack (eds.), *Cultural Plurality in Ancient Magical Texts and Practices: Graeco-Egyptian Handbooks and Related Traditions*, 276–297. Orientalische Religionen in der Antike 32. Tübingen.

Zellmann-Rohrer, M., 2019b, "The Woman Who Gave Her Breast for Hire: Notes on a Christian Wall-Painting from Tebtunis", *Journal of Egyptian Archaeology* 105, 297–303.

Zellmann-Rohrer, M., 2020a, "Notes on Magical Handbooks", *Zeitschrift für Papyrologie und Epigraphik* 215, 27–50.

Zellmann-Rohrer, M., 2020b, "The Text and Traditional Context of the 'Hay Cookbook' and Associated Magical Texts on Leather", in C. Graves (ed.), *BEC 4: Proceedings of the Fourth British Egyptology Congress, University of Manchester, 7–9 September 2018*, 169–179. London.

Zellmann-Rohrer, M., 2020c, "Tantalus and Hemorrhage: An Inscribed Hematite Gem and Its Tradition", in E. Mackil and N. Papazarkadas (eds.), *Epigraphy and Religion: Papers in Memory of Sara B. Aleshire from the Second North American Congress of Greek and Latin Epigraphy*, 310–334. Brill Studies in Greek and Roman Epigraphy 16. Leiden.

Zellmann-Rohrer, M., 2020d, "More on the Tradition of Amulet Pattern-Books in Post-Ancient Copies?", *Kernos* 33, 187–201.

Zellmann-Rohrer, M., 2020e, "A Lawsuit with a Headless Adversary: A Greek Incantation Motif", *Archiv für Religionsgeschichte* 21/22, 51–83.

Zellmann-Rohrer, M., 2021, " More on the 'Book of Protection' and the Syriac 'Charms:' New Texts and Perspectives for the Study of Magic and Religion", in S. Bhayro and M. Moriggi (eds.), *Studies in the Syriac Magical Traditions*, 77–140. Leiden.

Zellmann-Rohrer, M., and D. Martínez-Chico, 2021, "A Sicilian Amulet in Madrid and its Tradition", *Greek, Roman, and Byzantine Studies* 61, 62–72.

Ziegler, C., 2013, *Les tombes hypogées de basse époque, F 7, F 17, H, j1, Q, n1*. Fouilles du Louvre à Saqqara 2. Leuven.

Appendices

Concordance of Codex Page and Line Numbers with Worrell's Sequential Line Numbers

§	Page & Line Numbers	Worrell's Line Numbers
1	p. 2 ll. 1–9	1–9
2	p. 2 ll. 10–17	10–17
3	p. 2 l. 17–p. 3 l. 15	17–34
4	p. 3 ll. 15–19	34–38
5	p. 3 ll. 19–21	38–40
6	p. 4 ll. 1–12	41–52
7	p. 4 ll. 13–15	53–55
8	p. 4 ll. 16–19	56–59
9	p. 5 l. 1–p. 6 l. 5	60–84
10	p. 6 l. 6–p. 7 l. 11	85–110
11	p. 7 ll. 11–15	110–114
12	p. 7 l. 16–p. 8 l. 4	115–123
13	p. 8 ll. 5–13	124–132
14	p. 9 ll. 1–17 + p. 10 ll. 7–11	133–149 + 156–160
15	p. 10 ll. 1–6	150–155
16	p. 10 ll. 12–16	161–165
17	p. 10 ll. 16–19	165–168
18	p. 11 ll. 1–8	169–175
19	p. 11 ll. 9–15	176–182
20	p. 12 ll. 1–4	183–186
21	p. 12 ll. 4–11	186–193
22	p. 12 ll. 12–13	194–195
23	p. 12 ll. 13–16	195–198
24	p. 12 ll. 16–18	198–200
25	p. 12 ll. 18–20	200–202
26	p. 13 ll. 1–3	203–205
27	p. 13 ll. 3–5	205–207
28	p. 13 ll. 5–8	207–210
29	p. 13 ll. 8–10	210–212
30	p. 13 ll. 10–18	212–220
31	p. 14 ll. 1–20	221–240

Re-edition of Saqqara inv. F.17.10

As noted in **Transmitting Textual Traditions** and the excursus to §9, a re-edition of P.Saqqara inv. F.17.10 is provided here to reflect new readings and interpretation, now discussed at more length in a forthcoming article (Love and Zellmann-Rohrer fc.). While Favrelle's ed.pr. contained several unresolved problems, as well as grammatical and phonological peculiarities, and Müller's suggested corrections fell short of a re-edition of the text, the most recent edition by van der Vliet also contained some grammatical problems that were not addressed or resolved in the apparatus and textual commentary provided, and also fell short of providing a translation that made complete sense of the text.

Dimensions: 12.4 in height, 6.5 cm in width[815]
Condition: Complete. A number of horizontal creases are evident, but the exact number is hard to discern from the published photograph[816]
Date: c. 801–1000 CE (Favrelle in Ziegler 2013, 460); c. 951–1000[817] CE (Müller 2017, 130); c. 901–1100[818] CE (van der Vliet 2018, 146); c. 951–1100 CE is favored because paper was scarcely used in Egypt before the mid-10th century (Grob 2010)
Dialect: Sahidic (non-standard)
Phonetic features: Prevalence of long vowels, i.e. ⲱ for ⲟ;[819] absence of assimilation,[820] consider ⲛⲡⲉⲙⲁ (l. 10) yet ⲙⲡⲱⲟⲩ (ll. 10–11); doubling/ germination of ⲛ,[821] which—in our judgement—is erroneous; absence of superlineation[822]

ⲟⲩⲛⲧⲏⲟⲩ ⲙ̣ⲛⲧⲏⲟⲩ
ⲟⲩⲛϩⲱⲓⲙ ⲙⲛϩⲱⲓⲙ
ⲡⲉϩⲣⲱⲟⲩ ⲛⲥⲁϣϥⲉ
ⲛⲛⲁⲡⲏ ⲛ̣ϩⲱ̣ϥ̣ ⲁⲩⲉⲓ
ϩⲣⲁï ϩⲙ ⲡ̣ⲓ̣ⲱⲙ ⲉⲃⲟⲗ
ⲉⲃⲟⲗ ⲛϩⲱ̣ ⲛⲓⲙ ⲉⲧⲙⲏ-
ⲣ ϩⲛ ϫⲓⲥⲉ ϫⲉ ⲙⲛϩⲱϥ

[815] Favrelle in Ziegler 2013, 21; 460; Müller 2017, 130; van der Vliet 2018, 146.

[816] Three horizontal and one vertical creases (Müller 2017, 130); folded several times widthwise (van der Vliet 2018, 146).

[817] Based on the morphology of ⲙ, ⲟ, and ϕ.

[818] Van der Vliet did not provide any reasoning as to why he did not agree with Müller's more specific date.

[819] As noted in Favrelle in Ziegler 2013, 460; Müller 2017, 130–131; van der Vliet 2018, 146. For this, see *P.Bal.* I, §44.

[820] As noted in Favrelle in Ziegler 2013, 460; Müller 2017, 131.

[821] Favrelle in Ziegler 2013, 460; Müller 2017, 131. For this, see *P.Bal.* I, §80; §92.

[822] As noted in van der Vliet 2018, 146. For this, see *P.Bal.* I, §85.

ⲙⲏⲣ ⲙⲛϣⲉ ⲛⲁⲧⲱⲙ ϩⲛⲟ`ⲩ´-
ⲛ ϫⲓⲥⲉ ϫⲉ ⲁ̣ⲫⲱϥ ⲧ̣ⲃⲏⲗ
ϫⲱⲕ ⲕⲏ ⲛⲁⲕ̣ ⲛⲡⲉⲙⲁ ⲙ-
ⲡⲱⲟⲩ ⲉ̣̅ⲓ̅ⲁ̅ⲱ̣̅ ⲡⲉⲧⲃⲟⲗ
ⲙⲙⲱⲕ `ⲁ̣´ⲁ̣ⲱⲛⲉ ⲡⲉⲧ-
ⲕⲱ ⲙⲙⲱⲕ ⲉⲃⲟⲗ ⲉⲗ-
ϣⲉ ⲡⲉⲧ†ϩⲓⲏ ⲛⲁⲕ
ⲉⲛⲁϩⲙⲉⲕ ⲛⲧⲉⲓⲟⲩ-
ⲛⲟⲩ ⲇ̣ⲇ̣

[1] There is wind, there is no wind; [2] there is wave, there is no wave; [3] the seven voices [4] of the snake heads, they came [5] up from the sea (or, Fayum) to release [6] everything (or, every face) that is bound [7] in (the) knot, for nothing (or, no snake) is bound [8], no wood shall be sharp in [9] (the) knot, for the snake that is unbound [10] has completed another for you here [11] (and) today. It is Eiao who loosens [12] you. It is Adone who [13] releases you. It is Eloe [14] who gives (a) path for you [15] to save (or, preserve) yourself [16] immediately, (oh) NN.

2 ϩⲱⲓⲙ i.e. Sahidic ϩⲟⲉⲓⲙ (twice) **3** ⲡⲉ : ⲉ Favrelle ϩⲣⲱⲟⲩ i.e. Sahidic ϩⲣ(ⲟ)ⲟⲩ ⲡⲉϩⲣⲱⲟⲩ ⲛⲥⲁϣϥⲉ : ⲡⲉϩⲣⲱⲟⲩ ⲛ<ⲧ>ⲥⲁϣϥⲉ Müller "the sound of <the> seven" **4** ⲛⲛⲁⲡⲏ: l. ⲛⲁⲡⲉ Müller and van der Vliet "the sound of seven snake heads" ϩⲱϥ i.e. Sahidic ϩⲟϥ **5** ϩⲣⲁ̈ⲓ i.e. Sahidic ⲉϩⲣⲁ̈ⲓ (haplography) : ⲉϩⲣⲁ̈ⲓ Favrelle ⲓ̣ⲱⲙ i.e. Sahidic (ⲉ)ⲓⲟⲙ ⲉⲃⲟⲗ i.e. Sahidic ⲉ-ⲃⲱⲗ : l. "outside" Favrelle **6** ⲛϩⲱ l. Sahidic ⲙϩⲁⲁⲩ Favrelle ϩⲱ̣: l. ϩⲱⲃ (?) : ϩⲱ "face" Müller; van der Vliet ⲛⲓⲙ : ⲛⲓ̈ⲙ Müller **7** ϩⲱϥ: i.e. Sahidic ϩⲟϥ ϩⲛϫⲓⲥⲉ l. ϩⲛ<ⲟⲩ>ϫⲓⲥⲉ or ϩⲛ<ⲧ>ϫⲓⲥⲉ "aloft" or "in <a/the> back" Müller (where ⲧ is more likely than ⲟⲩ) : "in the spine" van der Vliet 8 ⲙⲏⲣ: i.e. Sahidic ⲙ̅ⲙⲏⲣ (haplography) ϣⲉ ⲛⲁⲧⲱⲙ ϩⲛⲟ`ⲩ´ : ϣⲉⲛⲁⲧ ⲱ ⲛϩⲛⲟⲩ Favrelle l. ϣⲱⲧ "cut" ⲟ+ "being" ⲛϩⲟⲩⲛ (?) "on the surface" : ⲱ ϩⲏ\ⲟⲩ/ l. ⲟ+ ⲛϩⲏⲟⲩ "is beneficial" Müller (but see ll. 8–9) ⲛⲁⲧⲱⲙ "shall be closed" van der Vliet (presumably thereby emending to ⲧⲏⲙ) **8–9** ϩⲛⲟ`ⲩ´ⲛϫⲓⲥⲉ : ϩⲛ\ⲟⲩ/ϫⲓⲥⲉ corrected from ϩⲛⲛϫⲓⲥⲉ Müller : ϩⲛⲟ`ⲩ´ⲛ ϫⲓⲥⲉ van der Vliet : l. Sahidic ⲛϩⲟⲩⲛ ⲛ (via haplography) (?) ⲙⲛϣⲉ ⲛⲁⲧⲱⲙ ϩⲛⲟ`ⲩ´ⲛ : "No wood/trees/mercy will be shut" Müller **9** ϫⲉ ⲁ̣ⲫⲱϥ ⲧ̣ⲃⲏⲗ : ϫⲉⲫⲱϥⲧ ⲃⲏⲗ "the thief is released" Müller (where ⲫ corrected from ϩ) or *ⲧⲃⲏⲗ causative of ⲃⲱⲗ Müller ⲁ̣ⲫⲱϥ : ⲫⲱϥ previous eds. ⲫⲱϥ ⲧ̣ⲃⲏⲗ : l. ⲡϩⲟϥ ⲉⲧⲃⲏⲗ "the snake is unbound" van der Vliet **10** ϫⲱⲕ "death" Favrelle : "head" Müller ⲛⲡⲉⲙⲁ: l. ⲙⲡⲉⲓⲙⲁ van der Vliet **10–11** ⲙⲡⲱⲟⲩ : ⲙⲡⲟⲟⲩ Favrelle **11** ⲡⲱⲟⲩ: i.e. Sahidic ⲡⲟⲟⲩ ⲉ̣̅ⲓ̅ⲁ̅ⲱ̣̅ : ⲉ̅ⲓ̅ⲁ̅ⲱ̅ van der Vliet : ⲉⲓⲁⲱ Muller **12** `ⲁ̣´ⲁ̣ⲱⲛⲉ : ⲁⲁⲱⲛⲉ Favrelle ⲙⲙⲱⲕ: i.e. Sahidic ⲙⲙⲟⲕ **13** ⲙⲙⲱⲕ: i.e. Sahidic ⲙⲙⲟⲕ ⲉⲃⲟⲗ : ⲉⲃ ⲟⲗ Favrelle (presumably typographical error) **16** ⲇ̣ⲇ̣ i.e. from Greek (ὁ/ἡ) δεῖνα τῆς δεῖνος

I. Comparing Readings of the Text

3–4 ⲡⲉϩⲣⲱⲟⲩ ⲛⲥⲁϣϥⲉ ⲛⲛⲁⲡⲏ ⲛ̣ϩⲱ̣ϥ̣ "the seven voices of the snake heads"[823]
All prior editors have amended the text here, reading "the voices of the seven snake heads", or similar. In our judgement, this is unnecessary and has also produced more grammatical problems than it has solved. Müller (2017, 131) rightly noted that if "seven" (ⲥⲁϣϥⲉ) corresponds to the "head" (ⲁⲡⲏ), the text must be amended to <ⲧ>ⲥⲁϣϥⲉ, not only because ⲁⲡⲏ is feminine, but also because a cardinal number is principally found determining another noun without the definite article only when it is the first position of an attributive construction.[824] This emendation allowed Müller to read "the voices of the heads of the seven snakes", but is unnecessary. Not heeding Müller's point on the grammar of cardinal numbers, van der Vliet read "the sound of seven snake heads", emending the text to ⲡⲉϩⲣⲱⲟⲩ ⲛⲥⲁϣϥⲉ ⲛ{ⲛ}ⲁⲡⲏ ⲛϩⲱϥ, but leaving the absence of the definite article before ⲥⲁϣϥⲉ uncommented, and thereby unresolved. Ultimately, the text can be understood grammatically in its present form, making even Müller's grammatically correct emendation unnecessary. Given that a cardinal number, while always defined in the singular, is always referred to as a plural when taken up subsequently, the "they" that arose from the sea, or Fayum, can be understood as either the voices or the snake heads—and perhaps both were meant or implied.[825]

5 ⲡ̣ⲓ̣ⲱⲙ "the sea (or, Fayum)"
The possibility that ⲡⲓⲱⲙ here is a specific, rather than generic, spatial reference was not considered by any prior editor. On that reading, there could be specific mythological associations underlying the reference whose latest reflexes still existed in the region around Saqqara at the late date at which the Saqqara text was copied.

5–6 ⲉⲃⲟⲗ ⲛϩⲱ̣ ⲛⲓⲙ ⲉⲧⲙⲏⲣ ϩⲛ ϫⲓⲥⲉ "to release everything (or, every face) bound in (the) knot"
While Favrelle's reading has several unresolved problems,[826] the first point of contention between our reading and interpretation and that of Müller and van der Vliet is the interpretation of ϩⲱ as either ϩⲱ for Sahidic ϩⲟ "face" or, given the later passages, as ϩⲱ(ⲃ) or ϩⲱ(ϥ) for Sahidic ϩⲱⲃ "thing" or ϩⲟϥ "snake",

[823] Could there be some relationship between the seven voices of the snake heads and the seven uraei from Egyptian tradition, as attested in *PT* 318, *CT* 85, 86, 87, and 310?

[824] Layton 2000, §66.

[825] Layton 2000, §66b.

[826] The translation "l'extérieur de toute tombe forclose de la surface" implies something like <ⲡ>{ⲉ}ⲃⲟⲗ <ⲙ>ⲛϩⲱ (i.e. Sahidic ⲙϩⲁⲁⲩ, cf. Akhmimic ⲙϩⲱ) ⲛⲓⲙ ⲉⲧⲙⲏⲣ ϩⲛ <ⲧ>ϫⲓⲥⲉ (Favrelle in Ziegler 2013, 460).

respectively. Müller and van der Vliet both read “face”[827] and did not comment on the possibility that ϥ renders Sahidic ⲃ nor that /v/ or /β/ is weak enough in closed syllables to be omitted in writing—especially around the Fayum, and at this late date.[828] The Fayumic influence in writing ϥ for ⲃ, and indeed the omission of ϥ, should not be ruled out given that the manuscript was excavated at Saqqara, north-east of the Fayum. As justified below, given that our interpretation differs substantially enough from that of Müller and van der Vliet as to mean that no body parts are mentioned in the text, in our judgement the most logical reading of ϩⲱ here is for Sahidic/Fayumic ϩⲱϥ “thing”. This seems all the more likely given that the second point of contention is the reading and interpretation of ϩⲛ ϫⲓⲥⲉ. How Favrelle reached the rendering “en surface” is unclear,[829] whereas Müller suggested that both “aloft” and “in <a/the> back” were possibilities,[830] as did van der Vliet.[831] Although van der Vliet also presented the possibility that ϫⲓⲥⲉ would render “knot” through “an entirely acceptable nominal formation” of the verb ϫⲱⲥ “to become hard/solid”, because such a form is not attested in Coptic, he did not find this reading and interpretation preferable.[832] Despite the fact that ϫⲓⲥⲉ for “knot” is not—*yet*, one might stress—attested in Coptic, in our judgement, this interpretation is to be favored due to the distinct lack of sense offered by the alternative translations.[833] To have a “face” bound in “the (or, a) spine” renders no immediate sense in translation. Thus, we also suspect that this would not make sense in Coptic both because of a distinct lack of known idioms in Egyptian-Coptic and of parallels for such a turn of phrase in any Coptic text. As noted by van der Vliet in his consideration of the possibility of ϫⲓⲥⲉ from *ṯꜣś.t* “knot”, the phenomenon of “knots” and “knotting” in Egyptian ritual—not just magical—practice is ubiquitous, as elaborated below.

7–8 ⲙⲛϩⲱϥ ⲙⲏⲣ “nothing (or, no snake) is bound [in (the) knot]”
Here, it seems likely that the copyist of this text, or a source text, omitted the following ϩⲛ ϫⲓⲥⲉ, otherwise paralleled in the preceding and following clause concerning something that is or is not bound. Given that this clause, where we

827 2017, 131 and 2018, 148, respectively.

828 A voiced labiodental fricative, or /β/ a voiced bilabial fricative: only in Bohairic was /b/ preserved as a voiced bilabial stop in word-final position (as suggested by orthographies alternating the use of ⲡ to indicate that bilabial stop), see Peust 1999, §3.12.5.

829 Favrelle 2013, 460.

830 Müller 2017, 131.

831 van der Vliet 2018, 138.

832 van der Vliet 2018, 150.

833 Compare “l’extérieur de toute tombe forclose de la surface” (Favrelle in Ziegler 2013, 460); “in order to release every face, which is bound aloft” (Müller 2017, 131); “in order to unbind every face bound in the spine” (van der Vliet 2018, 148).

understand Sahidic/Fayumic ϩⲱϥ "thing", rather than Sahidic/Bohairic ϩⲟϥ "snake",[834] follows directly the preceding, in our judgement the preceding ϩⲱ—preceding ⲚⲒⲘ, where ϩⲱϥ instead ends a line—is a rendering of the same word. Thus, there is a direct parallelism between the two clauses, which we consider preferrable to any further reference to snakes here. Indeed, it could even be considered that there is a deliberate pun on ϩⲱϥ "snake" and ϩⲱϥ as an orthographic variant of ϩⲱⲃ "thing" given the opening reference to snake heads in the mythological scene setting. That ϩⲱϥ "snake" and ϩⲱϥ "thing" would have been vocalized similarly follows from the above considerations, as well as that the realization of ⲃ and ϥ as /v/ or /β/ in those lexemes is borne out by their plural forms, Sahidic/Bohairic ϩⲃⲟⲩⲓ and Bohairic/Fayumic ϩⲃⲏⲟⲩⲓ respectively.[835]

8–9 ⲘⲚϢⲈ ⲚⲀⲦⲰⲘ ϩⲎⲞ`Ⲩ´Ⲛ[836] ϫⲒⲤⲈ "no wood shall be sharp in (the) knot" While Favrelle's interpretation once again contains several unresolved problems,[837] Müller's two grammatically possible suggestions—"no wood/trees (or, mercy) will be shut aloft"—, as he admits, render no immediate sense.[838] Van der Vliet, without discussing Müller's suggestions,[839] instead offers "no nose shall be closed in a spine".[840] The problems with van der Vliet's interpretation are firstly that ⲦⲰⲘ is a transitive verb, secondly that the offered translation implies ⲦⲎⲘ+, which is neither corrected nor explained, although given that this is ungrammatical, an "ingressive use" of the transitive infinitive (without a direct object) may be meant,[841] and thirdly that it once again does not offer any immediate sense—both "binding" and "releasing" a body part (whether face or nose) "bound" in "the (or, a) spine" is neither clear in translation nor with reference to any known Egyptian-Coptic idiom or parallel in any Coptic text. Given the problems with reading the verb as ⲦⲰⲘ "to shut" due to the absence of a qualitative form or direct object, the most likely interpretation is instead the verb ⲦⲰⲘ "to be sharp"—itself a transitive and intransitive verb, followed by an ad-

---

[834] The spelling with ⲱ for ⲟ prevents certainty, but this is true in both interpretations. Compare, "no snake is bound" (Favrelle in Ziegler 2013, 460; van der Vliet 2018, 148)—Müller did not correct Favrelle, and so presumably agreed with that reading and interpretation.

[835] Van der Vliet considered the "assonance" between ϩⲟ and ϩⲟϥ, but only in their interpretation as "face" and "snake" (2018, 149).

[836] As noted in the apparatus, ϩⲎⲞ`Ⲩ´Ⲛ ϫⲒⲤⲈ could be understood as a re-writing of ϩⲚ ⲞⲨϫⲒⲤⲈ, a rendering of ϩⲎⲚ for Sahidic ϩⲚ̄, where the indefinite article was added subsequently, or a reduced writing of Sahidic Ⲛϩⲟⲩⲛ Ⲛ "inside of".

[837] "pas de tranchet disponible en surface" (Favrelle in Zeigler 2013, 460).

[838] Müller 2017, 131.

[839] Van der Vliet 2018, 148.

[840] It is presumably from this clause that van der Vliet's title "Charming a Clogged Nose" derives.

[841] Layton 2000 §174. Layton (2000: 135) notes that for some transitive verbs ingressive meanings are frequent, whereas for others they are unattested.

verbial adjunct. With "nose" offering even less sense in relation to that verb, as Müller, ϣⲉ "wood" seems more likely—rendering a clear association between verbal subject and verbal action, as well as with the adverbial adjunct, the sharpness of wood, and the sharpness of wood in relation to a knot that could be cut, i.e. unbound.

9–11 ⲁ̣ϥⲱϥ ⲧ̣ⲃⲏⲗ ϫⲱⲕ ⲕⲏ ⲛⲁⲕ̣ ⲛⲡⲉⲙⲁ ⲙⲡⲱⲟⲩ "the snake that is unbound has completed another for you here (and) today"
No prior editor read a letter before ϥ. Although the paper is torn along the length of the vertical axis of ϥ, digital manipulation of the image demonstrates that the traces of ink along that vertical axis are too substantial to belong simply to the vertical stroke and left portion of ϥ. Furthermore, the morphology of the traces to the left of that tear are not only angular, and therefore inconsistent with the left portion of ϥ when compared to the right portion, they are closely comparable with those of ⲁ elsewhere upon the manuscript, where the tail was partially lost in that tear. This distinction also means that the reading and interpretation offered here further departs from that of all prior editors, with a past tense with object and adverbial adjunct instead understood—exactly the sort of performative announcement of what the ritual has already achieved expected in magical texts. "The snake that is unbound" is thus the subject of a following verb.[842] While ϫⲱⲕ was read "death" by Favrelle, presumably from ϫⲱⲕ "to complete", but "your head" by Müller,[843] followed by van der Vliet,[844] reading a noun is prevented by the presence of ⲁ before ϥⲱϥ. Here, the reference to one snake—or perhaps even "thing"—that has already been loosened, i.e. released, in turn having "completed another" for you, i.e. for the practitioner or client, in that place and during that same day relates directly to the juxtaposition presented earlier in the text between what is bound and what is not. This reading draws together not only the internal consistency of this interpretation, but also the punning between the "snake" of the mythological scene setting and the "thing" that is to be loosed or released, and therefore brought about, as the desired outcome of the ritual practice.

[842] Although understanding the syntax of ϥⲱϥ ⲧⲃⲏⲗ as Sahidic ⲡϩⲟϥ (ⲉ)ⲧⲃⲏⲗ, van der Vliet translated this erroneously as if a nominal sentence "the snake is unbound" (2018, 148).

[843] Müller (2017, 131) also ventured the possibilities of an unattested causative *ⲧⲃⲱⲗ or ϥⲱϥⲧ ⲃⲏⲗ "the theft is released".

[844] Favrelle in Zeigler 2013, 460; Müller 2017, 131; van der Vliet 2018, 148.

II. Knots and Knotting in Egyptian Tradition

The binding or tying and loosening or untying of the *ṯȝś.t* "knot", homophonous and cognate with the "knot-amulet" (*ṯȝś.t*), are ubiquitous in the Egyptian ritual tradition—whether in temple,[845] afterlife,[846] or magical[847] ritual texts. Used, as proposed here, in magical texts principally with a healing function, the reference to knots in such texts appears in practices to heal a headache,[848] poison,[849] and the womb,[850] as well as protect the womb when carrying a child,[851] protect a womb from the negative influence of a deceased or deity,[852] protect from the influence of an "enemy" or deceased on the head or any body part of a patient,[853] protect from snakes,[854] and even protect from plague.[855] The efficacy of the

---

845 P.Brook. 47.218.50 (ed. Goyon 1972), dating to c. 600–551 BCE, a composition that served to confirm royal power at the new year, discussed in the excursus to §10, features the pectoral of the "great seat" that is to be tied around the neck of the king with 60 knots (1/9).

846 From the Pyramid Texts onwards, consider the passage from the pyramid of Pepi II discussed in the excursus to §9. Elsewhere in that pyramid, the "lords of Nun" are described as being the ones who "loosen (*wḥ'*) the knots (*ṯȝś.t*)" for the deceased king (*PT* 358). By comparison, the "day of tying the knot" (*hrw n smn.t ṯ(ȝ)ś.t*) is attested in *BD* 50, where the deceased are described as having a knot tied around them in the sky. For the "knots" utilized in the ritual of *Mummification*, see the relevant passages in Töpfer 2015.

847 Consider the numerous examples cited in the following footnotes.

848 In the tenth recipe of the formulary bookroll of magical texts P.Leiden I 348, ed. Borghouts 1971, the invocation is to be recited while an amulet of seven knots is tied before being hung around the patient's neck (recto 4/5–9). Similar are those prescribed in the eighth (recto 3/8–4/3) and fourth (recto 2/9–3/2) recipes, which are instead to be tied to the left foot and large toe respectively.

849 Consider the 11th recipe of the formulary bookroll of magical texts P.Brit.Mus. EA 10687 (P.Chester Beatty VII), where the invocation is to be recited over the material to be tied into seven knots and applied directly to the sting (5/5–6/1). In the sixth recipe (3/7–4/4), the knots are described as surrounding the poison; similarly the 18th recipe (7/7–8/8).

850 In the 29th recipe from the formulary bookroll of medical texts P.Brit.Mus. EA 10059, ed. Leitz 1999, 51–84; pls. 26–46, the invocation is to be recited over the knotting of the threads that produce the amulet, which is then inserted into the womb of the suffering woman (9/14–10/1).

851 In the 28th recipe from the aforementioned P.Brit.Mus. EA 10059, the invocation is to be recited over two types of thread that are then to be knotted together four times; each time a knot is tied, the invocation is to be repeated, and given to the back, or behind, of the patient to prevent any bleeding and to strengthen the "egg" (*swḥ.t*) (9/9–14).

852 In the 30th recipe from the aforementioned P.Brit.Mus. EA 10059, the invocation is to be recited after two knots have been tied in particular threads and inserted into the patient's womb (10/1–2).

853 Consider the second recipe in the formulary bookroll of magical texts P.Budapest 51.1961, ed. Kákosy 1971, where the invocation is to be recited over the threads tied into four knots and given to the head of a patient (1/5–2/6). Similar is found in the sixth (3/8–4/3) and third (2/7–3/1) recipes, where the latter case also concerns the sleeplessness of the patient—the eighth (4/4–4/7) recipe, also against a headache, is instead to be given to the patient's foot.

854 In a recipe to "protect the body from any male and any female snakes" from the formulary bookroll of magical texts P.Brit.Mus. EA 10763 (P.Ramesseum 10), ed. Altenmüller 1979, the

number seven, also featured in P.Saqqara inv. F.17.10, and the number of knots idealized in an amulet are also found in common combination.[856] Among the latest pre-Coptic Egyptian magical texts, the *PDM*,[857] one recipe for finding a thief in P.Brit.Mus. EA 10588 recto 6/1–16 (*PDM* lxi. 79–94), dating to the end of the 2nd or beginning of the 3rd century CE, also prescribes the production of a "knot" (*ṯꜣś.t*).[858] Consequently, and given the absence of any appropriate idiom in Egyptian-Coptic or parallel in the ritual tradition for phraseology concerning "binding" or "loosening" body parts within a "spine", in our judgement the Saqqara text preserves not just the latest reflexes of a mythological scene setting with a millennia-long history and deep cosmogonic references—as discussed at length in the excursus to §9—but also evidence in the tradition of Coptic magical texts for the continued association of knotting with magical and medical ritual practices concerning the healing of particular ailments.[859]

---

invocation is to be recited over a thread tied in two knots and then given to the right hand of the patient (1/1–2/2). Similar is the third recipe of the formulary bookroll of magical texts P.Brit.Mus. EA 9997+10309, ed. Leitz 1999, 3–30; pls. 1–11 (3/12–5/4).

[855] In the first recipe of the formulary bookroll of magical texts P.Leiden I 348, ed. Borghouts 1971, the seven-times knotted amulet of finest linen, inscribed with images of deities, is said to protect from the "plague" (*ỉꜣd.t rnp.t*) (1/1–2/4).

[856] In the 5th recipe of the formulary bookroll of magical texts P.Berl. inv. 3027, ed. Erman 1901, a recipe to protect a newborn child, the invocation is to be recited seven times over the ritual paraphernalia that are to be produced as part of the practice, one of which is an amulet (*ṯꜣś.t*) of seven knots to be made and tied around the child's neck (verso 6/1–7). Earlier on in the same recipe, the mythological precedent whence these amulets of seven knots came is described directly, in which they are those "spun (*sšn*) by Isis", "twisted (*msn*) by Nephthys", in making a "knot" (*ṯꜣś.t*), i.e. *ṯꜣś.t*-amulet, of "divine chord" (*nṯr.i*)–compare with the latest example in Demotic, described below. This is one of seven recipes utilizing a "knot" (*ṯꜣś.t*) in the compilation of recipes upon this manuscript.

[857] Introduced and discussed in **Transmitting Textual Traditions**.

[858] "When you want to discover a thief: you should bring a chord/thread of flax; you should recite a text to it; you should say the names of every single man, one by one; you should make a knot and draw it together. If he is the one who stole it, he speaks while you tie the knot. (6/5–8). The invocation follows, and features a mythological precedent referring Isis making a knot with a strip of flax "until he [i.e. the strip, or perhaps Seth] revealed (it) to Horus in the papyrus-thicket", where an analogy is drawn between the strip of flax used by the contemporary practitioner and that used by Isis, the divine protagonist in the mythological precedent (6/11–16).

[859] Demotic *ṯśi̯*, the verbal predecessor to Coptic ϫⲱⲥ, is still attested with meanings relating to "tying" or "binding" in afterlife ritual texts. Consider *P.Harkness*, where a "garland of justification" will be "tied" (*ṯśi̯*) for the deceased (5/8) or *P.Rhind 1* and *P.Rhind 2* where certain amulets (*śꜣ.w*) will be "bound" (*ṯśi̯*) for the deceased (8/d2 and 8/d3 respectively).

III. The Purpose of the Text

Although van der Vliet's suggestion of the releasing or loosening of a clogged nose is a possible purpose for inscribing or reciting the text, no parallels in specifically textual amulets were presented in his study, nor are any known to us. There are parallels in medical texts of recipes for the opposite, that is, staunching nosebleeds and runny noses, but all of those are delivered orally (or with some topical application of writing, such as writing in the discharge from the nose on the patient's forehead), but not as durable amulets. In our judgement, a clogged nose is too ephemeral and minor an issue to go to the trouble to write or commission a textual amulet.[860] The repeated mention of "binding" in conjunction with "snakes" and the fact that ϣⲉ can also be "wood" might point in another direction (if "thing" can be accepted in l. 6 in place of "face", based on the parallel ϩⲱ̣ ⲛⲓⲙ ⲉⲧⲙⲏⲣ [ll. 6–7] and ϩⲱϥ ⲙⲏⲣ [ll. 7–8]): in many medieval Greek texts "binding" is a way of conceiving male impotence as the result of sorcery, and the terminology used to describe its remedy is similar, "releasing", "loosening", and "unbinding".[861] This would be a more serious problem and give more justification to a semi-permanent amulet that a client would want to carry around, while there would be fitting analogies between unbound snakes, "sharp" unknotted wood, and erections. Further, this might also give some sense to the locution "the snake that is unbound has completed another for you today"—i.e., the one (cosmic) snake helps the other (fleshy) one.

The mythological scene setting of P.Saqqara inv. F.17.10 is paralleled in other Coptic, Demotic, and hieratic magical texts discussed at length in the excursus to §9. There, its use in all of these parallels highlighted a thematic comparison: each recipe exhibits the pairing of blockage and its resolution in unblocking. In all cases but the Saqqara text, this association is also reflected explicitly in the desired outcome of the practices, where unblocking results in healing (from poison, from a lack of menstrual flow, or from a difficult childbirth). The interpretation of the creative resonances of these motifs as discussed in the excursus to §9 entails an expression of the tension between existence (of a poison or a blockage in the body) and absence (of menstrual flow or delivery), between creation (the life-giving associations of menstruation and childbirth) and its opposite (death from poison or an illness caused by blockage), as well as explicitly in some cases between sealing and the releasing of such sealing. The result, in all cases, involves bringing something out of the body, which can be brought into focus within the suggested purpose of the text as proposed here.

---

860 A more literal application to driving away snakes from the named bearer is found in the tradition of Coptic magical texts, e.g. *P.Ryl.Copt.* 104.8–18 [§4] and P.CtYBR inv. 1792, ed. Parássoglou 1974.

861 Zellmann-Rohrer 2018, 121 with n. 1.

Indices

Word Lists

Egyptian-Coptic

ⲙⲓⲕⲉ "to rest"
ⲙⲟⲕⲉ+ (14/5)
ⲙⲕⲁϩ "to be in pain" (10/12)
ⲙⲟⲭϩ+ (13/4)
ⲙⲟⲩⲗⲁϩ "wax" (4/15; 14/2)
ⲙ(ⲛ)ⲛ-/ⲙⲛⲧ(ⲉ)⸗ "not to be"
ⲙ̄ⲛ̄- (5/1; 5/2)
ⲙⲛ̄-/ⲛⲙ̄ⲙⲁ⸗ "and", "with"
ⲙⲛ̄- (10/13; 12/3; 12/10)
ⲙ̄ⲛ̄- (2/3; 2/8; 9/7; 9/8; 9/10)
ⲙⲉⲛ- (5/17)
ⲛ̄ⲙ̄ⲙⲁ⸗ (7/17; 9/12; 9/16)
ⲙⲏⲛⲉ "midday"
ⲙ̄ⲙⲏⲛⲉ "daily"
ⲙ̄ⲏⲛⲉ (9/12)
ⲙ̄ⲙⲏⲛⲉ (10/11)
ⲙⲟⲟⲛⲉ "to pasture" (6/8)
ⲙⲁⲥⲉ "bull", "calf" (12/13; 13/2; 13/5; 13/7; 13/8)
ⲙⲓⲥⲉ "to give birth to" (5/18)
ⲙⲁⲥ "offspring" (6/4)
ⲙⲟⲧⲉ "neck", "shoulders" (12/13)
ⲙⲁⲩ "there"
ⲙ̄ⲙⲁⲩ "there" (adverb) (6/2; 14/14)
ⲙⲁⲁⲩ "mother" (6/6)
ⲙⲟⲟⲩ "water" (11/14; 12/8)
ⲙⲟⲩ- (10/8)
ⲙⲉ(ⲉ)ⲩⲉ "thought"
ⲙⲉⲩⲉ (7/9)
ⲙⲏϩⲉ "feather" (12/4; 12/11)
(ⲉ)ⲙϩⲓⲧ "north"
ⲉⲙϩⲓⲧ (7/6)
ⲙⲁⲁϫⲉ "ear" (13/1; 13/2)

ⲛ̄- (attributive marker)
ⲛ̄- (3/17; 3/18; 3/20; 3/21; 4/13; 4/14; 4/16; 5/1 [twice]; 5/13; 5/15; 5/16; 5/20; 6/10; 6/18; 7/2 [thrice]; 7/3 [twice]; 9/3; 9/4; 9/5; 9/9; 9/11; 9/12; 9/13; 9/16; 10/4; 10/7; 10/8; 10/9; 10/10 [twice]; 10/13; 10/14 [twice]; 10/15; 10/18 [twice]; 11/8; 11/10; 11/11 [twice]; 11/12; 11/13; 12/2 [thrice]; 12/4; 12/6 [thrice]; 12/9; 12/16 [twice]; 12/19; 13/1; 13/1; 13/4; 13/5; 13/6; 13/7 [twice]; 13/8; 13/11; 13/12; 13/13; 13/14; 13/14; 13/15; 13/16; 14/2; 14/3; 14/4 [twice]; 14/6)
ⲛ- (12/8)
ⲛ̄ⲛ̄- (dittography) (10/15)
ⲛ̄ⲛ- (dittography) (12/7; 14/16)
ⲉ- (5/18)
ⲙ̄- (12/2; 12/13; 12/18)
ⲛ̄- (attributive or preposition: instrumental)
ⲛ̄- (6/14 [twice]; 6/15)
ⲛ̄-/ⲙ̄ⲙⲟ⸗ (object marker)
ⲛ- (2/7)
ⲛ̄- (5/11 [twice]; 5/19; 7/9; 10/13)
ⲙ̄- (5/19; 6/3; 10/11)
ⲙ̄ⲙⲟ⸗ (9/6; 9/9; 12/3–4; 12/10–11; 12/20; 13/18; 14/12; 14/16)
ⲙⲙⲟ⸗ (14/17)
ⲛ-/ⲛⲁ⸗ (preposition: dative)
ⲛⲁ⸗ (7/20; 10/13)
ⲛ-/ⲛ̄ⲧⲉ- (preposition: genitive)
ⲛ̄- (5/2; 5/9; 6/1; 6/6 [twice]; 6/11; 7/6; 8/1 [twice]; 8/2; 9/1; 9/3; 9/4; 9/5; 9/8; 9/9; 10/17; 12/8; 12/19)
ⲙ̄- (6/5; 6/17; 7/1; 7/9; 9/2; 10/4; 12/5)
ⲛⲧⲉ- (5/7)
ⲛ̄ⲧⲉ- (13/11)
ⲛ- (preposition: instrumental)
ⲛ̄- (5/20; 6/4; 6/18; 7/1; 7/20; 9/11; 9/12; 12/4; 12/11; 12/12; 12/13; 13/18)
ⲙ̄- (5/3; 5/4 [twice]; 11/2; 11/15; 13/8)
ⲛⲁ "to go" (5/6)
ⲛ(ⲉ)- (definite article)
ⲛ̄- (2/2; 2/7; 5/9; 6/7)
ⲛ- (2/6)
ⲛ- (4/17; 5/11 [twice]; 11/1)
ⲛⲉ- (2/8)
ⲉⲛ- (?) (5/17)
ⲙ̄- (7/9)
ⲛⲁï (demonstrative pronoun) (2/2; 2/7)
ⲛⲉ⸗ (possessive article)
ⲛⲁ (5/10)
ⲛⲉⲕ (6/20; 9/14)
ⲛⲉϥ (4/13; 4/15; 13/3)
ⲛⲉⲩ (6/16; 9/7; 9/10; 12/3; 12/10)
ⲛⲉ (copula) (2/2)
ⲛⲱ (possessive prefix/pronoun)
ⲛⲁ- (5/10)
ⲛⲏⲩ+ "to be coming", "come" (5/3; 5/4; 5/15)
ⲛⲁⲁⲕⲉ "pains"
ϯⲛⲁⲁⲕⲉ "to be in pain" (5/16)
(ⲉ)ⲛⲕⲟⲧⲕ "to sleep"
ⲛ̄ⲕⲟⲧ̄ⲕ̄ (14/19)

⸗ⲥ (suffix pronoun)
⸗ⲥ (5/16; 5/18; 6/2; 7/9; 10/15; 10/17 [twice]; 10/19; 12/5; 12/9; 12/14 [twice]; 12/15; 12/19; 12/20; 14/8; 14/14)
⸗ⲥ̅ (12/14; 13/17; 14/9)
⸗ø (haplography) (14/14)
ⲥⲁ "side"
ⲛ̅ⲥⲁ- "behind", "after" (8/4)
ⲛ̅ⲥⲱ⸗ (7/8; 9/6)
ⲙⲛ̅ⲛ̅ⲥⲱⲥ "afterwards"
ⲙ̅ⲛ̅ⲛ̅ⲥⲱⲥ (9/17)
ⲥⲁⲣⲏⲥ "south(ern side)" (7/8)
ⲥⲁϩⲏⲧ "north(ern side)"
ϭⲁϩⲏⲧ (7/8)
⸗ⲥⲉ (suffix pronoun) (9/14; 9/15; 9/16)
ⲥⲱ "to drink"
ⲥⲉ- (9/13; 10/7; 10/8; 10/11)
ⲥⲟⲟ⸗ (10/19)
ⲥⲏⲃⲉ "reed"
(ⲉ)ⲣ-ⲥⲏⲃⲉ "to sprout"
ⲣ̅ⲥⲏⲃⲉ (6/13)
ⲥⲓⲃⲧ "hill"
ⲥⲓⲃⲓⲧ (5/7)
ⲥⲱⲕ "to draw"
ⲥⲉⲕ-
ⲥ̅ⲕ̅- (14/8)
ⲥⲓⲙ "radish" (14/4)
ⲥⲙⲓⲛⲉ "to prepare", "establish"
ⲥⲙⲛ-
ⲥ̅ⲙ̅ⲛ̅- (6/3)
ⲥⲙⲛⲧ⸗
ⲥⲙ̅ⲛ̅ⲧ⸗ⲉ (6/3)
ⲥⲙⲟⲧ "form", "character" (5/4)
ⲥⲟⲛ "brother" (7/7)
ⲥⲛⲧⲉ "two (f.)"
ⲥ̅ⲛ̅ⲧⲉ (5/6)
ⲥⲛⲁⲩ "two (m.)" (5/6; 7/7; 14/5)
ⲥⲛⲟϥ "blood" (3/20; 3/21)
ⲥⲡⲗⲏⲗⲓⲛ "poultice"
ⲥⲡⲗⲉⲗⲓⲛ (13/11)
ⲥⲏⲩ "day", "time"
ⲥⲟⲩ (5/16)
ⲥⲓⲟⲟⲩⲛ "bath"
ⲥⲉⲟⲟⲩⲛ (14/20)
ⲥⲟⲟⲩⲧⲛ "to stretch"
ⲥⲟⲩⲧⲱⲛ⸗
ⲥⲟⲩⲧⲱⲛ̅⸗ (14/19)
ⲥⲟⲟⲩϩⲉ "egg" (5/12; 5/13)
ⲥⲁϣ "sore" (12/17)
ⲥⲓϣⲉ "gall" (12/13; 13/1)
ⲥⲁϣϥ "seven (m.)"
ⲥⲁϣϥ̅ (9/13; 12/6)
ⲥⲁϣ̅ϥ̅ (10/7; 10/8–9; 10/9–10)
ⲥⲁϣϥⲉ "seven (f.)" (9/16)
ⲥϩⲁï "to write" (2/7)
ⲥⲁϩ⸗ (2/6)
ⲥⲁϩ̅⸗ (11/8)
ⲥϩⲃⲏⲏⲧⲉ "foam" (4/14)
ⲥϩⲓⲙⲉ "woman" (10/12; 10/16)
ⲥⲁϩⲧⲉ "to kindle" (13/16–17)

ϯ "to give", "put"
ϯ (4/14; 9/5; 12/15; 12/17; 14/7)
ⲧⲁⲁ⸗ (6/1; 9/7; 10/14; 10/18; 12/9; 12/15; 13/2; 13/16; 14/10)
ⲧⲱ+ (5/18)
ⲙⲁ- (imperative) (11/6)
ⲙⲁϯ (7/20)
ⲧ(ⲉ)- (definite article)
ⲧ- (6/5; 6/6 [thrice]; 6/9; 7/20; 9/13; 9/17; 10/7; 12/1; 14/13; 14/14)
ⲧⲉ- (8/1; 13/10)
ⲧⲁï (demonstrative pronoun)
ⲧⲉⲓ- (demonstrative article)
ⲧⲉï- (5/7; 11/2)
ⲧⲉ⸗ (possessive article)
ⲧⲟⲩ (6/3)
ⲧⲉⲥ (6/1; 10/12)
ⲧⲉ (copula) (5/17; 10/17; 14/14)
ⲧⲱⲱⲃⲉ "brick"
ⲧⲱⲃⲉ (5/17; 14/20)
ⲧⲃⲛⲏ "domestic animal"
ⲧ̅ⲃ̅ⲛⲏ (7/4; 7/10)
ⲧⲃⲛⲟⲟⲩⲉ "domestic animals"
ⲧ̅ⲃ̅ⲛⲛⲟⲟⲩⲉ (6/7)
ⲧⲕⲁⲥ "pain"
ϯ-ⲧⲕⲁⲥ "to give", "have pain" (10/17)
ⲧⲓ-ⲧⲕⲁⲥ (12/18; 13/1)
ⲧⲁⲗⲟ "to raise", "mount"
ⲧⲁⲗⲟ⸗ (11/12)
ⲧⲁⲗⲁ⸗ (14/11)
ⲧⲁⲗⲏⲩ+ (5/7)
ⲧⲙⲉⲥⲓⲟ "to cause to give birth"
ⲧⲙⲁⲥïⲟ (5/10–11)
ⲧⲱⲛ "where?" (5/3; 5/15)
ⲧⲱⲛⲟⲩ/ⲧⲟⲛⲟⲩ "very"
ⲧⲟⲛⲟⲩ (3/19)

ϣⲟⲙ̅ⲛ̅ⲧ (10/10)
ϣⲟⲙⲛ̅ⲧ̅ (9/12)
ϣ̅ⲙ̅ⲛ̅ⲧ̅- (5/2)
ϣⲟⲙⲧⲉ “three (f.)” (13/14)
ϣⲟⲙⲛ̅ⲧ̅ⲧⲉ (dittography) (14/15–16)
ϣⲙϣⲉ “to serve”
ϣ̅ⲙ̅ϣⲉ (6/3)
ϣⲱⲛⲉ “to be sick” (11/1; 14/13)
ϫⲱⲛⲉ (11/6)
ϣⲱⲡⲉ “to be(come)” (12/17)
ⲉϣⲱⲡⲉ “if”, “when” (10/16; 12/12; 13/5)
ϣⲱⲡⲉ “cucumber” (6/11–12)
ϣⲏⲣⲉ “child” (6/4; 7/5; 7/11)
ϣⲉ- “child of” (10/6)
ϣⲱⲥ “shepherd” (6/14; 6/16; 6/19)
ϣⲱⲱⲧ “to cut”, “slay”
ϣⲁ(ⲁ)ⲧⲛ- “except”
ϣⲁⲧ̅ⲛ̅- (5/12–13)
ϣⲓϯ “to gush”
ϣⲓⲧ(ⲉ) (5/12)
ϣⲁⲩ “use”, “value”
(ⲉ)ⲣ-ϣⲁⲩ “to be useful”, “prosperous”
ⲣ̅-ϣⲁⲩ (5/12)
ϣⲁϥⲉ “to swell”
ϣⲁϥⲃⲉ (4/16)
ϣⲁϫⲉ “to speak” (14/15; 14/17)

⸗ϥ (suffix pronoun)
⸗ϥ (3/18; 4/17; 4/18 [twice]; 4/19; 5/8; 5/13; 5/14; 5/17; 6/1; 6/12; 6/13; 6/14; 6/15; 6/18; 7/18; 9/10; 10/18 [twice]; 10/19; 11/12; 11/14; 12/7; 12/9; 12/12; 12/16; 12/17; 13/2; 13/3; 13/6; 13/8; 14/4; 14/11)
⸗ϥ̅ (2/1; 6/13; 6/17; 7/1; 10/5; 11/8; 11/14; 13/4; 13/9; 14/12)
ϥⲱ “hair”
ⲃⲱ (10/14)
ϥⲛⲧ “worm”
ⲃⲛⲧ (6/11)
ϥⲧⲟⲟⲩ “four (m.)” (5/16; 10/4)
ϥⲧⲟ “four (f.)” (12/2)

ϩⲁ- (preposition) (6/17; 7/1; 13/3)
ϩⲁⲣⲟ⸗ (5/8; 13/17; 14/20)
ϩⲉ “manner”
ⲛ̅ⲑⲉ ⲛ̅- “in the manner of” (11/13)
ⲛ̅ⲧⲉⲓϩⲉ “in this way” (12/14)
ϩⲏ “forepart”
ϩⲏⲧ⸗ (preposition) (5/14; 6/17 [or ϩⲏⲧ⸗ “tip”, “edge”])
ϩⲏⲧ̅⸗ (7/1)
ϩⲏ “belly”
ϩⲏⲧ⸗ (9/14)
ϩⲏⲧ̅⸗ (13/4)
ϩⲓ- (preposition)
ϩⲓ “and”, “with” (3/18 [twice]; 3/21; 4/18; 7/4; 12/14; 12/15)
ϩⲓ- “on”, “at”, “in”, “from” (12/6; 12/17; 14/19)
ϩⲓ “and”, “with” or “on”, “at”, “in”, “from” (12/17)
ϩⲟ “face” (8/3; 8/4; 12/5)
ⲛⲁϩⲣⲛ-/ⲛⲁϩⲣⲁ⸗ “before”
ⲛ̅ϩⲣ̅ⲛ̅- (8/2)
ⲛⲁϩⲣⲛ- (8/3)
ϩⲱⲃ “thing” (10/5)
ϩⲓⲃⲱⲓ “ibis”
ϩⲓⲃⲱϊ (12/4; 12/11)
ϩⲉⲗⲕⲓⲉⲙⲁ (?) (see commentary to p. 13/14)
ϩⲗⲗⲱ “old woman”
ϩⲉⲗⲱ (10/14)
ϩⲗⲟϭ “to be sweet”
ϩⲟⲗϭ+
ϩⲟⲗ̅ϭ̅ (10/18)
ϩⲟⲉⲓⲙ “wave”, “flood”
ϩⲟϊⲙⲉ (5/1; 5/2)
ϩⲙⲟⲩ “salt” (3/19; 4/16)
ϩⲙⲙⲉ “to be hot”
ϩⲏⲙ+ (12/19)
ϩⲙⲙⲉ “heat” (11/13)
ϩ̅ⲙ̅ⲙⲉ (9/17; 10/8)
ϩⲙⲟⲟⲥ “to sit”
ϩⲙ̅ⲟⲟⲥ (10/15)
ⲙⲁ-ⲛ̅ϩⲙⲟⲟⲥ “seat”, “backside”, “anus”
ⲙⲁⲛⲉϩⲙⲟⲟⲥ (12/17)
ϩⲙϫ “vinegar”
ϩ̅ⲙ̅ϫ (3/18)
ϩⲙ̅ϫ (12/9; 12/14; 13/13; 14/3)
ϩⲛ̅- (preposition)
ϩⲛ̅- (9/13)
ϩ̅ⲛ̅- (5/10; 6/5; 10/5; 14/6)
ϩ̅ⲙ̅- (5/20; 10/13; 11/10; 11/14; 12/5; 13/10; 14/12)
ⲛ̅ϩⲏⲧ⸗ (4/17; 14/9)
ϩⲉⲛ- (indefinite article)
ϩⲉⲛ- (3/19; 13/18; 14/10)

ⲁ- (12/17)

Circumstantial Converter
ⲉⲣⲉ-/ⲉ⸗
ⲉ- (4/14; 4/17; 5/1; 5/2; 5/8; 6/12 [twice]; 6/13; 10/17; 14/14; 14/15)
ⲉ⸗ (3/18; 4/16; 6/17; 6/18 [twice]; 6/19; 7/7 [twice]; 7/8; 10/10; 10/11; 10/12; 10/17; 10/18; 11/2; 11/9; 12/5; 12/7; 12/9 [twice]; 12/12; 12/15; 12/16; 12/17; 12/18; 12/19; 13/1; 13/3; 13/6; 13/8; 13/18 [twice]; 14/4; 14/7; 14/16; 14/17 [twice]; 14/19)
ⲉ(ⲉ)⸗ (10/5)
(ⲉ)⸗ (5/17)
ⲉⲣⲉ- (3/21; 5/9; 6/20; 14/20)

Focalizing Converter
ⲉⲣⲉ-/ⲉ⸗
ⲉ⸗ (5/3; 5/4; 5/7; 5/10; 5/11; 5/12; 5/15; 5/16)

Relative Converter
ⲉⲧ-/ⲉⲧ(ⲉ)⸗
ⲉⲧ- (5/11 [twice]; 7/17; 10/1; 11/1; 11/6; 12/1; 14/13)
ⲉⲧⲉ- (7/18)
ⲉⲧ̄⸗ (2/2; 14/14)

Imperfect Converter
ⲛⲉ-/ⲛⲉ⸗
ⲛⲉ⸗ (5/8)

Conjugations (Tripartite System)
Perfect I +ve & -ve
ⲁ-/ⲁ⸗
ⲁ⸗ (5/13; 5/14; 6/7; 6/8; 6/15; 10/17)
ⲙ̄ⲡⲉ⸗
ⲛⲡⲉ⸗ (4/14)
ⲙ̄ⲡⲉ⸗ (5/18 [twice]; 5/19)
ⲙⲡ⸗ (14/7; 14/17)
ⲙ̄ⲡ⸗ (14/8; 14/17)
ⲙⲡ̄⸗ (14/15)

Completive ("not yet")
ⲙ̄ⲡⲁⲧⲉ-/ⲙ̄ⲡⲁⲧⲉ⸗
ⲙⲡⲁⲧⲉ⸗ (6/12)
ⲙⲡⲁⲧ̄⸗ (6/13)

Aorist +ve & -ve
ϣⲁⲣⲉ-/ϣⲉ⸗
ϣⲁⲣⲉ- (10/12; 11/2)
ϣⲁ⸗ (2/6; 4/17; 14/14)
ⲙⲉⲣⲉ-/ⲙⲉ⸗
ⲙⲉ⸗ (6/13; 6/14)
ⲙⲁ⸗ (6/15)

Future III +ve & -ve
ⲉⲣⲉ-/ⲉ⸗×-ⲉ-
ⲉⲣⲉ- (7/10)
ⲉⲣⲁ- (6/7–8; 6/9)
ⲛ̄ⲛⲉ-/ⲛ̄ⲛⲉ⸗
ⲛ̄ⲛⲉ⸗ (3/20)

Imperative
ⲙⲁ- (11/6)

Causative Imperative
ⲙⲁⲣⲉ-/ⲙⲁⲣⲉ⸗
ⲙⲁⲣⲉ- (7/3–4)
ⲙⲁⲣⲉ⸗ (10/15; 10/19)

Causative Infinitive
ⲧⲣⲉ-/ⲧⲣⲉ⸗
ⲧⲣⲉ- (4/13; 5/12)
ⲧⲣⲉ⸗ (11/3; 11/9)

Subordinate Clause Conjugations
Conjunctive
ⲛⲧⲉ-/ⲛ⸗
ⲛ̄⸗ (2/1; 6/1; 6/2; 7/9; 9/5; 9/6; 9/7; 9/9; 9/10; 9/11; 9/12; 9/14 [twice]; 9/15; 9/16; 9/17; 10/7 [twice]; 10/8; 10/9 [twice]; 10/10; 11/15; 13/15; 13/16; 14/9; 14/11; 14/15; 14/18)
ⲛ⸗ (14/11; 14/18)

Limitative
ϣⲁⲛⲧⲉ-/ϣⲁⲛⲧ⸗
ϣⲁⲛⲧ⸗ (11/14)
ϣⲁⲛⲧ̄⸗ (4/18–19; 14/12)
ϣⲁⲛⲧⲉ⸗ (7/6–7)
ϣⲁⲧ̄⸗ (13/17)

Conditional
ⲉⲣⲉ-/ⲉ⸗
ⲉ⸗ (5/18; 12/14)

Greek Lemmata as Loanwords in Egyptian-Coptic

* φυλλάννησον “anise-leaf” (?)
  ⲫⲓⲗⲁⲛⲓⲥ (9/2)

χαλβάνη “galbanum”
  ⲭⲁⲗⲃⲁⲛⲏ (11/10)
χαίρειν “to hail” (lit. “rejoice”)
  ⲭⲁⲓⲣⲉ (7/17 [twice]; 7/18 [twice]; 7/18–19; 7/19; 7/19–20)
χαρακτήρ “sign”
  ⲭⲁⲣⲁⲕⲧⲏⲣ (2/8)
χάρις “grace”
  ⲭⲁⲣⲓⲥ (8/2)
χαριτήσιον “Favor-procedure”
  ⲭⲁⲣⲓⲧ︦ⲩ (7/16)

ψιμύθιον “white lead”
  ⲡⲥⲓⲙⲓⲑⲓⲟⲩ (13/15)
  ⲥⲓⲙⲓⲑⲓⲟⲛ (13/8–9)

Select Greek Words in Monolingual Greek-language Texts

As the morphology and orthography of the monolingual Greek texts are of relatively less linguistic significance than their Coptic counterparts, this index focuses instead on phrase-context. The definite article, δέ, ἤ, καί, and pronouns are omitted.

ἀβασάνιστος “without torment”
  ’βασανίστως (3/12)
αἷμα “blood”
  κάτεχε τὸ αἷμα ἐν ποιῷ μέλει τοῦ ΔΔ (7/13–14)
ἀκίνδυνος “without peril”
  ἀκίνδυν{ω}ων (3/11–12)
ἅμμα “knot”
  ποίησον ζ̅ ἅμμα (4/8)
ἀνατολή “east”
  εἰς τὶν ἀνατολὴ βλέψας (4/8–9)
ἀναχωρεῖν “to withdraw”
  ἄψ τε ἀνεχώρησσεν (4/4)
ἀνιστάναι “to stand up”
  παλίνορσος ἀνέντη (4/2)
ἀπό “from” (3/16)
ἀργύρεος “silver”
  γρ(άφε) εἰ ἀργυρᾶν (2/12)
ἀφλέγμαντος “without inflammation” (3/11)

ἄψ “backward”
  ἄψ τε ἀνεχώρησσεν (4/4)

βάλλειν “to place”
  βάλε ὑποκάτω αὐτῆς (3/14)
βάπτειν “to wet”
  βάψον μαλλὸν ἐρίδη λευκοῦ (3/13)
βασιλεύειν “to rule”
  βασιλεύουσα ἐν τῷ τελείῳ μέλανι (2/18–19)
βῆσσα “glen”
  οὔρεος ἐν βήσσῃς (4/2–3)
βλέπειν “to look”
  εἰς τὶν ἀνατολὴ βλέψας (4/8–9)

γένεσις “origin”
  οὐρανοῦ γένεσι (3/1)
γίγνεσθαι “to become” (3/10)
γράφειν “write”
  γρ(άφε) εἰ ἀργυρᾶν (2/12)
  εἰς κασσίτερ(ον) γρ(άφε) (8/6–7)
γυῖον “limb”
  ὑπό τε τρόμος ἔλλαβε γυῖα (4/3–4)

δεῖν “to tie”
  ζ̅ χορδὰς ἢ στήμονος ἢ κρόκης δήσας (4/6–8)
δεῖνα (placeholder for personalization)
  ἐν ποιῷ μέλει τοῦ ΔΔ (7/14)
  τῆς δεῖ(νος) ἣν ἔτεκαν ἡ δεῖ(να) (3/9)
  τὸ ΔΔ (4/5)
δέσποινα “mistress”
  δέσποινα θεῶν (2/19–3/1)
δόκιμος “proven”
  δόκιμον ἔμπλαστρον (3/16)
  πρὸς ποδάγραν δόγιμον (2/10)
δράκων “snake”
  δράκοντα ἰσὼν (4/1–2)

εἶναι “to be” (3/11)
εἰπεῖν “to say”
  εἰπὲ γ̅ (4/9)
εἰς “in(to)”, “on(to)” (3/10; 4/8; 8/6)
  εἰ (2/12)
ἔμπλαστρον “plaster”
  δόκιμον ἔμπλαστρον (3/16)
ἐν “in” (2/18; 4/3; 7/14)
ἐνεργής “effective”
  λείαν ἐνεργές (2/15)

σελήνη "moon"
  σελήνη ληγούσης (2/12–13)
σπληνῖτις "splenitis"
  σπλην(ῖτιν) (3/15)
στήμων "warp"
  ζ̅ χορδὰς ἢ στήμονος ἢ κρόκης δήσας (4/6–8)
στόμαχος "stomach(-ache)" (8/5)

ταχύ "quickly"
  ἤδη β̅ ταχὺ β̅ (3/12–13)
  ἤδη β̅ ταχὺ ταχύ (4/5–6)
τε "and" (4/1) (4/3) (4/4)
τέλειος "perfect"
  βασιλεύουσα ἐν τῷ τελείῳ μέλανι (2/18–19)
τίκτειν "to bear (a child)"
  τῆς δεῖ(να) ἣν ἔτεκαν ἡ δεῖ(να) (3/9)
τις "someone" (4/1)
* τρίτε "thrice" (4/4)
τρόμος "trembling"
  ὑπό τε τρόμος ἔλλαβε γυῖα (4/3–4)

ὑποκάτω "beneath" (3/14)
  βάλε ὑποκάτω αὐτῆς (3/14)
ὑπολαμβάνειν "to seize"
  ὑπό τε τρόμος ἔλλαβε γυῖα (4/3–4)

φυλακτήριον "amulet"
  φυλακτήρ(ιον) πρ(ὸς) στόμαχον καὶ καφαλλαλγίαν (8/5–6)
φύσις "nature"
  τὸ κατὰ φύ(σιν) (3/10)

χλιαρός "warm"
  θαλάσσης χλιαρᾷ καταντλῶν (2/13–14)
χορδή "strings"
  ζ̅ χορδὰς ἢ στήμονος ἢ κρόκης δήσας (4/6–8)

ὥρα "hour"
  ἕως ὅ(ρας) ϛ τῆς ἡρέρας (3/17)
ὡς "as"
  ὅς δ᾽ ὅτε (4/1)

Divine Names (Theonyms)
ⲁⲃⲣⲁⲥⲁⲝ "Abrasax" (8/1)
ⲁⲙⲟⲩⲛ "Amun" (5/2; 5/3; 5/14; 6/6)
Γαβριήλ/ⲅⲁⲃⲣⲓⲏⲗ "Gabriel"
  Γαβριήλ (4/5; 4/10 [twice]; 4/11)
  ⲅⲁⲃⲣⲓⲏⲗ (7/19)
Δαμναμενεύς "Damnameneus" (7/15)
ⲏⲥⲉ "Isis" [see also s.v. ˀΙσις]
  ⲏⲥⲉ̅ (5/15)
ⲑⲟⲟⲩⲧ "Thoth" (5/9; 5/14)
ⲓⲁⲱ "Iao" [see also Magical Names (voces magicae) under ⲓ̈ⲁⲥⲁⲃⲁⲱ̅ⲑ̅]
  ⲓⲁⲱ (7/5)
  ⲓ̅ⲁ̅ⲱ̅ (8/1)
ˀΙσις "Isis" (2/18) [see also s.v. ⲏⲥⲉ]
ⲙⲓⲭⲁⲏⲗ "Michael" (7/19)
ⲡⲟⲣⲧⲟⲩ "The Great of Five" (5/10)
ⲥⲁⲃⲁⲱⲑ "Sabaoth" (7/5; 8/2) [see also Magical Names (voces magicae) under ⲓ̈ⲁⲥⲁⲃⲁⲱ̅ⲑ̅]
ϩⲱⲣ "Horus" (6/4)

Place Names (Toponyms)
ⲉⲃⲱⲧ "Abydos"
  ⲉⲃⲱⲧ (5/6)
  ⲁⲃⲱⲧ (7/6)
ⲧⲓⲛ "Thinis" (7/6)

Magical Names and Words (*voces magicae*)
ⲁⲃⲁⲑⲁⲓ̈ (3/8)
ⲁⲇⲱⲛⲁⲓ (10/3)
ⲁⲏ (3/8)
ⲁⲑⲉⲣⲛⲉⲃⲟⲩⲛⲓ (3/2)
αμακουμ (2/12)
ⲁⲛⲁⲝ (2/3)
ανουσφ (7/12 [four times]; 7/13)
ανουσφιβιαχ (7/13)
ⲁⲡⲏⲙⲉⲛⲱⲛ (2/4)
αρδαβαι (2/11)
ⲁⲭⲣⲁ (3/8)
ⲃⲁⲑⲁⲑ (3/7)
ⲃⲁⲥⲧⲁⲓ̈ (3/4)
ⲃⲓⲃⲓⲟⲩ (10/2 [thrice])
ⲃⲟⲣⲁⲩ (2/4)
ⲑⲁⲑ (3/7)
ⲑⲁⲣⲑⲁⲑⲁⲃⲁⲁⲑⲑⲁ (3/6–7)
ⲑⲉⲣⲏⲥⲓⲃⲁⲧ (3/5)
ⲓ̈ⲁⲥⲁⲃⲁⲱ̅ⲑ̅ (10/2)
ⲓ̈ⲟⲥⲫⲏ (10/1 [thrice])
ⲓⲥⲓ (3/3)
ⲓ̈ⲱⲃⲁⲥⲧ (3/4)

Magical Vowels

Numerals & Abbreviations

Manuscript Sources

References to the commentary (of the form, e.g., "comm. 3/1") point to lemmata by page and line number of the Michigan codex.

Papyrological

Epigraphic

Western medieval codices

Modern archival documents

Literary and sub-literary texts with a manuscript tradition

Biblical texts

Select Greek and Coptic words discussed in the commentary (not in the Michigan codex)

Subject Index

Plates

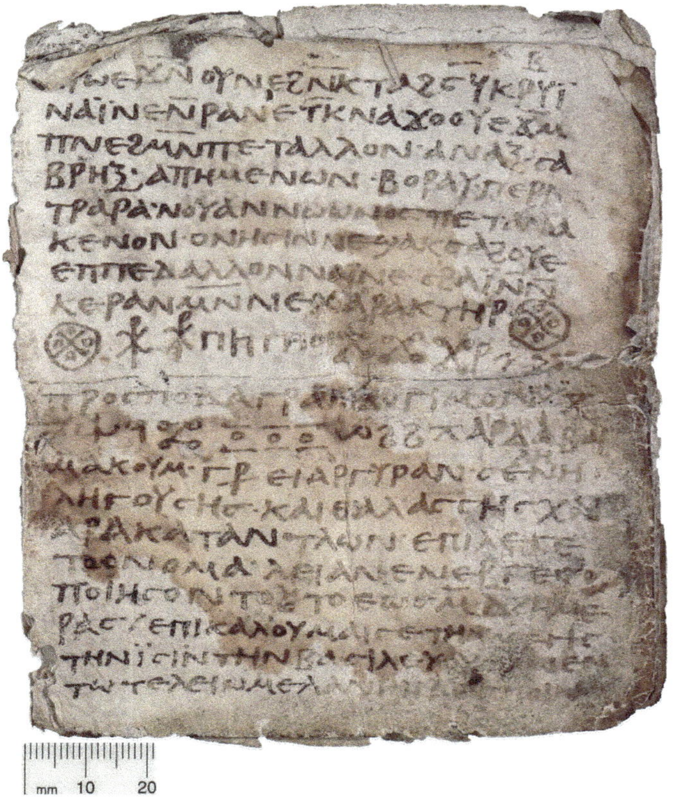

Michigan Ms. 136, p. 2

Plate II

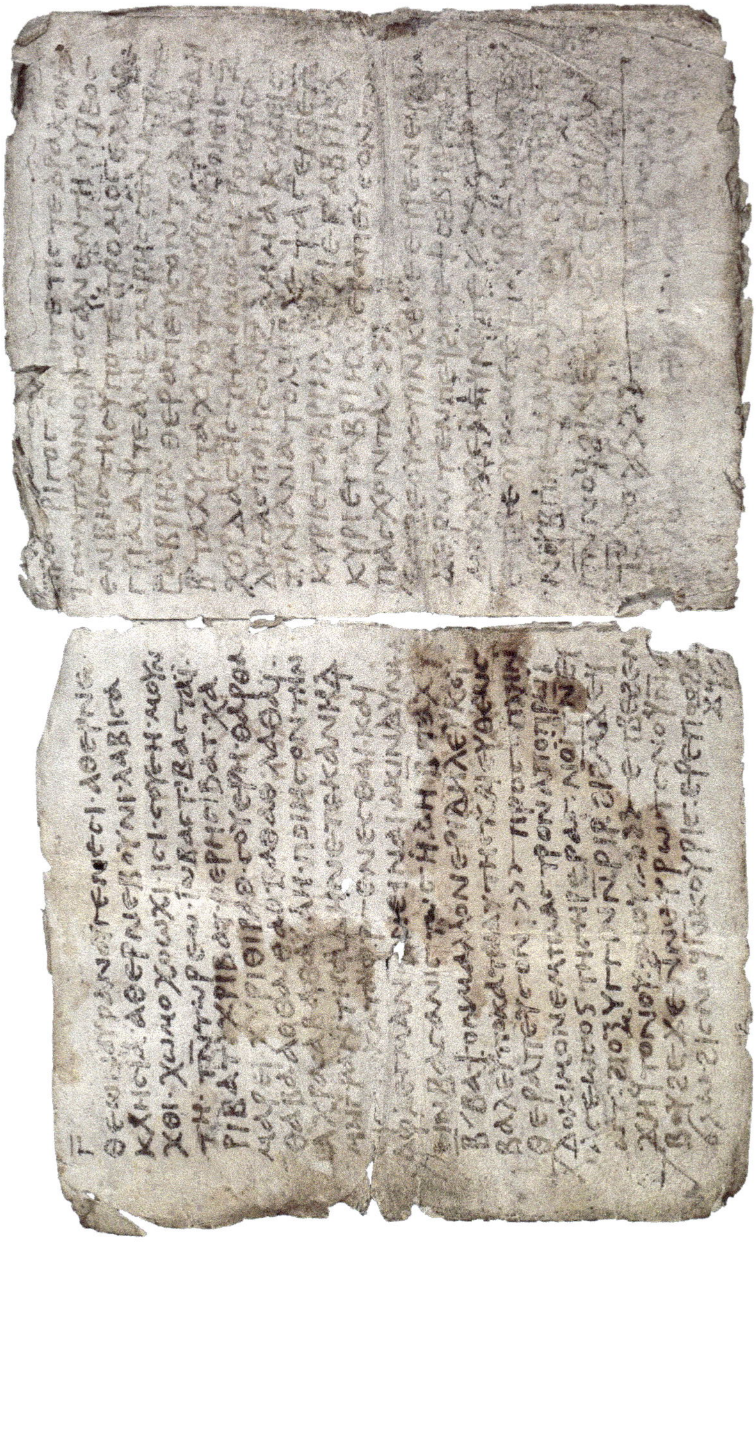

Michigan Ms. 136, pp. 3–4

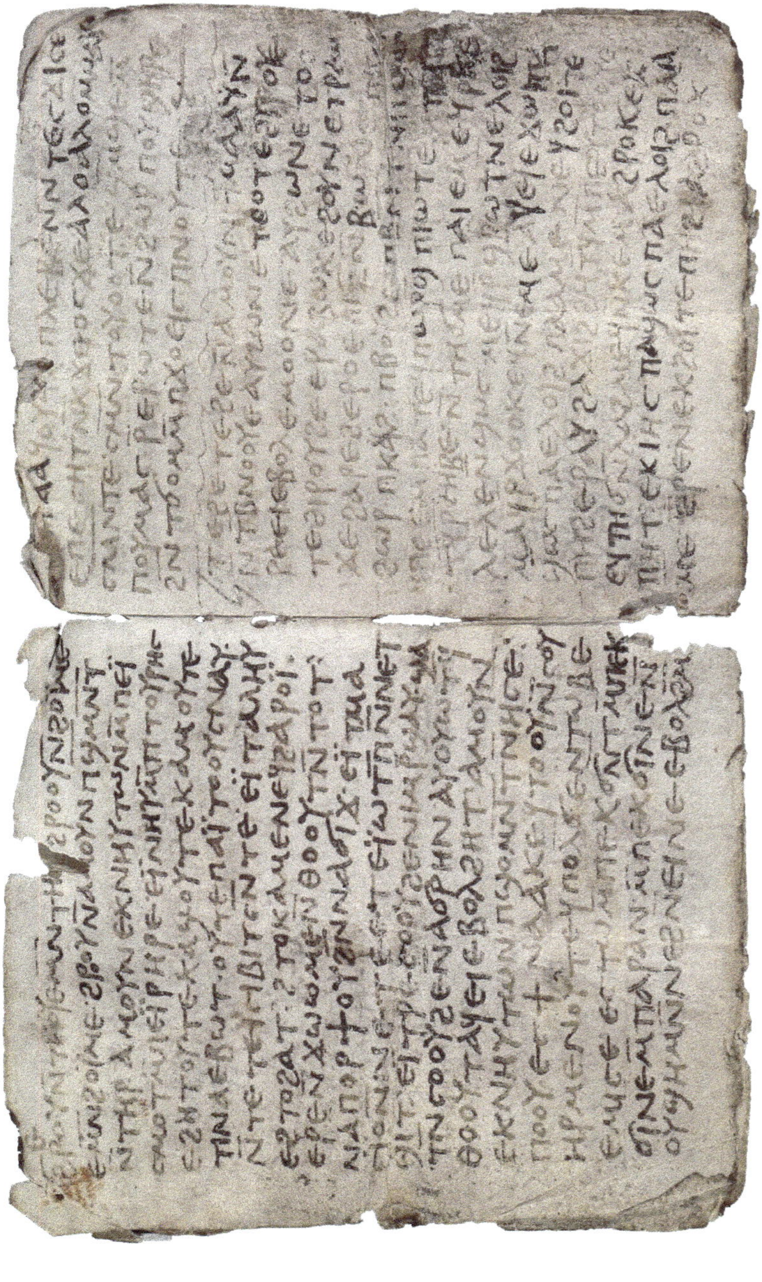

Michigan Ms. 136, pp. 5–6

Plate IV

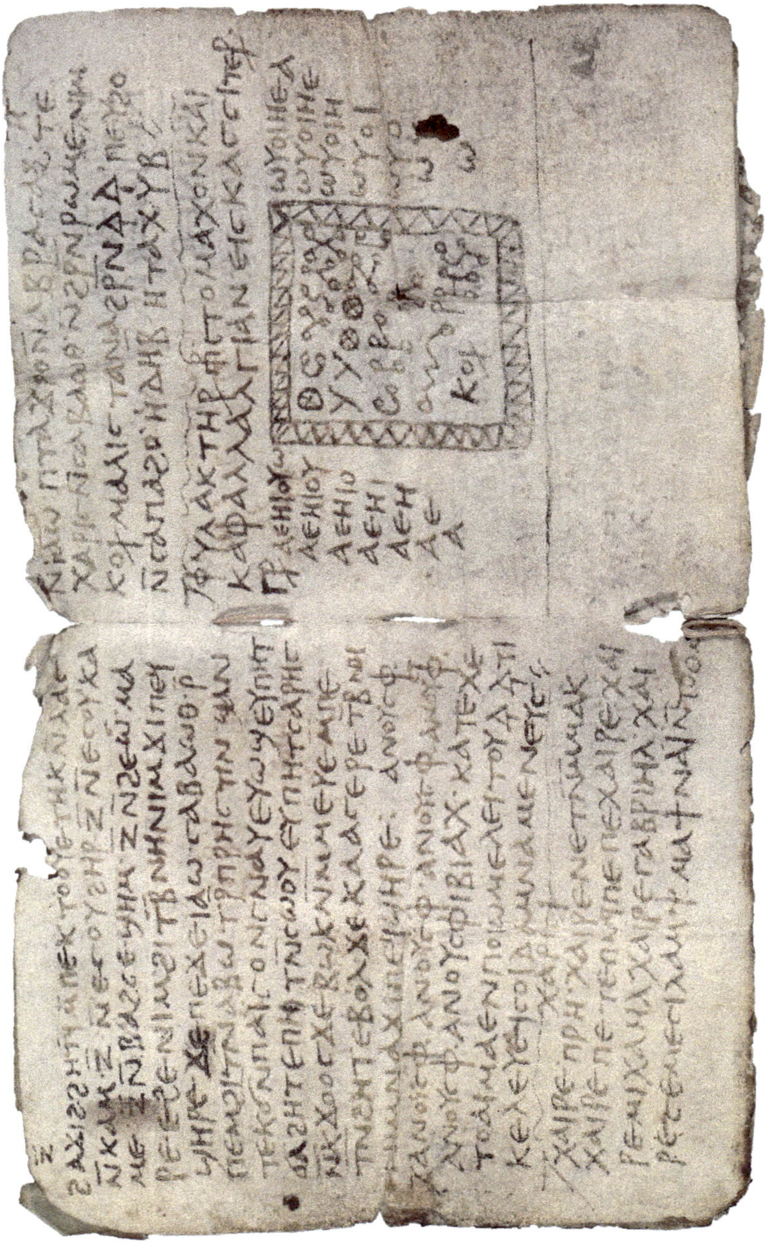

Michigan Ms. 136, pp. 7–8

Plate V

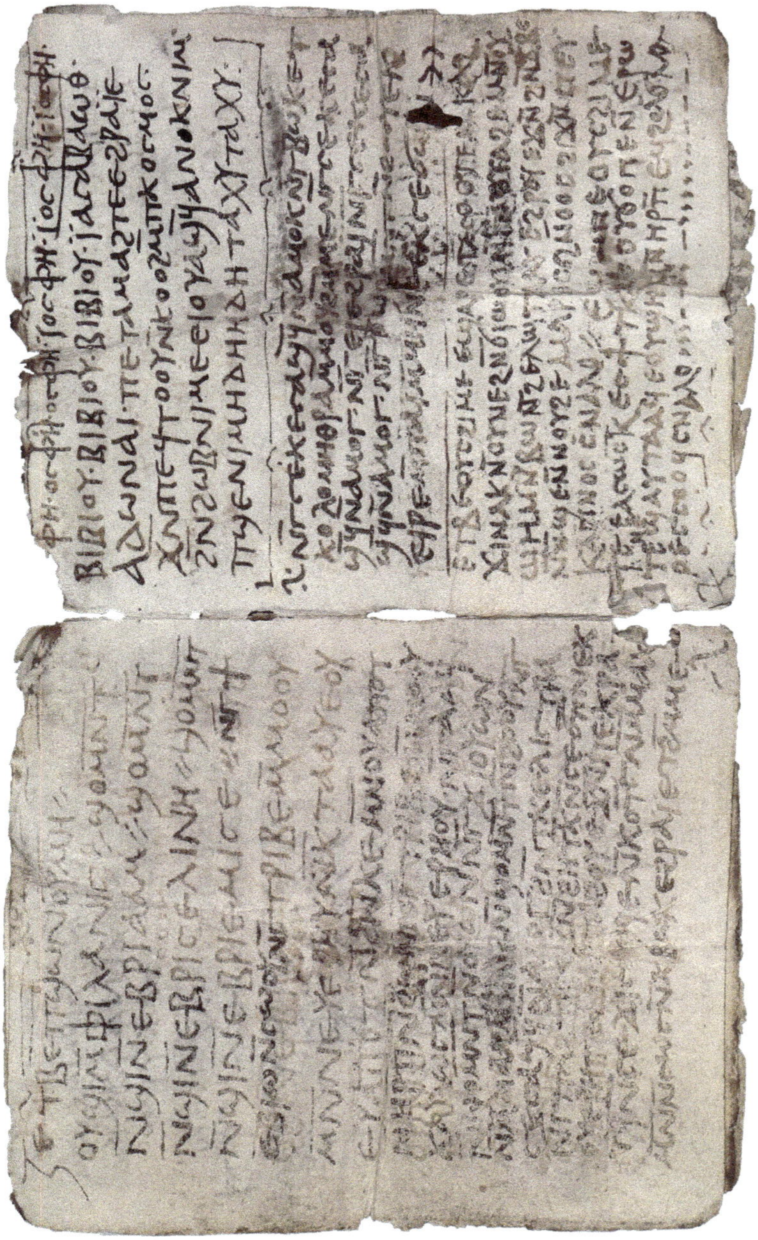

Michigan Ms. 136, pp. 9–10

Plate VI

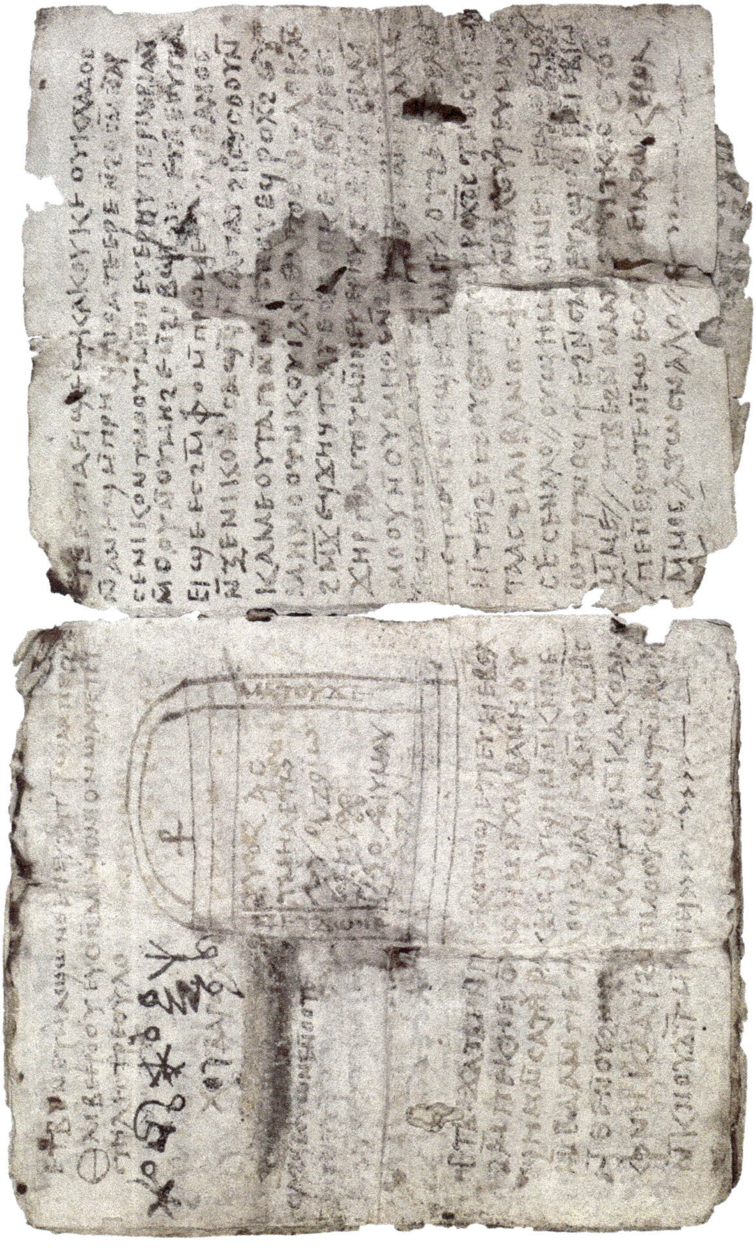

Michigan Ms. 136, pp. 11–12

Plate VII

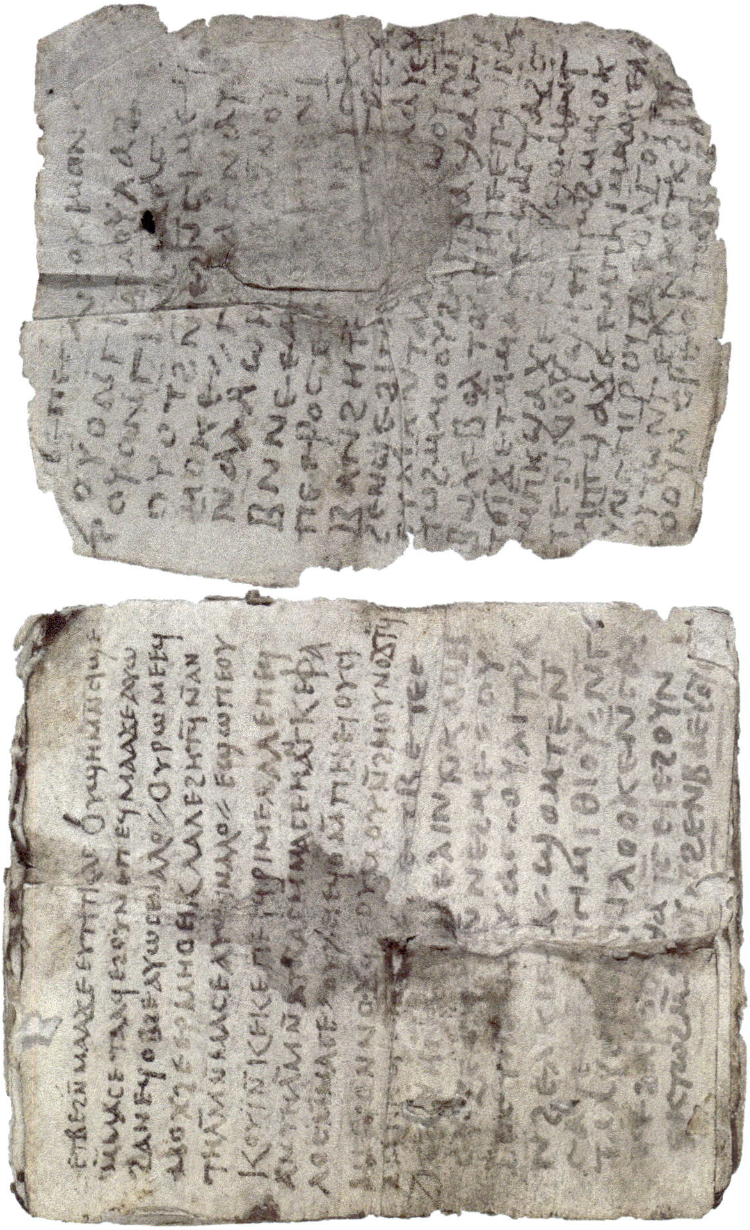

Michigan Ms. 136, pp. 13–14

Plate VIII

Michigan Ms. 136, back cover

www.ingramcontent.com/pod-product-compliance
Ingram Content Group UK Ltd.
Pitfield, Milton Keynes, MK11 3LW, UK
UKHW052008051026
15624UKWH00004B/627

9 783110 778755